BETTER LIVING

BETTER LIVING WITH DEMENTIA

Implications for Individuals, Families, Communities, and Societies

Laura N. Gitlin, Ph.D. FAAN
Adjunct Professor, Johns Hopkins University Distinguished University Professor Dean, College of Nursing and Health Professions Drexel University, Philadelphia, PA, USA

Nancy A. Hodgson, Ph.D., RN, FAAN
Anthony Buividas Endowed Term Chair in Gerontology Associate Professor, Biobehavioral Health Sciences Department Program Director, Hillman Scholars Program in Nursing Innovation University of Pennsylvania School of Nursing, Philadelphia, PA, USA

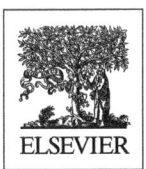
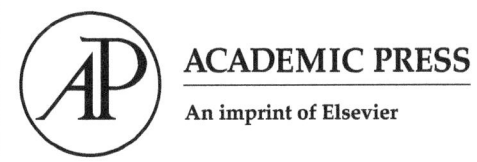

Academic Press is an imprint of Elsevier
125 London Wall, London EC2Y 5AS, United Kingdom
525 B Street, Suite 1650, San Diego, CA 92101, United States
50 Hampshire Street, 5th Floor, Cambridge, MA 02139, United States
The Boulevard, Langford Lane, Kidlington, Oxford OX5 1GB, United Kingdom

Copyright © 2018 Elsevier Inc. All rights reserved.

No part of this publication may be reproduced or transmitted in any form or by any means, electronic or mechanical, including photocopying, recording, or any information storage and retrieval system, without permission in writing from the publisher. Details on how to seek permission, further information about the Publisher's permissions policies and our arrangements with organizations such as the Copyright Clearance Center and the Copyright Licensing Agency, can be found at our website: www.elsevier.com/permissions.

This book and the individual contributions contained in it are protected under copyright by the Publisher (other than as may be noted herein).

Notices
Knowledge and best practice in this field are constantly changing. As new research and experience broaden our understanding, changes in research methods, professional practices, or medical treatment may become necessary.

Practitioners and researchers must always rely on their own experience and knowledge in evaluating and using any information, methods, compounds, or experiments described herein. In using such information or methods they should be mindful of their own safety and the safety of others, including parties for whom they have a professional responsibility.

To the fullest extent of the law, neither the Publisher nor the authors, contributors, or editors, assume any liability for any injury and/or damage to persons or property as a matter of products liability, negligence or otherwise, or from any use or operation of any methods, products, instructions, or ideas contained in the material herein.

British Library Cataloguing-in-Publication Data
A catalogue record for this book is available from the British Library

Library of Congress Cataloging-in-Publication Data
A catalog record for this book is available from the Library of Congress

ISBN: 978-0-12-811928-0

For Information on all Academic Press publications visit our website at https://www.elsevier.com/books-and-journals

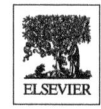 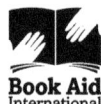 Working together to grow libraries in developing countries

www.elsevier.com • www.bookaid.org

Publisher: Nikki Levy
Acquisition Editor: Dennis McGonagle
Editorial Project Manager: Michelle Kubilis
Production Project Manager: Priya Kumaraguruparan
Cover Designer: Matthew Limbert

Typeset by MPS Limited, Chennai, India

Transferred to Digital Printing in 2018

To my wonderful supportive family - my husband, Eduardo, and sons, Keith and Eric. Como siempre, with profound love, gratitude, and honor. - **Laura Gitlin**

To my family, especially my mother, brother, sister, and daughter for their deep love and support. - **Nancy Hodgson**

To our dedicated global and local collaborators who share our passion for better dementia care through research, practice, and education.

To the inspiring individuals, families, and caregivers living with dementia that fuel our mission to find better ways. - **Laura Gitlin and Nancy Hodgson**

Contents

About the Authors — xi
Written Commentaries — xv
Foreword — xvii
Preface — xxi
Acknowledgments — xxvii
Introduction: A Framework for Understanding Impacts of Dementia and Supporting Quality of Life With Disease Progression — xxix

PART I
ABOUT THE PERSON LIVING WITH DEMENTIA

1. How the Brain Is Affected — 3

Pathophysiology of Dementia — 4
The Challenge of Diagnosis — 8
Role of Biomarkers in Diagnosis — 11
The Trajectory of Dementia — 13
Changing Needs — 15
Key Points — 17
References — 18
Further Reading — 21

2. Lived Experiences of Individuals With Dementia — 23

Principles for Understanding Lived Experiences — 25
The Good Life Model — 26
Differential Needs of People Living With Dementia — 27
Daily Challenges — 33
Practical Implications for Dementia Care — 43
Key Points — 44
References — 47
Further Reading — 52

3. Breaking the Cycle of Despair — 53

Three Buckets of Research — 54
Paradigm of Despair — 57

Assumptions For Developing a System for
Care and Supportive Services   60
Conclusion   62
References   63

4. Making Life Better for Individuals Living With Dementia   65

Treatment Goals   66
What Can We Do Now?   69
Ethical Dilemmas Providing Care and Supports   85
Why Individuals Living With Dementia Do Not Receive
Evidence-Based Care, Services and Supports   87
Key Points   88
References   89

PART II
ABOUT THE CAREGIVER

5. Family Member as Care Partner   97

Who Are Family Caregivers?   98
What Do Caregivers Do?   100
What Are the Consequences of Caregiving?   103
What Do Caregivers Need?   105
Research Implications   106
The Future of Caregiving   107
Key Points   107
References   108

6. How We Can Support Families   113

Assumptions for Providing Care and Services to Families   114
Pathways for Supporting Family Caregivers   116
Looking Backwards to Move Forward   119
Begin With Assessment   121
Evidence-Based Approaches: What Works?   127
Exemplars   129
Lessons Learned   142
Do All Caregivers Need Support?   145
Ethical Considerations   146
Key Points   147
References   148

7. Formal Caregivers: The Role of the Interprofessional Team   155

What is an Interprofessional Approach to Formal Caregiving?   158
Why Is Interprofessional Care Important?   161

What Skills Do Formal Caregivers Need to Practice as Part of an Interprofessional Care Team?	163
Conclusion	165
Key Points	166
References	166
Further Reading	168

PART III
ABOUT LIVING ENVIRONMENTS

8. The Physical Home Environment: A Neglected Therapeutic Context	171
Critical Drivers of Home as an Epicenter for Dementia Care	171
Impact of Home Environments on Daily Life	174
Home Safety Considerations	177
The Health Provider Perspective	180
Environmental Assessments	181
Environmental Modifications	187
When to Stay Put and When to Leave?	189
Unintended Negative Consequences of Staying Home	189
Conclusion	190
Key Points	192
References	192
Further Reading	195
9. Living in the Community	197
The Need for Security and Belonging	198
Dementia-Friendly Communities	200
Key Points	208
References	209

PART IV
ABOUT SOCIAL SYSTEMS AND POLICIES

10. Services and Settings of Care	213
What Is Person- and Family-Centered Care?	215
Service Needs Across the Dementia Trajectory	218
Best Practices in Setting Design and Programming	220
Examples of Person-Centered Service Models	221
Conclusions	223
References	224

11. Global Efforts and National Plans 227

Dementia by the Numbers Globally 228
Global Disease Burden 228
National Plans and Their Impact 230
Gaps in Global Efforts 241
Key Points 242
References 244
Further Reading 245

12. Transforming Dementia Care 247

Movement Towards a Social–Medical Comprehensive
Dementia Care Model 247
Individual Level 249
Caregivers 250
Living Environment 251
Neighborhood and Community 252
Health and Human Services 253
Social Policy 258
Putting It All Together 260
Conclusion 260
References 262

PART V
TAKING ACTION

13. Developing and Implementing an Action Plan 267

14. Putting It All Together: Synthesis and Future Directions 273

Index 281

About the Authors

Laura N. Gitlin, PhD, is an applied research sociologist. At the time of writing this book, she was the Isabel Hampton Robb Distinguished Professor in the Department of Community Public Health in the School of Nursing with joint appointments in the Department of Psychiatry and Division of Geriatrics and Gerontology, School of Medicine, at Johns Hopkins University. She was also the founding director of the Center for Innovative Care in Aging at Johns Hopkins University School of Nursing. As of February 1, 2018, she became the Distinguished University Professor and Dean of the College of Nursing and Health Professions of Drexel University. Also, as of October 2017, she became the Chair of the Advisory Council on Alzheimer's Research Care and Services which advises the Secretary of the Department of Health and Human Services (HSS) on federal programs affecting people with Alzheimer's disease and related dementia and continue development and progress on the National Plan to address dementia by HHS, Veterans Affairs, the Department of Defense, and the National Science Foundation. She is also a member of Medical Scientific Advisory Board of the US National Alzheimer's Association.

For over 30 years, she has been involved in developing, evaluating, disseminating, and implementing many innovative programs to improve the lives of older adults and their families and specifically persons and families living with dementia. She works collaboratively with health and human service professionals, community agencies, and healthcare organizations in advancing comprehensive and social ecologically sound dementia care that supports the physical, social, and emotional functioning of people with dementia and their family caregivers. Specifically, she is nationally and internationally recognized for her work in nonpharmacological approaches. As a well-funded researcher, she has received continuous funding from federal agencies and private foundations to test interventions throughout her career. Interventions developed with her collaborators in dementia care such as New Ways for Better Days: Tailoring Activities for Persons with Dementia (TAP), Skills$_2$Care^R, Caring for Persons with Dementia in their Living Environment (COPE), Project ACT (Advancing Caregiver Training), Resources for Enhancing Alzheimer's Caregiver Health (REACH I and II) are in varying stages of translation and implementation worldwide. With colleagues, she has also developed an online platform, the

WeCareAdvisor™, currently being tested and designed to help families manage behavioral symptoms (Gitlin, Kales, Marx, Stanislawski, & Lyketos, 2017; Kales et al. 2016).

She has published extensively in peer-reviewed journals. She has also written numerous books including a research text (DePoy & Gitlin, 2015), a grant writing book (Gitlin & Lyons, 2014), book on the Skills$_2$Care^R program for occupational therapists (Gitlin & Corcoran, 2005), a book on behavioral intervention research for researchers (Gitlin & Czaja, 2016), and a guide book for families concerning preventing and managing common behavioral symptoms in persons with dementia (Gitlin & Piersol, 2014).

A theme throughout her research is applying a social ecological perspective and person-directed approach as well as collaborating with community organizations and health professionals to maximize the relevance and impact of her programs. She is the recipient of numerous awards including the 2009 Eastern Pennsylvania Geriatric Society, Charles Ewing Presidential Award for outstanding contribution to geriatric care, the 2010 United Way Champion Impact Award for Healthy Aging at Home, the 2010 National Institute of Senior Centers Award with Center in the Park, the 2010 MetLife Award for translating the Skills$_2$Care^R Program (a dementia caregiver intervention program) with Fox Rehabilitation (a home health agency), the 2011 John Mackey Award for Excellence in Dementia Care, from Johns Hopkins University, the 2014 M. Powell Lawton Award from the Gerontological Society of America, an Honorary Fellow of the American Academy of Nursing (FAAN) in 2015, and the 2017 American Occupational Therapy Foundation Research Leadership Award.

Nancy A. Hodgson, RN, PhD, FAAN, is an associate professor in the Department of Biobehavioral Health in the University of Pennsylvania School of Nursing. Her 30 + year nursing career has been dedicated to improving the end of life experiences for cognitively and physically frail older adults. She earned her graduate degrees in nursing from the University of Pennsylvania (MSN-1988; PhD-1999). After completing her postdoctoral training at Johns Hopkins School of Public Health in 2001, she was the first nurse researcher to be named as Senior Research Scientist at two nationally renowned gerontology institutes (the Polisher Research Institute at the Philadelphia Geriatric Center where she was Interim Director, followed by the Thomas Jefferson University Center for Applied Research in Aging and Health). At both institutes, she served as a bridge between the scientific knowledge base and clinical decision-making. Her work in designing and implementing one of the first nursing home–based palliative care programs at the Abramson Center for Jewish Life (formerly the Philadelphia Geriatric Center) had direct impact on the care of over 3000 nursing home residents in

Pennsylvania, and received the Archstone Foundation and the American Public Health Association Award for Excellence in Program Innovation.

She is a nationally recognized nurse researcher in applied gerontology. Her highly collaborative and productive program of research is focused on the development, testing, and dissemination of person-centered and family-centered interventions for cognitively and physically frail older adults and their family caregivers. This work has helped to inform care practices for persons living with dementia and their caregivers through the development of palliative care protocols that address the leading symptoms in dementia that cause distress or impair quality of life.

As a clinician and educator, she seeks out innovative ways to foster academic–community partnership by linking research and practice in order to move evidence-based findings into dementia care practice. She was formerly the Associate Director of Implementation Research at the Center for Innovative Care in Aging at Johns Hopkins University where her research and scholarly practice was focused on the translation of proven interventions in community settings to improve access to evidence-based care for frail older adults. A few of her awards include the 2013 Excellence in Research Award from the Gerontological Advanced Practice Nurses Association, and the 2013 Outstanding Pathfinder Award from the Maryland Nurses Association. She is a Fellow in the American Academy of Nursing and the Gerontological Society of America.

Collectively, Drs. Gitlin and Hodgson have close to 60 years of experience working with individuals and families living with dementia as well as health and human service professionals to change the landscape of dementia care. For the past 15 years, they have collaborated on numerous research programs specific to dementia care. Their successful Massive Online Open Course (MOOC) on Living with Dementia, currently available on demand through Coursera (https://www.coursera.org/), involves five modules that moves participants through an understanding of the impact of dementia on individuals, families, communities, and society. Researchers, providers, administrators, and families from over 169 countries have taken the course with over half million individuals viewing the video lectures. This book was inspired in large part by this MOOC, participants request for written materials to accompany lectures, and to the overwhelming global and local need to advance an understanding of the nuances and multiple facets of living with dementia and how it affects persons themselves, their care partners, families, communities, and society at-large.

References

DePoy, E., & Gitlin, L. N. (2015). *Introduction to research: Understanding and applying multiple strategies* (5th ed.). Amsterdam: Elsevier/Mosby Year Book.

Gitlin, L. N., & Corcoran, M. (2005). *Occupational therapy and dementia care: The home environment skill-building program for individuals and families.* Bethesda, MD: American Occupational Therapy Association.

Gitlin, L. N., & Czaja, S. J. (2016). *Behavioral intervention research: Designing, evaluating and implementing.* Berlin: Springer Publishing Company.

Gitlin, L. N., Kales, H. J., Marx, K., Stanislawski, B., & Lyketos, C. (2017). A randomized trial of a web-based platform to help families manage dementia-related behavioral symptoms: The WeCareAdvisor™. *Contemporary Clinical Trials.* Available from https://doi.org/10.1016/j.cct.2017.08.001.

Gitlin, L. N., & Lyons, K. J. (2014). *Successful grant writing: Strategies for health and human service professionals* (4th ed.). Berlin: Springer Publishing Company.

Gitlin, L. N., & Piersol, C. V. (2014). *A caregiver's guide to dementia: Using activity and other strategies to prevent, reduce, and manage behavioral symptoms.* Philadelphia, PA: Camino Books, Inc.

Kales, H. C., Gitlin, L. N., Stanislawski, B., Marx, K., Turnwald, M., Watkins, D., & Lyketsos, C. G. (2016). WeCareAdvisor™: The development of a caregiver-focused, web-based program to assess and manage behavioral and psychological symptoms of dementia. *Alzheimer Dementia and Associated Disorders.* Available from https://doi.org/10.1097/WAD.0000000000000177.

Written Commentaries

Jean Gagardo, OTR, PhD: Jean Gajardo is an assistant professor in the Department of Occupational Therapy and Occupational Science, University of Chile, Santiago, Chile. He is an occupational therapist with a PhD in public health. His professional and research focus is on public health policies in aging and the promotion of nonpharmacological interventions addressing dependency in older adults. He has been part of the design, implementation, and evaluation of Community Centers for People with Dementia and has been part of the Commission for the elaboration of Chile's First National Dementia Plan by the Ministry of Health. He has broad experience in training individuals, families, health and human service professionals in dementia care, and older adult care in Chile.

Helen C. Kales, MD: Dr. Kales is Professor of Psychiatry at the University of Michigan and a research investigator in the Center for Clinical Management Research (CCMR) and the Geriatric Research Education and Clinical Center (GRECC) in the VA Ann Arbor Health System. She is also the founding director of the UM Program for Positive Aging (PPA), a multifaceted UM program established in 2009. As a fellowship-trained, board-certified geriatric psychiatrist, her research program is directly informed by her clinical work and experiences with patients, families, providers, and systems to diminish the barriers to effective and high-quality care for older patients with dementia or with mental health issues.

Jason Karlowish, MD: Jason Karlawish is Professor of Medicine, Medical Ethics and Health Policy, and Neurology at the University of Pennsylvania. He is the Codirector of the Penn Memory Center and the Director of the Healthy Brain Research Center. His research focuses on ethical and policy issues encountered by older adults with cognitive disorders such as Alzheimer's disease and cognitive aging. He developed the ACED, an instrument to assist in decisional capacity assessment, and the concept of "whealthcare," a novel model to promote cognitive health and maintain wealth with a particular focus on the banking and financial services industries (www.whealthcare.org).

Constantine Lyketsos, MD, MHS: A world expert in the care and treatment of patients with dementia, Dr. Lyketsos leads efforts to disseminate state-of-the-art dementia care to the community. His clinical and research interests are integrated in the Johns Hopkins Memory and

Alzheimer's Center which he founded in 2007 as a collaborative partnership between three departments to offer comprehensive evaluation and innovative treatment for conditions that affect cognition and memory. He is the recipient of several awards including the American College of Psychiatrists' 2018 *Geriatric Research Award*. He has authored over 350 peer-reviewed articles, as well as several chapters, commentaries, and five books. Castle-Connolly has named Dr. Lyketsos as one of *America's Top Doctors* every year since 2001.

Esther Oh, MD, PhD: Dr. Oh is an associate professor in the Division of Geriatric Medicine and Gerontology (Department of Medicine) at the Johns Hopkins University, and the associate director of the Johns Hopkins Memory and Alzheimer's Treatment Center. She is also a faculty member in the Department of Psychiatry and Behavioral Sciences, and in the Division of Neuropathology. Her clinical expertise is in evaluation and management of memory disorders. She has an extensive experience in evaluating memory disorders in older adults with multiple chronic diseases, and takes an integrative approach in the treatment of memory disorders.

James Pickett, PhD: Dr. James Pickett is Head of Research at Alzheimer's Society, overseeing a large portfolio of research across the spectrum from studies of single molecules to studies of healthcare systems. He develops new partnerships and initiatives to deliver Alzheimer's Society research strategy. Previously he worked for Diabetes UK and worked as a journal editor in *Nature Reviews*. He completed his PhD in molecular pharmacology from the University of Cambridge in 2006.

Quincy M. Samus, PhD: Dr. Quincy M. Samus is an associate professor in the Department of Psychiatry and Behavioral Sciences and an applied gerontologist, trained in behavioral health services research and epidemiology. With over 15 years of experience as PI and coinvestigator on a number federally funded grants (R01s, K01, CMMI HCIA), her research focuses on understanding and improving the care and delivery of health and supportive services to persons with dementia and their families, both in community and residential care settings. She is the Director of the Translational Aging Services Core (TASC) and is committed to advancing the development-, evaluation- and practice-based implementation of pragmatic evidence–based interventions and delivery models that identify and address the diverse needs of persons with dementia and their families.

Foreword

Becoming Dementia Ready

This book is about you; it is also about me. This book is about your parents, my parents, their parents, our siblings, our partners, our friends, our children, and our children's children. Dementia touches every family, every community, and every nation. This book is about all of us because dementia knows no boundaries. This book is for all of us because to fight a disease that knows no boundaries we need an effort that knows no boundaries. Persons suffering from dementia get lost in the shadow of the boundaries in our current fragmented systems of care, research, and policies, and so do the family members, professional providers, and community service agencies who seek to help them.

Today, millions of our families and our neighbors are suffering and feeling alone in the shadow of dementia. Millions more of us will face this disease and the financial cost is already measured in the hundreds of billions. Big numbers are important, but so are the individual faces of the persons living with dementia. Our families, our health systems, and our communities are underprepared. Only recently we are beginning to understand that we are all in the path of this terrible disease and we are all part of the solution in learning how to live well in the face of dementia. We will not learn to live well with dementia until we shine some light into the shadows, until we turn the stigmatizing whispers into caring conversations, and until we break down the boundaries in our social institutions.

How do we find ourselves in a century that will be dominated by so many persons living with dementia? We find the answer in a simple irony. By far, the biggest risk factor for dementia is living a long life. Thus, if we successfully avoid premature death before our seventh decade, we increase the likelihood that we will face dementia as we age. Like aging, dementia is a journey. For some of you, you are already well on your way along this challenging journey. For others, the journey is still in your future. Like any journey, wonderful or daunting, the path is made more understandable by a roadmap. We can gain understanding by the advice of the travelers who have gone before us. This book offers understanding. This book also offers a plan for action. Whether you are a baby boomer, the parent of a baby boomer, or the child of a baby boomer, it is time to become dementia ready.

How do we find ourselves underprepared? We have known for at least 65 years that the number of older adults in the world was going to increase dramatically. All of the people who are now 65 years and older have already been alive for 65 years—we have been able to count them and plan for their aging into adulthood and older ages for at least 65 years. By extension, we also knew that in reaching older ages, many of these people would be living with chronic conditions, disability, and dementia. Over the past 65 years, however, we have had a very difficult time redesigning our health care system, our social system, and our communities to accommodate all of these older adults. Imagine that you are a 30-year-old person with an uncomplicated pneumonia. There is a very good chance that you will be accurately diagnosed and treated and that you will completely recover if you seek medical advice in a timely fashion. As you recover, you won't need much more than a few days of help from your family and the only home- and community-based services you will need is your own bed. Our system of care works very well for this condition that used to kill many people in centuries past. To someone living in the 19th century, this care would be miraculous. Now imagine you are an 80-year-old person with dementia. There is a very good chance that you will not be accurately diagnosed and treated, you will most definitely not completely recover, you may live with the disabling condition for 10–15 years, and you will need hundreds of unpaid hours of support from your daughter to maintain a decent quality of life. To someone living in the 19th century, this care would be the standard for the day. Sadly, it is still the standard in the 21st century.

Why have we not made more progress in the care of this condition? The easiest answer is that despite the investment of billions of dollars, our research and development did not produce a magic bullet. A more painful answer is that while striving for the magic bullet, we did not simultaneously invest in building the systems of health care and community supports that people would need to live with this disease absent a cure. The absence of a cure may also produce a more insidious injury: despair on the part of patients and nihilism on the part of providers. Primary care providers represent the foundation of health care in the United States and many other countries. These providers are dedicated professionals working under difficult conditions and in a system that does not support the care they would like to provide for persons living with dementia. They cannot prescribe an antibiotic for dementia care. Currently, diagnosis is too often delayed, education and guidance is too shallow, and patients and families feel lost and unsupported. We can do better, we know how to do better, but we have not found the will to declare the current system unacceptable. We have not become dementia ready.

This book, and the approach the authors espouse, differs for three reasons. First, the approach completely and finally embraces the reality that our communities will indeed include many friends, neighbors, and family members with failing brains. No technology or magic bullet or mass denial will change this reality. Family caregivers will be the main workforce providing day-to-day care for these people living with dementia. Second, the authors propose a socio-ecological model that shows us how to breech the walls and span the boundaries of our fragmented efforts to design care for persons living with dementia. A socio-ecological model helps us understand that persons living with dementia interact with caregivers, families, and social networks who interact with complex health systems, home- and community-based services, and social institutions that in turn interact in ever larger and ever more complex social networks and national environments. We all live and grow and interact within this socio-ecological framework—we shape it and it shapes us. Third, this book offers the hope that comes from learning that there is something that we can do to help persons living with dementia. The recommendations presented here build from a solid foundation of research and science.

Wherever you find yourself in our social fabric and in your personal journey of dementia, you will find action items here that help all of us become dementia ready.

Christopher M. Callahan, MD
Regenstrief Institute, Inc., Indianapolis, IN, United States

Preface

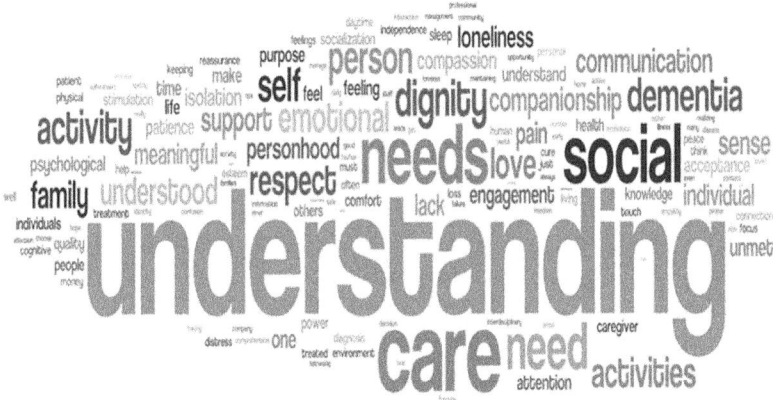

Wordle, generated from a Massive Online Open Course, involving over 169 countries and more than 50,000 respondents to the question, "What do persons living with dementia need?"

Alzheimer's disease and related disorders are one of the most disabling and burdensome health conditions worldwide, making it one of the most daunting and significant global health challenges of our day. With over 47 million people in the world currently living with dementia and 135 million expected to have this condition by 2050, are we prepared to effectively prevent, treat, and manage this impending challenge to individuals, families, communities, and societies?

Despite gallant and ongoing efforts to search for underlying mechanisms of the dementias from which to identify a cure and/or treatments to delay progression, there are no medical therapeutics to date nor are there expected to be any in the near future. Additionally, few countries have adequate systems of care to address the daily realities that individuals living with this chronic, progressive, and terminal condition and their care partners and communities confront. This is particularly the case in the United States in which dementia is the sixth leading cause of death and one of the most feared conditions, now surpassing cancer. Regardless of the expected increase in prevalence, disease burden, and public fear, we are not dementia "ready" nor do we have a uniform evidence-informed comprehensive approach to dementia care.

Unlike other conditions and diseases, such as heart disease, stroke, or cancer, in which treatments have improved longevity and quality of life, there are no equivalents to date that can prevent or slow disease progression in dementia nor which can adequately support families providing care across the trajectory of decline. Even in the unlikely case of a preventive or disease modifying breakthrough in the next few years, millions of individuals and their families and communities in the United States and worldwide will still be living with the long march of dementia—this is the case in the foreseeable future and forthcoming decades. Dementia must command our careful attention and we must strive for transformative, sweeping changes in our responses, health care, human services, and policies to enable families to live with life quality, dignity, and without stigma throughout the disease process. A premise of this book is that such transformative change is possible now.

This book examines the local and global challenges of living with all-cause dementias—Alzheimer's disease, vascular disease, Lewy body disease, frontotemporal, and other variants—and the implications of the dementias for individuals, families, communities, and societies. We highlight the evidence to date and importantly offer specific positive actions—in the home, community, healthcare context, national policy levels—that can be implemented now for bettering lives.

There are many books on dementia. We recognize that our book enters a crowded field. Our book differs however from others in several critical ways. First, most books focus solely on dementia as a disease process of the brain. But this is a partial truth as dementia is not just about the brain. Although its root causes are not yet known, there is evidence to suggest this complex condition is an outcome of multiple and interactive processes including individual genetics, health, and life choices, as well as societal forces such as access to education and resources. For example, as low-income countries compared to high-income countries, and in the United States, African Americans, and Latinos compared to whites, have higher prevalence rates, socioeconomic forces, and living contexts including education level appear to enhance individual vulnerability or susceptibility to dementia in some ways that are of yet not completely understood. Furthermore, the evidence suggests that the brain cannot be implicated alone so to speak and that other aspects of health and well-being as well as the physical, social, and policy environments may be important contributors to pathological pathways and also the dementia experience. Additionally, as the disease affects all aspects of functioning including memory, behaviors, new learning, physical functioning, ability to interact, socialize, and engage—to name a few—understanding the individual living with dementia in this totality including the manifold consequences of degeneration, adaptive mechanisms, and informal resources is vital so that we can effectively address the multitude of changing needs and derive a just right supportive environment at home, in the community, and within social and medical contexts as the disease progresses. A focus solely on brain processes ignores the context in which individuals live their lives and experience dementia, the relationship of brain function to daily function, the social stigma that comes with a dementia diagnosis, and the social, psychological, physical, environmental, community, health care, and policy solutions that can, should, and must be implemented. Furthermore, a focus solely on the brain impedes our ability to search for potential solutions, given the limited treatment options to impact the disease at the brain level. Thus a broader vision is essential. Most guides to dementia have focused on caregiver support and education among others. What has been overlooked is that dementia is also fundamentally a societal problem, and that it also impacts every sector, employers, and communities and in turn we must engage all of these stakeholders in coming up with solutions.

Second, other books assume a segmented market approach; that is, the book is written for or geared toward one slice or subdivision of the "market" affected by dementia such as family caregivers (e.g., Mace and Rabins, *36 Hour Day*), health practitioners (e.g., Rabins and Lyketsos, *Practical Dementia Care*), or researchers (e.g., Boltz and Galvin, eds., *Dementia Care: An Evidence-Based Approach.* Switzerland: Springer International Publishing). Although these books offer critical and important contributions to the landscape of and dialogue concerning dementia, a segmentation approach (a common marketing strategy) does not allow for an aerial, 360-degree perspective of the full scope of the issues that all societies aging with dementia confront and from which to more fully prepare for and address multilayered and interrelated needs and challenges by all stakeholders involved in this disease (from the individual, to family members, the community, service providers, policy makers, and researchers). Our book provides foundational knowledge to all stakeholders but from a different perspective than that offered thus far by others.

In contrast to a segmented approach, our book assumes an "all-in" perspective. This book is for anyone and everyone touched or affected by or involved with dementia. This includes scientists in any field of study (gerontology, nursing, neurology, psychiatry, sociology, social work, occupational therapy, creative arts therapies, physical therapy, speech therapy, neuroaesthetics, and anthropology), health and human service providers, policy makers, administrators, students, advocacy groups, formal and informal caregivers, and persons with dementia. As dementia affects all of us and every aspect of life from the individual to community to national policy level, the book is based on the fundamental premise that we are "all in" this together and that we need to involve the voices, experiences, knowledge, and practices of all stakeholders to develop a common foundational understanding of needs and necessary actions to improve care and services. Thus, we must learn from each other and move forward together to advance evidence-informed, evidence-based policy, societal, community, familial and individual responses, and "dementia-ready" practices that positively support families and individuals and assure a sustained and stigma-free, quality of life.

Our ultimate goal is to make a real and transformative difference in the lives of individuals living with dementia and their families by providing foundational knowledge along with specific proven strategies for action on each of the topics that are covered in this book. Thus, we seek to use print medium to expand and enhance knowledge about dementia and from which to derive transformative behavioral, organizational, and societal changes that we all recognize must occur now. We believe that by expanding knowledge of all stakeholders, we have an opportunity to impact on skills, daily contexts, and possibly policy.

To this end, we boldly envision this book as a call to action. We examine issues from different vantage points in order to move all readers forward to identifying how to make a difference in changing dementia care in their particular life space—whether that be as an individual with dementia, providing care at home, engaging families in the community, assuring attention to and support of individuals and family caregivers in medical and healthcare encounters, or researching treatment strategies, therapeutics, and supportive services. We seek to change the way all readers understand dementia; this includes researchers, family members, service providers, administrators, and decision and policy makers.

Lastly, our book is grounded in a set of principles about dementia and dementia care that cross-cut all chapters and which are based on the best evidence to date. These basic principles are summarized in Box 1. Foremost is the need to attend to the differential impact of dementia including disparities in rates between men and women and race/ethnic groups, time to diagnosis, and access to needed resources must command our attention in the design of new services and policies related to dementia care at the local, regional, and national levels. Also, we assume a perspective that recognizes the long haul of the disease process and that disease stages are punctuated with different needs, conditions, concerns, resources, strengths, and possibilities. As the trajectory of the disease process is interposed by changes in cognition, function, behavioral symptoms, and well-being of affected individuals and these changes occur over time, discussion of any care challenge must be located within this trajectory as well as within the context of etiology, race, ethnicity, culture, gender, setting, and so forth.

Furthermore, there are disparities in the consequences of dementia for individuals, families, and communities depending upon disease stage as well as other equally important factors including social determinants (e.g., resources, financial stability, education, geographic

> **Box 1**
> **Principles Underlying this Book**
>
> - Dementia is experienced differentially depending upon gender, race, ethnicity, culture, socio-economic status, geographic location, resources
> - The course of the disease is highly individuated; individuals will experience different types of losses at different times depending upon etiology, comorbidities and other factors
> - Dementia care must be person and family-centered and family-directed
> - One size does not fit all – there is not a singular solution, approach, care or service; rather many different strategies, programs and solutions and their coordination are needed
> - Flexibility and nimbleness in policies and practices are required to address different constellation of factors shaping the experience of living with dementia
> - Dementia has medical, social, financial, emotional, physical and environmental impacts which must be simultaneously addressed (not just the medical).

location, literacy, race/ethnicity, and gender). Strategies or practices adopted for one disease stage/etiology and set of characteristics of individuals, families, and environments may not be appropriate or effective for another disease stage/etiology and different constellation of factors, thus requiring nimbleness, flexibility, and responsiveness in our policies, systems of care, and concrete practices. Hence, the topics covered in this book are explored in terms of their location along the disease trajectory and other manifold factors. For example, stigma experienced by individuals initially diagnosed and in an early stage of the disease may affect work and social participation; stigma experienced in a later disease stage may affect how health providers interact with individuals and treatment options that are offered (e.g., rehabilitation therapies may be withheld with the belief that they require the capacity for new learning versus trying different strategies to provide individuals what they need).

So, who should read this book? In keeping with our "all-in" approach, we target our writing to all constituents—health and human service professionals (physicians, nurses, occupational therapists, physical therapists, counselors, creative arts therapists, physician assistants, speech therapists, social workers, and care managers), researchers, students, family caregivers, friends of persons with dementia, individuals with dementia, policy makers, and administrators—that is, anyone interested in learning about dementia, who is directly or indirectly involved in dementia care, and who seeks and needs foundational knowledge. As dementia affects all segments of society, we believe we all need to be "dementia ready." Thus, this book seeks to offer introductory knowledge from a more holistic perspective than previous books and discussions have provided along with identifying specific actions and evidence that can be deployed in a variety of contexts in which persons living with dementia and their families reside, interact in, and are offered care and services.

The book is organized according to our social–ecological perspective (see Introduction, Fig. 1), moving from the impact of the disease on individuals outwards to family, providers, home and community, health and human service settings, and to society as a whole and back down again to the individual. We summarize evidence to date and derive specific actions based on the state of knowledge to date, keeping in mind the disease trajectory and social–ecological level that can be impacted. Specifically, each chapter:

- weaves research evidence and theories with practical know-how;
- offers evidence-informed recommendations for research, practice, policy, and how to make things better at home, in the community, in healthcare and service settings, and through national policies;
- provides local and global exemplars of what works; and
- provides case vignettes to illustrate key points with live examples.

Subsequently, based on the knowledge gained, we encourage readers to develop an "action plan" (see Chapter 13: Developing and Implementing an Action Plan) directed at making a difference in the particular setting and/or context (or level of the social-ecological model) in which one lives or works; whether that be adopting a new way of supporting an individual living with dementia at home, addressing home safety or home repair concerns, advocating for a dementia-friendly community in a locale, implementing an evidence-based program in a community-based agency, to identifying missing gaps in knowledge and pursuing them through rigorous scientific investigation.

As we are all in this together—we welcome you to this exploration and encourage you to read and then take action to improve dementia care in your context.
Let's Get Started!

Acknowledgments

We would like to extend our sincere appreciation to numerous individuals who helped with the preparation of this book. In particular, we would like to recognize Daniel Scerpella, research assistant, who conducted thorough literature searches and reviewed chapters for reference accuracy; and Jennifer Wells Smith, Senior Administrator, for working on references and chapter formatting, both of whom are at the Center for Innovative Care in Aging, Johns Hopkins University School of Nursing.

Our heartfelt gratitude to Dennis McGonagle, Acquisitions Editor, Academic Press/Elsevier, who understood, valued and believed in the importance of this book project, and for the astute attention of the editorial team who helped to make this book the best it could be.

We would also like to extend our sincere gratitude to the many federal and foundation sponsors who have supported in part through grant funding our research and translational efforts in dementia care. These include the National Institute on Aging, National Institute of Nursing Research, National Institute of Mental Health, the Alzheimer's Association, the Retirement Research Foundation, Administration on Community Living, and the Veteran's Administration.

Introduction: A Framework for Understanding Impacts of Dementia and Supporting Quality of Life With Disease Progression

> When people say, "You have Alzheimer's," you have no idea what Alzheimer's is. You know it's not good. You know there's no light at the end of the tunnel. That's the only way you can go. But you really don't know anything about it. And you don't know what to expect... ***Nancy Reagan, former First Lady of the United States.***

This book is about illuminating "the tunnel." It starts at the point in which individuals and families receive a diagnosis or recognize there is a dementia, and where current health and social systems of care typically stop and indicate to families that "nothing can be done." Although most families do not receive a formal diagnosis of a dementia[1] (Alzheimer's Disease International, 2015), those who do, have similar experiences as Mrs. Reagan—they receive a diagnosis, but no roadmap, information, or direction for moving forward, for understanding how to live with dementia. This remains particularly the case in the United States as well as for most parts of the world,[2] even though more and more countries are adopting national plans to develop a roadmap (see Chapter 11: Global Efforts and National Plans). Upon receiving a diagnosis, families are typically left with many unanswered questions and needs:

---

[1]The World Alzheimer's Report (Alzheimer's International, 2015) indicates that approximately 50% of individuals with dementia are not diagnosed in high-income countries. The rate of diagnosis drops to an estimated 10%–20% in low- and middle-income countries.

[2]Some countries such as England and Scotland have successfully implemented major policy initiatives and national campaigns to improve access to diagnosis resulting in incremental increases in diagnostic rates. In turn, increases in diagnostic rates create new and more demands for treatments and care pathways. Thus, countries must be prepared for improving care and services simultaneously as they seek to improve access to diagnosis.

"What does the diagnosis mean? What should we do next? How shall we prepare for the future? Where do we go for help; what kind of help do and will we need? How do we support each other as a family? How can my community support us? What will happen if I am unable to care or become sick? How do I work, take care of the kids and take care of mom? Do I tell my employer, neighbors, or children and how do I tell them? Will I get the disease?"

Similarly, health and human service professionals confront many clinical challenges for which they are poorly prepared to manage including providing the diagnosis and supporting families thereafter.

"How do I explain the disease to this patient? The wife looks worse than her husband who has the dementia but she is not my patient—do I ask her how she is doing? This person lives by himself and I don't know how he will be able to keep his doctor's appointments. The caregiver is overwhelmed and I am more concerned about him than my patient."

Most health and human service professionals lack even basic knowledge about dementia and its long-term management,[3] effective approaches for involving individuals with dementia and families in care decision-making, and evidence-based care and supportive programs and strategies that can be offered (Marx et al., 2014). This is the case across most care settings and countries, particularly in the United States.

Furthermore, organizational and financial systems of care are not designed to effectively support the management of chronic conditions in older adults in general,[4] and dementia specifically. As dementia is a terminal and long-term disorder, and evidence-based and evidence-informed care strategies have received little main stream attention or integration into routine care, health and human service professionals, administrators, policy makers, and other stakeholders normally extricate themselves from its management (Khanassov, Pluye, & Vedel, 2014; Koch & Iliffe, 2010; Sampson, 2006). This structural blind eye in turn places an undue additional financial and other care burdens upon individuals living with dementia and their family caregivers (Jutkowitz et al., 2017a; Jutkowitz et al., 2017b; Taylor & Quesnel-Vallée, 2016). The

---

[3]Although major medical organizations in the United States and other countries have published numerous treatment guidelines and there are a few quality measures that serve as indicators of effective clinical practices with persons with dementia, these are not well integrated or widely used in clinical practices and care settings.

[4]As discussed in *Reinventing American Health Care*, Emanuel (2014) describes the current healthcare systems inability to care for chronic disease and mental illness and identifies the need for programs of care that keep chronically ill persons in the community out of the emergency room and hospital, thereby decreasing the frequency of avoidable complications and rate of hospitalization, associated costs, and personal decline.

explicit assumption and expectation is that the family will assume responsibility for all care-related matters.

Despite significant limitations in our understandings of the neurobiology of dementia and the mechanisms underlying its core clinical features, such as functional decline and behavioral and psychological symptoms, its consequences on everyday living and society at-large are beginning to be documented. Moreover, although more research is critically needed, there is sufficient evidence and know-how concerning the forms of care and services that can improve the lives of people with dementia and their caregivers now and to help individuals remain living at home or in their place of choice with quality of life. Although, the evidence to date does not address all issues, concerns, and challenges of disease management and individual and caregiver needs and preferences, it does provide a roadmap for helping families to "live well"[5] or better than they are now presently able to do because of the wide chasm between what we know and what we actually do.

How we support quality of life and better living with dementia and organize for comprehensive care and services will require nothing short of a paradigm shift—a transformation in every sector of society—from how we educate/train and support health and human service professionals and administrators, to the organization and reimbursement of care, to housing options and community setup, to the quality, type, and availability of services that provide continuous education, skills, and support to individuals and all members of families affected. Such a transformation is intricately linked to, and not dissimilar from, other calls for action for dramatic changes in healthcare systems and supports, particularly in the United States, as it concerns long-term care and services for older adults in general, and particularly for individuals 80 years and older who experience increasing frailty (US Senate Commission on Long-Term Care, 2013) and require chronic disease management (Clarke, Bourn, Skoufalos, Beck, & Castillo, 2017; Institute of Medicine, 2012). Transformation will also need to include the integration of social and medical care and full involvement of family caregivers (National Academies of Sciences, Engineering, & Medicine, 2016).

This book seeks to provide a framework for how to think about and act upon such a transformation. It also provides concrete steps that can be taken by individuals, caregivers, researchers, communities, health and human service professionals, as well as decision and policy makers to make life better for families now as we continue to move forward with big transformative changes which may take more time and political and societal will power.

---

[5]England's National Dementia Strategy of 2009 entitled "Living Well with Dementia," viewed dementia as a chronic illness that can be managed. The report strived to develop approaches to make life better for individuals with dementia and their carers.

WHY CARE ABOUT CARE?

It may seem unnecessary to have to justify a focus on care. Unfortunately, a rationale is necessary at this historical juncture to capture the attention and imagination of key stakeholders including policy makers and funders. The limited research attention and research funding granted to dementia worldwide and particularly in the United States[6] has typically been earmarked for the discovery of pharmacological therapeutics to prevent, reverse or slow disease progression, the neurobiology, and finding a cure.[7] The search for drugs that prevent, delay onset, or slow disease progression or cure has not been successful to date, albeit a paucity of funding has been provided even in these favored areas compared to other conditions such as cancer and heart disease. Drug development has been found to be very challenging with either no difference found with placebo or with life-threatening side effects, or extreme adverse events including unacceptable levels of toxicity. A review of clinical trials conducted between 2002 and 2012, for example, found high trial attrition and an overall failure rate of 99.6% (Cummings, Morstorf, & Zhong, 2014).

While it goes without saying that cure is everyone's goal, this singular, myopic focus has nevertheless left millions of individuals and their families in the dark to fend for themselves and figure out how to manage the daily challenges that typify the disease process. As the disease transpires over a protracted trajectory and upwards of 20 plus years, the no-care situation is unacceptable. A focus on research oriented to examining causal mechanisms of the disease and its cure must be balanced with research on ways to assure quality of life. Furthermore, with the current concern with identifying disease processes earlier through biomarkers and the discovery of drug therapies to delay onset or disease progression, more individuals will be identified as symptomatic and may be living with the disease longer. Hence, even more individuals will be in need of care planning, care, services, and supports. Of critical importance is that there are signals that with appropriate care, services, and supports, we may be able to condense disability, and slow disease progression.

---

[6]In the United States, Congress over the past few years has passed bills to increase funding to the National Institutes of Health for dementia research which has been an important step forward in generating new knowledge.

[7]An example is in the United States, in which the National Institutes of Health directed only an estimated 3% of its dementia funding towards advancing care-oriented research.

Comprehensive dementia care may slow disease progression and compress disability and disease burden to a shorter time frame. This is a critical empirical question that research must shed light on — how does care, services, supports impact the course of the disease biologically, psychologically, financially, emotionally.

Until very recently has any action been taken in the form of policies, national plans, reorganizing of care, and incentives to address the multitude of care challenges that individuals/families confront (see Chapter 11: Global Efforts and National Plans, on national plans). A fundamental premise of this book is that a focus on cure must be equally balanced with an emphasis on care. Some argue that the balance should be tipped more to the favor of care for several key reasons including the numbers of people affected, the complexities and burdens imposed by the disease, and economic and moral considerations.

The Numbers Imperative

The numbers alone are cause for grave societal concern for and support of the need for serious and immediate attention to developing, evaluating, and widely implementing care and supportive strategies. In the United States, over 5 million individuals are living with Alzheimer's-type dementia (Alzheimer's Association, 2016), 3 million with vascular or multi-infarct dementia, and another 1.4 million individuals with Lewy Body Dementia. Worldwide, estimates are as high as 47 million individuals living with dementia. These numbers may be much higher as the vast majority of individuals do not receive a diagnosis as mentioned above (Alzheimer's Disease International, 2015).

Numbers appear to vary considerably worldwide with an estimated 58% of persons with dementia living in low- and middle-income countries and 28% living in the world's seven richest countries (Alzheimer's Disease International, 2015). The projected numbers into the future are stunning as well; an estimated 74.5 million are expected to have a diagnosis of all-cause dementia by 2030 and 131.5 million by 2050 (Alzheimer's Disease International, 2015).

Of public importance is that recent reports indicate a slight decline in age-specific dementia incidence rates. This appears to be occurring in some countries such as the United Kingdom (Matthews et al., 2013), the United States (Langa et al., 2008), Spain (Lobo, Launer, & Fratiglioni, 2000, 2007) Canada, Sweden (Qiu, von Strauss, Backman, Winblad, & Fratiglioni, 2013), Denmark (Christensen et al., 2013), and the

Netherlands (Schrijvers et al., 2012), but not others such as China (Jia et al., 2014; Ji et al., 2015; Wu et al., 2014) and Japan (Dodge et al., 2012; Okamura, Ishii, Ishii, & Eboshida, 2013) in which there are reported increases in incidence. It is unclear as to the reasons for these trends although strong evidence points to the role of better education, as well as diet, and lifestyle improvements as explanatory factors contributing to the lowering of dementia risk. However, as aging remains the most significant risk factor for dementia and all countries are experiencing population aging, moving forward, incidents and prevalence rates may actually be higher than currently projected. Furthermore, with the emergence of new diagnostic criteria and emphasis on early identification, an even greater number of people are expected to be diagnosed and living longer with the disease (Jack et al., 2011).

> By the sheer numbers alone that are and will be affected (individuals and families), dementia presents as one of the greatest global challenges for care and services of the 21st century that must be addressed.

The Disease Burden Imperative

Another strong motivation to seriously focus on the care and service needs of families is the imperative imposed by the unprecedented disease burden presented by dementia. The World Health Organization declares that dementia contributes to the greatest disease burden worldwide (World Health Organization, 2016). Dementia is the number one feared disease among adults, surpassing cancer in recent surveys (Alzheimer's Association, 2014; Cantegreill-Kallen & Pin, 2012). Individuals with dementia typically cease employment in the mild stages and experience a wide range of financial, physical health, and emotional consequences throughout the disease process that significantly impact their life quality (see Chapter 2: Lived Experiences of Individuals With Dementia, for further discussion).

Additionally, although there is an increasing number of persons with dementia who live alone (Alzheimer's Association, 2016; Miranda-Castillo, Woods, & Orrell, 2010), most remain in their long-term residences or that of their families and are cared for by family members throughout the trajectory of the disease. In the United States, there is an estimated 15 million families who provide care to persons with dementia (Alzheimer's Association, 2016). Although rates worldwide are difficult to discern, speculation suggests similarly that a large number of families are providing some form of care for people living with dementia. This is particularly the case in low-income countries. In these countries, there may be an even greater reliance on informal or unpaid family members than in high resourced countries. As such, these countries tend to experience high disease burden due to limited resources and access to care (Alzheimer's Disease International, 2015).

The needs of individuals with dementia increase exponentially with disease progression. They may include but are not limited to the need for assistance with daily intimate forms of assistance with everyday living needs of bathing, dressing, toileting, feeding, ambulating, and managing medications, as well as assuring safety, well-being and quality of life, coordinating care and care transitions, negotiating unwieldy and disjointed health and human service systems, accompanying doctor visits, and advocating, protecting, supporting, and comforting the person with dementia, particularly in healthcare encounters, and juggling this all-inclusive care with other familial and employment responsibilities (Gaugler & Kane, 2015). The disease burden on families—including financial, physical, and psychological—are well substantiated (see also Chapter 5: Family Member as Care Partner). Nevertheless, many (but not all) of the manifestations of the disease (e.g., functional decline, behavioral symptoms) and their impact on individuals and caregivers can be ameliorated in part through evidence-based and/or evidence-informed practices, strategies, programs, and clinical know how. Helping families manage dementia may lessen the burden of symptoms and enhance the family's ability to effectively manage day to day and effectively cope throughout the disease trajectory. Also, we do not know whether providing care that reduces behavioral symptoms enhances quality of life and has a physiological impact such that it slows or alters the course of disease progression; this is an untested empirical question but one that should be examined. Although there is insufficient evidence to date that addresses all symptoms, challenges, and concerns associated with dementia (e.g., communication disorders, fall risk, sensory impairments), there is much that is known that can ease disease burdens.

> Disease burden coupled with the fact that there are common sense and evidence-based approaches to ease this burden make it an imperative to transform dementia care. Care and services may reduce burdens as well caused by our unresponsive systems of care and factors over and above that which the disease itself imposes.

The Economic Imperative

The economics of dementia and dementia care are staggering for nations, individual, and families and are cause alone for refocusing on attempts to make care better. At the societal level, the global cost of dementia is estimated at US $818 billion, a total of 1.09% of the global gross domestic product (Alzheimer's Disease International, 2015). These costs are projected to increase such that by 2015 they will reach US $1 trillion and by 2030, they will reach US $2 trillion (Alzheimer's Report, 2016). In the United States, 50% of spending ($117 billion) in Medicare is for dementia; 18% of spending ($43 billion) in Medicaid is for dementia. Medical costs include but are not limited to hospitalizations, nursing home placements, medications, and home health.

Costs incurred by families obviously vary by country. In the United States, the cost of informal or family caregiving versus direct medical costs is estimated at US $92.3 billion vs US $61.1 billion,[8] dramatically highlighting how significantly families are economically affected and take on the brunt of disease costs. Besides lost time in employment and social security benefits, specific aspects of caring for persons with dementia incur increased costs. For example, even a one-unit change in functional dependence is associated with $24.68 (95% confidence interval (CI): $1.11−$48.25) additional out-of-pocket spending per month or $296.16 per year for family caregivers. Also, a one-unit increase in functional dependence is associated with a 0.05 (95% CI: 0.01−0.09) increase in the probability of having out-of-pocket nursing home expenditures (Jutkowitz et al., 2017a). Additionally, families absorb the most costs even more than Medicare and Medicaid (Jutkowitz et al., 2017b).

Behavioral symptoms have also been implicated in driving up costs of care. Having more behavioral symptoms has been associated with the need for increased caregiver supervision and time spent in direct care (Jutkowitz et al., 2017a). Additionally, an estimated 30% of the costs associated with caring for persons living with dementia at home and in the community have been associated with behavioral management (Schnaider Beeri, Werner, Davidson, & Noy, 2002).

Extraordinary costs of care, mostly absorbed by families, may be due in part to the lack of comprehensive and proactive dementia care and services. By caring for and supporting individuals and families and preventing/managing dementia manifestations, we may prevent unnecessary hospitalizations, premature nursing home placement, and caregiver burnout and poor health, thus lowering

---

[8]For a breakdown of costs by countries, see the World Alzheimer's Report of 2015.

costs to society, individuals and families. Moreover, we must achieve a better balance between familial and societal responsibilities of care as well as the costs.

The Moral Imperative

The moral/ethical dimension of dementia care is rarely discussed (Barber & Lyness, 2001). Nevertheless, one can apply any number of common ethical frameworks to support the imperative to provide care and support to individuals with dementia and their caregivers. For example, a consequentialist/utilitarian framework suggests that strategies must be pursued that produce the greatest happiness for the greatest number of persons or for which the best results for all concerned are achieved (Barrow, 2016). This ethical framework advocates for assessing individual and caregiver needs as it would do the greatest good for all persons. A deontological/Kantian approach similarly supports reaching out to individuals with dementia and their caregivers suggesting that there is a moral, humanitarian duty to do so (Steinbock, London, & Arras, 2013). In other words, we should care about care because we should.

One can also query as to the ethics of not providing individuals living with dementia and their caregivers care and services and the best evidence available to support daily life (Gitlin & Hodgson, 2016). Not doing so may result in the experience of "moral distress," among health and human service providers and family caregivers due to "when one knows the right thing to do, but institutional constraints make it nearly impossible to pursue the right course of action" (Jameton, 1984, p. 6). Not providing adequate care also contributes to inequalities for older adults in general and specifically between those aging with dementia and those aging without. Ethical frameworks suggest that collectively, individual researchers, health and human service professionals, caregivers, communities, and society must have a moral sensitivity to the needs of individuals living with dementia and family caregivers and move forward with implementing the know-how, we have concerning better care and services.

We have a collective moral imperative and obligation to assure the health, wellbeing and safety of individuals living with dementia and their families.

CONCEPTUAL FRAMEWORK FOR DEMENTIA CARE

Inspired by others such as the personhood movement (Kitwood, 1997), our approach to understanding and transforming dementia care, services, and supports is guided by a classic social—ecological framework, particularized for the dementia context. This framework, shown in Fig. 1, conceptualizes comprehensive dementia care as encapsulating and cutting across six interrelated and interacting spheres. These spheres include individuals living with dementia, their living environment, the family and immediate social network, the neighborhood and community, healthcare systems, and society at-large.

Each sphere in turn consists of multiple interactive factors influencing daily quality of life. For example, key factors at the individual level consist of those related to the disease process (neurobiological), health, behavioral and psychological profiles, and social well-being. Key factors at the living environment level consist of its safety, security, maintenance, and supportive features of function and well-being including accessibility, presence of adaptive equipment, repair needs, level of stimulation, and number of persons. At the caregiver level, factors may include caregiver's location in their own life course and human development, their own physical, emotional, and cognitive health, their relationship and closeness to the person with dementia, their knowledge, skills, and motivations, their employment and financial status, as well as their values, beliefs, and approaches to or style of caregiving (Corcoran, 2011). Next is the neighborhood and community composed of issues related to access to transportation, shopping, medical care, and community service agencies (senior centers, adult day) as well as spiritual opportunities, safety, and security. The health and human service organizations are yet another layer of important consideration with factors including the training and competences of health and human service professionals, organization and payment structure of care influencing well-being of families. The final sphere of importance concerns the national level including policies and plans, research support, government agencies, oversight structures, whether healthcare is organized as a right or privilege and associated payment models.

This social—ecological model provides a comprehensive framework for zeroing in on particular spheres and factors without losing an understanding of all spheres and factors impacting people living with dementia and families. The model emphasizes the interactivity of factors within and between spheres. It helps us to NOT lose sight that what may appear as distal such as health and social policies have a direct impact on daily lives. As dementia is a very complex condition, so too is the provision of care, services, and supports, necessitating this

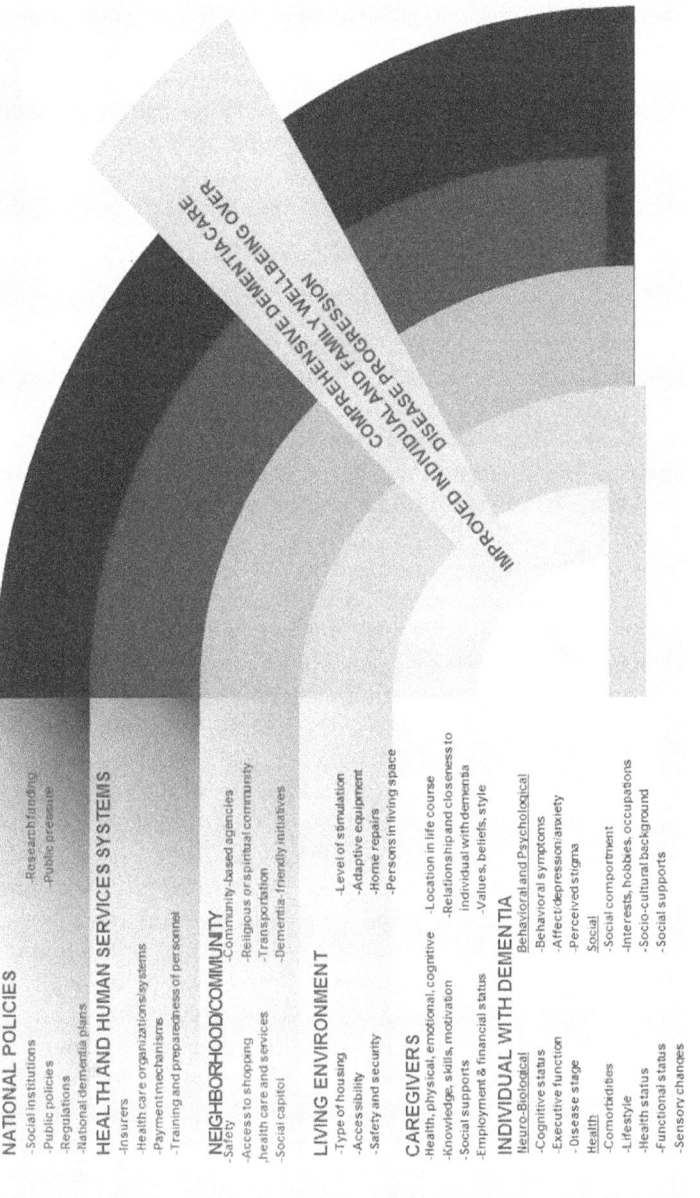

FIGURE 1 Socio-ecological model for developing and implementing comprehensive dementia care.

type of framework that can allow for a focused, zeroed-in effort on a particular problem, challenge, sphere, and factor without losing sight of the whole. Thus, a person's life space is impacted by all factors, spheres, and each must be considered when designing comprehensive dementia care. Yet even this model does not encapsulate other considerations. For example, cutting across this ecology is the concept of life course—that is the stage in a person's life course in which diagnosis occurs and the stage in a family member's life course in which care begins.

Our approach can be understood through the case snapshot of Mrs. B.

Case Snapshot – Mrs. B

Mrs. B is a 78 year old African American, diagnosed with Alzheimer's disease 4 years ago. A widow for 8 years, she lives alone in a small neat city row home. At the moderate disease stage, Mrs. B also has diabetes and hypertension and some difficulties ambulating. Her daughter and her husband and two young sons live in the same neighborhood a few blocks away. Her daughter works full time and checks in on her mom after work. She shops, prepares light meals and assures Mrs. B takes her medications nightly. The daughter also calls Mrs. B daily at noon to remind her to eat the sandwich she prepared for her the evening before. Mrs. B is no longer able to manage the trip and stairs to her church. Church members visit regularly but depend upon the daughter to arrange. Mrs. B is still able to use the telephone to talk to her daughter but she can become easily confused when others call her. She also has on occasion opened the door to strangers and been a victim of scams by telephone and mail. While she does not leave the home generally, one day neighbors found her walking up the block. She had fallen in her home having tripped over a frayed rug, resulting in a scraped knee. She became frightened and unsure how to handle her bleeding knee, prompting her to leave the house to seek help. Her daughter also noticed Mrs. B was occasionally wearing her bathroom or when dressed, she was putting on inappropriate clothing, and also spending more time in her bedroom. The daughter was increasingly taking more time off from work to check in on her, arrange for and attend her doctor appointments and assure her safety in addition to attending to her other familial responsibilities. Her employer has begun to notice her erratic schedule and expressed concern. With nothing to do all day but watch TV, Mrs. B is bored, fearful listening to the news all day and easily agitated. She wants her daughter to be with her but also worries about being a burden to her. Her daughter is becoming increasingly anxious and having difficulty taking care of two households and working. She has had to miss her own doctor and dentist appointments and Mrs. B's doctor has only offered medications to address Mrs. B increasing anxiety that had side effects and were subsequently discontinued.

This case snapshot illustrates how each sphere and their associated factors as well as the point in which dementia occurs in the life course of family members affect the well-being of Mrs. B and her family members. At the individual level, her health, problem-solving and executive abilities are declining affecting her ability to carry out instrumental and basic self-care and participate in valued activities (going to church) that have meaning to her. In the home environment, there are physical barriers, including fall hazards, and stairs which make it difficult for Mrs. B to get around. At the caregiver level, her daughter, the primary caregiver, is now the "woman in the middle"—a point in her life course where she finds herself having to balance care of an aging parent with caring as a mother to her children as well as full time employment (Brody, 2006). Her own physician and employer are unaware of her situation. At the neighborhood/community level, there are helpful neighbors but no volunteer or neighborhood watch group or social services nearby such as adult day (e.g., see Chapter 10: Services and Settings of Care, for a discussion of the Village concept). At the healthcare organization level, neither her own physician nor that of her mother has asked her how she is doing, what she needs, or addressed the wide range of needs of Mrs. B and her daughter. Mrs. B's physician is unaware of the local Alzheimer's Association number or their resources nor does she have time to spend inquiring about the daughter's well-being. At the national level, in the United States, there is no coordinated plan to help Mrs. B and her family as she progresses through the disease process. She lives in a state that has not received demonstration funds to evaluate caregiver supportive programs, and the daughter remains unaware of possible resources or how to access them.

The needs of Mrs. B and the care responsibilities of her daughter and other family members reflect a family contending with moderate dementia. Their needs would be somewhat different at the preclinical stage, moderate–severe stage, or at the end of her life. As dementia progresses,[9] the time dimension with its associated disease-based decrements and other complexities associated with comorbidities and aging add complexity to the social—ecological framework and treatment goals and must be considered in and a driver of the design and delivery of care and services.

> A social-ecological framework is a heuristic to organize how we can understand and manage the disease processes, integrate actionable treatments/approaches for assuring quality of life and personhood of individuals throughout the disease trajectory (from diagnosis to end of life and bereavement of families), to enabling all sectors of society to effectively interact and support individuals and their families.

Using this social—ecological framework, several guiding principles for comprehensive dementia care be derived (Callahan et al., 2014; ICHOM, 2017; Odenheimer et al., 2014). First, the experience of dementia must be understood as occurring within a complex web of interactive factors and multiple levels involving the individual him/herself and their unique experiences of the disease and associated processes, the living environment, family, the home and community, healthcare systems, and national policies. Each of these levels serve as barriers or supports to the health and well-being of individuals with dementia and their families independently and in combination. Also, there is the dimension of time—needs, abilities, and values will change with disease progression. Thus, one important principle is to recognize and accept the complexity presented here. There is not going to be one size that fits all in terms of the approaches, interventions, programs, services, and/or strategies that are employed. Rather, tailoring or customizing to specific characteristics at any given time will be necessary.

Second, as there are significant interactions among levels of the model, dementia care and services are more likely to be effective if the characteristics of each level and the interactions among them are considered. In other words, delivery of care and services cannot be designed and implemented in isolation or in a vacuum and solely focus on individual level determinants of health and behaviors, which is typically the approach. Rather, programs, strategies, and delivery systems must consider the independent and joint influences of determinants at all of

---

[9] Although average time to death from diagnosis is estimated as 4—6 years, individuals can live upwards to 20 + years. Also, the average is changing upward as individuals are diagnosed early in the disease process with improved disease detection technologies.

the specified levels of our social—ecological figure. Levels may be proximal or distal to the immediate outcomes sought; however, at some point in the delivery of a care/service, each level will need to be actively considered and activated. For example, designing a fall reduction program for Mrs. B by having her exercise at home and also take walks will depend upon the availability of her daughter or other individual to supervise her, the safety of her neighborhood for walking, the training of physical therapists in designing a balance and strengthening program for persons living with dementia, and reimbursement policies for physical therapy to also provide training and education for the person's care partners. Thus, the second principle is that a care program/approach/service/strategy at one level may be affected by factors in other levels, therefore, always requiring a holistic approach to deriving the best fit or care and supportive strategy.

Third, the levels and their interactions are dynamic, and determinants may change with disease progression along with changes in other spheres over time. Therefore, any system for delivery of dementia care and services must be extremely nimble and adaptable to these potential changes and dynamic relationships over time.

These principles are interwoven throughout this book and taken as a whole suggest that we need new ways of thinking about and acting upon the design, evaluation, and implementation of care/services/interventions/programs/strategies/policies.

CHALLENGES

There are critical and unique challenges in transforming the landscape of dementia care at each sector as shown in Fig. 1. We recognize that a transformation requires economic investments in research, service delivery, education, and training of health and human service professionals, and as such, retooling may not be accomplished immediately although we also believe it is unethical to ask families to wait and only have hope for small incremental improvements! We also recognize that how we transform our response to and actions for dementia will be driven by political, economic, and social forces, as well as societal values and by families and people living with dementia themselves. We introduce this book into the fray to help provide clarity and identify our choices.

There are various challenges to transformation that will necessitate careful and ongoing deliberations but which this book in itself cannot address or solve alone. First is the challenge of language. Dementia brings with it significant linguistic challenges. The label itself has been called into question as stigmatizing and (see Chapter 2: Lived Experiences of Individuals With Dementia) possibly inaccurate from a neuro-biologic perspective. Previously, different labels have been applied to persons with dementia reflecting inadequacies of our knowledge of the disease mixed with cultural mythologies. Also, it remains unclear if dementia or its variants, are a singular disease, disorder, condition, syndrome or illness. Although we recognize that "dementia" may not be the preferred term or it may be proven to be inaccurate in the future, we do defer to its use in this book at this historical juncture in our understandings — yet always referring to persons first and then the disease.

Yet another challenge is how we identify and refer to family members assisting, supporting, and helping people living with dementia. Although we us the term "caregiver" broadly as encompassing fictive kin, neighbors, friends, and blood relatives, the term itself is not necessarily recognized by those who assume this role. Also, it is unclear when a person becomes a caregiver; family members may begin by providing episodic care and may not view advocacy, transportation, coordination, and these responsibilities within the purview of "caregiving." Furthermore, varying terms may be ascribed to family members. In the medical encounter, for example, a family member may be considered as the proxy, key informant, or companion. Many families do not recognize their extraordinary efforts as caregiving. The lack of self-identification as a "caregiver" poses a challenge to service provision as access to resources may be dependent upon self-recognition. Part of a transformative approach to dementia care will have to attend to language and understanding effective approaches to reaching out to and involving families who are providing assistance.

Another critical challenge is bridging the gaps between research, practice, policy, and education of health and human service professionals. The chasm between what we know and what we do negatively impacts the experience of dementia. As we move forward with clinically relevant research, mechanisms for disseminating and implementing evidence is paramount to changing the landscape of dementia care and services (Gitlin & Czaja, 2016). How is a clinician to decide which supportive care approach to provide and where to find information about evidence-based programs? What level of evidence is needed for knowledge transfer to occur as it concerns care and services and what is the pipeline (e.g., how does evidence wind its ways through scientific evaluations to being accessible to clinicians, health providers, and families)? Moreover, what competencies and evidence-informed approaches should be introduced in the education of health and human service professionals?

As we do not have a pipeline and government oversights for developing, testing, and implementing care strategies comparable to what presently exists for the advancement of pharmacological treatments, moving the available evidence to end users continues to be complex and challenging. Nevertheless, we cannot wait for all of these to be sorted out. We have to start now in integrating what we know in educational programs to prepare a workforce, in communities to make them dementia capable and health and human service delivery.

> Despite gaps in knowledge and known challenges, we must act now to transform care and services for individuals living with dementia and their families.

ROADMAP

In considering these complexities, this book seeks to sort out and provide best practices at each level of the social–ecological framework and provide a thoughtful and systematic guide to designing and implementing better living and community environments and national policies. A wide array of topics are covered that we consider fundamental in this field and of high relevance to being dementia aware. By improving knowledge, we hope we can impact the state of dementia care and services. We try here to be part inspirational, part practical, and part change agent.

Organized by our framework, we start in Part I, About the Person Living With Dementia, and focus on the individual. Here we first examine neurobiology and disease pathology and then evaluate the impact of the disease process on the person, considering day-to-day living experiences, valuation and quality of life, the role of stigma and strive for continued personhood. In Part II, About the Caregiver, we focus on families and examine roles, needs, risks, and supportive approaches. Part III, About Living Environments, discusses the home as the primary living environment and characteristics that are supportive of daily engagement and overall well-being. Part IV, About Social Systems and Policies, is all about social systems and policies. Here we explore exemplars, criteria for dementia-capable communities, national plans and their implications for changing the landscape of dementia care and supportive services. We also examine healthcare and its organization and explore issues related to training current and next generations of health and human service providers, current payment mechanisms, and what makes a dementia-friendly hospital system. We also discuss the role of national plans and their impact on the organization of care and services and human rights of individuals with dementia and caregivers.

Finally, in Part V, Taking Action, we put it all together, summarizing major points and asking readers to act within their own environments in a way that may make a difference to individuals, families, and/or communities. As to the latter and in chapter 13, we encourage readers to develop an action plan to address a care challenge specific to his/her context—whether that be caring at home, identifying ways to effectively involve the preferences of a person living with dementia, or providing meaningful activity, to involving family members in medical encounters, modifying curricula to assure appropriate education in dementia and basic competencies in supporting families, advocating for policies to support comprehensive dementia care and inclusion of families and individual preferences, to redesigning our communities, or making hospitals more dementia friendly.

Throughout this book, we discuss possible practical solutions based on the evidence to date and clinical know-how and also present considerations for research, for clinical action, service provision, or what family caregiver/individuals and other stakeholders can do. While our primary focus is on the United States, we believe our basic premises and discussions are relevant elsewhere. We explicitly call upon exemplars worldwide and discuss some of the key challenges for delivery and implementation of effective approaches in care and services in low-, middle-, and high-income resourced countries.

This book is meant as a challenge and poses two essential questions:

- What can we do better now at each social−ecological level to support the well-being of Mrs. B and her family and as she progresses through the disease trajectory?
- What do we need to accomplish now with regard to research, social policies, educating a workforce and providing services to make life better for Mrs. B and her family?

> A focus on care/services can transform the landscape of dementia − we can improve the wellbeing of individuals with dementia and their family caregivers, possibly change the course of the disease trajectory, and reduce disease burden on individuals, families and societies. We can do this now, although unquestionably, more research to assure better care and services, better policies and workforce preparation are all urgently needed.

KEY POINTS

- Dementia impacts not only individuals but also families, communities, and society at-large.
- It is a myth that nothing can be done.
- Justification for focusing on care at this historical juncture is still necessary but is increasingly being recognized as equally important as finding a cure.

- Dementia is one of the most feared diseases now surpassing cancer.
- Dementia is extremely complex and progresses over time affecting all persons and contexts of daily life.
- With disease progression, disease presentation changes and hence the needs of individuals and families change.
- A social–ecological framework provides an holistic approach to understand ways to support individuals and families at any given point in the disease process.
- A social–ecological framework allows for a zeroed-in focused examination of any one factor or aspect of a person's daily life without losing the larger context and complexities in which it occurs.
- There is and will not be one "magic pill" or program or approach—rather, we need multilayered and multidimensional strategies in research, policy, and practice to provide effective care and support.
- This book is about the practices, research, and policies that can be implemented now and into the near future to make daily life better for individuals and their caregivers from the time of diagnosis to the end of life.

References

Alzheimer's Association. (2014). *2014 Alzheimer's disease facts & figures.* Retrieved from https://www.alz.org/downloads/facts_figures_2014.pdf.

Alzheimer's Association. (2016). *2016 Alzheimer's disease facts & figures.* Retrieved from https://www.alz.org/documents_custom/2016-facts-and-figures.pdf.

Alzheimer's Disease International. (2015). *World Alzheimer report 2015: The global impact of dementia.* Retrieved from https://www.alz.co.uk/sites/default/files/pdfs/world-alzheimer-report-2015-executive-summary-english.pdf.

Barber, C., & Lyness, K. (2001). Ethical issues in family care of older persons with dementia: Implications for family therapists. *Home Health Care Services Quarterly, 20*(3), 1–26. Available from https://doi.org/10.1300/j027v20n03_01.

Barrow, R. (2016). *Utilitarianism: A contemporary statement.* New York: Taylor & Francis.

Brody, E. (2006). *Women in the middle: Their parent-care years* (2nd ed). New York: Springer Publishers.

Callahan, C. M., Sachs, G. A., LaMantia, M. A., Unroe, K. T., Arling, G., & Boustani, M. A. (2014). Redesigning systems of care for older adults with Alzheimer's disease. *Health Affairs, 33*(4), 626–632. Available from https://doi.org/10.1377/hlthaff.2013.1260.

Cantegreil-Kallen, I., & Pin, S. (2012). Fear of Alzheimer's disease in the French population: Impact of age and proximity to the disease. *International Psychogeriatrics, 24,* 108–116.

Christensen, K., Thinggaard, M., Oksuzyan, A., Steenstrup, T., Andersen-Ranberg, K., Jeune, B., et al. (2013). Physical and cognitive functioning of people older than 90 years: A comparison of two Danish cohorts born 10 years apart. *The Lancet, 382*(9903), 1507–1513. Available from https://doi.org/10.1016/s0140-6736(13)60777-1.

Clarke, J. L., Bourn, S., Skoufalos, A., Beck, E. H., & Castillo, D. J. (2017). An innovative approach to health care delivery for patients with chronic conditions. *Population Health Management, 20*(1), 23–30. Available from https://doi.org/10.1089/pop.2016.0076.

Corcoran, M. A. (2011). Caregiving styles: A cognitive and behavioral typology associated with dementia family caregiving. *The Gerontologist*, *51*(4), 463–472. Available from https://doi.org/10.1093/geront/gnr002.
Cummings, J., Morstorf, T., & Zhong, K. (2014). Alzheimer's disease drug-development pipeline: Few candidates, frequent failures. *Alzheimers Res Ther*, *6*(4), 37. Available from https://doi.org/10.1186/alzrt269.
Dodge, H., Buracchio, T., Fisher, G., Kiyohara, Y., Meguro, K., Tanizaki, Y., & Kaye, J. (2012). Trends in the prevalence of dementia in Japan. *International Journal of Alzheimer's Disease*, *2012*, 1–11. Available from https://doi.org/10.1155/2012/956354.
Emanuel, E. J. (2014). *Reinventing American health care: How the Affordable Care Act will improve our terribly complex, blatantly unjust, outrageously expensive, grossly inefficient, error prone system*. New York, NY: PublicAffairs.
Gaugler, J., & Kane, R. (2015). *Family caregiving in the new normal*. London: Elsevier Academic Press.
Gitlin, L., & Czaja, S. (2016). *Behavioral intervention research: Designing, evaluating, implementing*. New York: Springer Publishing Company.
Gitlin, L. N., & Hodgson, N. A. (2016). Who should assess the needs of and care for a dementia patient's caregiver? *AMA Journal of Ethics*, *18*(12), 1171–1181. Available from https://doi.org/10.1001/journalofethics.2016.18.12.ecas1-1612.
Institute of Medicine. (2012). *Living well with chronic illness: A call for public health action*. Washington DC: National Academies of Science Press.
International Consortium for Health Outcomes Measurement (ICHOM). Dementia. http://www.ichom.org/medical-conditions/dementia/. Accessed April 19, 2017.
Jack, C. R., Albert, M. S., Knopman, D. S., McKhann, G. M., Sperling, R. A., Carrillo, M. C., ... Phelps, C. H. (2011). Introduction to the recommendations from the National Institute on Aging-Alzheimer's Association workgroups on diagnostic guidelines for Alzheimer's disease. *Alzheimer's & Dementia*, *7*(3), 257–262. Available from https://doi.org/10.1016/j.jalz.2011.03.004.
Jameton, A. (1984). *Nursing practice: The ethical issues* (p. 331) Englewood Cliffs, NJ: Prentice-Hall.
Ji, Y., Shi, Z., Zhang, Y., Liu, S., Liu, S., Yue, W., et al. (2015). Prevalence of dementia and main subtypes in rural northern China. *Dementia and Geriatric Cognitive Disorders*, *39*(5–6), 294–302. Available from https://doi.org/10.1159/000375366.
Jia, J., Wang, F., Wei, C., Zhou, A., Jia, X., Li, F., et al. (2014). The prevalence of dementia in urban and rural areas of China. *Alzheimer's & Dementia*, *10*(1), 1–9. Available from https://doi.org/10.1016/j.jalz.2013.01.012.
Jutkowitz, E., Kuntz, K. M., Dowd, B., Gaugler, J. E., MacLehose, R. F., & Kane, R. L. (2017a). Effects of cognition, function, and behavioral and psychological symptoms on out-of-pocket medical and nursing home expenditures and time spent caregiving for persons with dementia. *Alzheimer's & Dementia*, *13*(7), 801–809. Available from https://doi.org/10.1016/j.jalz.2016.12.011.
Jutkowitz, E., Kane, R. L., Gaugler, J. E., MacLehose, R. F., Dowd, B., & Kuntz, K. M. (2017b). Societal and family lifetime cost of dementia: Implications for policy. *Journal of the American Geriatric Society*. Available from https://doi.org/10.1111/jgs.15043.
Khanassov, V., Pluye, P., & Vedel, I. (2014). Case management for dementia in primary health care: A systematic mixed studies review based on the diffusion of innovation model. *Clinical Interventions in Aging*, *9*, 915–928. Available from https://doi.org/10.2147/cia.s64723.
Kitwood, T. (1997). *Dementia reconsidered: The Person comes first*. Buckingham, United Kingdom: Open University Press.

Koch, T., & Iliffe, S. (2010). Rapid appraisal of barriers to the diagnosis and management of patients with dementia in primary care: A systematic review. *BMC Family Practice*, *11*(1), 52. Available from https://doi.org/10.1186/1471-2296-11-52.

Langa, K., Larson, E., Karlawish, J., Cutler, D., Kabeto, M., Kim, S., & Rosen, A. (2008). Trends in the prevalence and mortality of cognitive impairment in the United States: Is there evidence of a compression of cognitive morbidity? *Alzheimer's & Dementia*, *4*(2), 134−144. Available from https://doi.org/10.1016/j.jalz.2008.01.001.

Lobo, A., Launer, L. J., & Fratiglioni, L. (2000). Prevalence of dementia and major subtypes in Europe: A collaborative study of population-based cohorts. Neurologic diseases in the elderly research group. *Neurology*, *54*(11), 4−9.

Lobo, A., Saz, P., Marcos, G., Dia, J., De-la-Camara, C., Ventura, T., et al. (2007). Prevalence of dementia in a southern European population in two different time periods: The ZARADEMP Project. *Acta Psychiatrica Scandinavica*, *116*(4), 299−307. Available from https://doi.org/10.1111/j.1600-0447.2007.01006.x.

Matthews, F. E., Arthur, A., Barnes, L. E., Bond, J., Jagger, C., Robinson, L., & Brayne, C. (2013). A two-decade comparison of prevalence of dementia in individuals aged 65 years and older from three geographical areas of England: Results of the Cognitive Function and Ageing Study I and II. *The Lancet*, *382*(9902), 1405−1412. Available from https://doi.org/10.1016/S0140-6736(13)61570-6.

Marx, K., Stanley, I., Van Haitsma, K., Moody, J., Alonzi, D., Hansen, B., & Gitlin, L. (2014). Knowing versus doing: Education and training needs of staff in a chronic care hospital unit for individuals with dementia. *Journal of Gerontological Nursing*, *40*(12), 26−34. Available from https://doi.org/10.3928/00989134-20140905-01.

Miranda-Castillo, C., Woods, B., & Orrell, M. (2010). People with dementia living alone: What are their needs and what kind of support are they receiving? *International Psychogeriatrics*, *22*(04), 607−617. Available from https://doi.org/10.1017/s104161021000013x.

National Academies of Sciences, Engineering, and Medicine. (2016). *Families caring for an aging America*. Washington, DC: National Academies Press.

Odenheimer, G., Borson, S., Sanders, A. E., Swain-Eng, R. J., Kyomen, H. H., Tierney, S., ... Johnson, J. (2014). Quality improvement in neurology: Dementia management quality Measures. *Journal of the American Geriatrics Society*, *62*(3), 558−561. Available from https://doi.org/10.1111/jgs.12630.

Okamura, H., Ishii, S., Ishii, T., & Eboshida, A. (2013). Prevalence of dementia in Japan: A systematic review. *Dementia and Geriatric Cognitive Disorders*, *36*(1−2), 111−118. Available from https://doi.org/10.1159/000353444.

Qiu, C., von Strauss, E., Backman, L., Winblad, B., & Fratiglioni, L. (2013). Twenty-year changes in dementia occurrence suggest decreasing incidence in central Stockholm, Sweden. *Neurology*, *80*(20), 1888−1894. Available from https://doi.org/10.1212/wnl.0b013e318292a2f9.

Sampson, E. (2006). Differences in care received by patients with and without dementia who died during acute hospital admission: A retrospective case note study. *Age and Ageing*, *35*(2), 187−189. Available from https://doi.org/10.1093/ageing/afj025.

Schnaider Beeri, M., Werner, P., Davidson, M., & Noy, S. (2002). The cost of behavioral and psychological symptoms of dementia (BPSD) in community dwelling Alzheimer's disease patients. *International Journal of Geriatric Psychiatry*, *17*(5), 403−408. Available from https://doi.org/10.1002/gps.490.

Schrijvers, E., Verhaaren, B., Koudstaal, P., Hofman, A., Ikram, M., & Breteler, M. (2012). Is dementia incidence declining? Trends in dementia incidence since 1990 in the Rotterdam Study. *Neurology*, *78*(19), 1456−1463. Available from https://doi.org/10.1212/wnl.0b013e3182553be6.

Steinbock, B., London, A., & Arras, J. (2013). *Ethical issues in modern medicine.* New York: McGraw-Hill.

Taylor, M., & Quesnel-Vallée, A. (2016). The structural burden of caregiving: Shared challenges in the United States and Canada. *The Gerontologist, 57,* 19–25. Available from https://doi.org/10.1093/geront/gnw102.

US Senate Commission on Long-Term Care,. (2013). *Report to the Congress.* Washington DC. Retrieved from http://ltccommission.org/ltccommission/wp-content/uploads/2013/12/Commission-on-Long-Term-Care-Final-Report-9-26-13.pdf.

World Health Organization. (2016). *Dementia.* Retrieved from http://www.who.int/mediacentre/factsheets/fs362/en/.

Wu, Y., Lee, H., Norton, S., Prina, A., Fleming, J., Matthews, F., & Brayne, C. (2014). Period, birth cohort and prevalence of dementia in mainland China, Hong Kong and Taiwan: A meta-analysis. *International Journal of Geriatric Psychiatry, 29*(12), 1212–1220. Available from https://doi.org/10.1002/gps.4148.

Further Reading

Khachaturian, A. S., Hoffman, D. P., Frank, L., Petersen, R., Carson, B. R., & Khachaturian, Z. S. (2017). Zeroing out preventable disability: Daring to dream the impossible dream for dementia care. Recommendations for a national plan to advance dementia care and maximize functioning. *Alzheimer's & Dementia, 13*(10), 1077–1080. Available from https://doi.org/10.1016/j.jalz.2017.09.003.

PART I

ABOUT THE PERSON LIVING WITH DEMENTIA

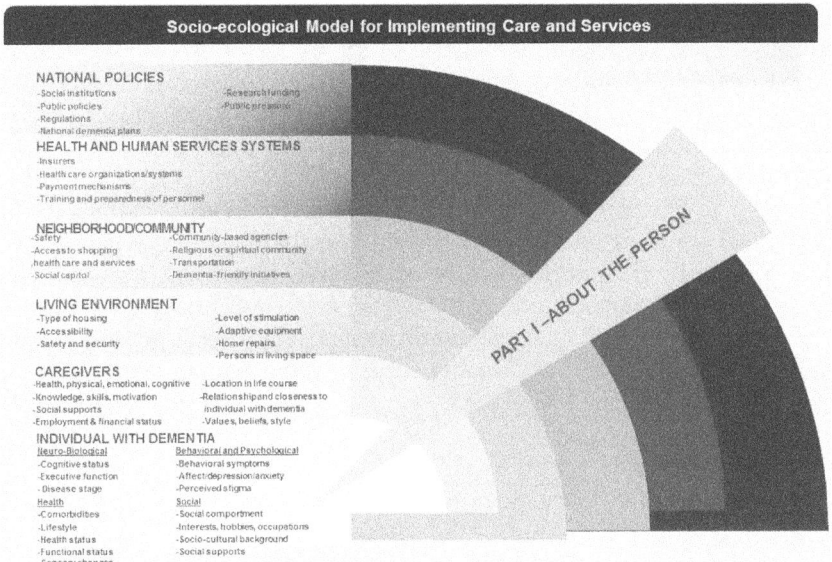

In Part I, we examine the impact of dementia on individuals living with this disease. We start by providing a broad strokes understanding of what is currently known about the pathophysiology and different etiologies of dementia (see Chapter 1: How the Brain Is Affected), and the search for biomarkers for early diagnostic purposes. We then move on to discuss some of the most salient experiences of living with dementia for affected individual. Although there is limited research which includes the perspective of individuals themselves who are living with a diagnosis, we discuss what we do know and tackle key concerns of individuals such as when and how to disclose one's diagnosis, perceived and structural stigma, ongoing biographical management and strive for maintaining a sense of self-identity with disease progression (see Chapter 2: Lived Experiences of Individuals With Dementia). Furthermore, we offer a multifaceted model to understand factors contributing to quality of life (which we also refer to as the "good life," in keeping with the originator of the model, Dr. M. Powell Lawton). The model provides a comprehensive framework that can guide an understanding of different domains affected by the disease, as well as ways to consider intervening to support/improve quality of life.

In Chapter 3, Breaking the Cycle of Despair, we discuss a structural form of stigma we refer to as a "cycle of despair." We argue that a cycle of despair is inadvertently imposed upon individuals and families by most healthcare system's exclusive curative stance and acute care organizational structure. This stance promotes a set of negative communications that are relayed with a diagnosis of disclosure, e.g., "nothing can be done," leading to a sense of despair and inaction. In turn, we discuss how this cycle of despair is buttressed by six factors that pose as barriers to comprehensive dementia care (lack of diagnosis, unprepared workforce, fragmented care systems and payments structures, social determinants and disparities, cultural beliefs and stigma, lack of knowledge and access).

Finally in Chapter 4, Making Life Better for Individuals Living With Dementia, we examine the evidence to date that suggests what can be done presently to support quality of life. We identify various proven approaches/programs/strategies which suggest ways to make life better.

Taken as a whole, Part I is about the person—biological processes, psychosocial considerations, and quality of life improvement opportunities.

CHAPTER 1

How the Brain Is Affected

I've forgotten what it's like to remember. I've lost the mindless confidence that a moment, an idea, a thought will be there for me later, the bravado of breezing through experience in the certainty that it will become part of my self, part of my story. **Floyd Skloot, American poet, novelist, and memoirist.**

Let us start where dementia begins and resides—the brain. This chapter focuses on the initial, individual-level, factors that impact persons living with dementia including the underlying changes that occur in the brain, the diagnostic process, and the pharmacologic treatment options currently available. We focus on these particular aspects in order to provide basic foundational knowledge for understanding the experience of dementia as it progresses.

Case Snapshot—Ms. H.

Ms. H. is age 77. She is divorced and has been living alone for many years as a vital and active member of her community. Lately her daughter, Julia, has been noticing that her mom has been missing dates with friends, and that there are unpaid bills and clutter in her normally clean and organized home. Last week Ms. H. became lost in her neighborhood and became shaken by the experience. Today Ms. H. and Julia just completed a visit with the neurologist. Her diagnosis was confirmed. Dementia. Ms. H. looks to you, then her daughter, and says plainly and sadly, "I am not sure what to do."

This case snapshot of Ms. H illustrates the challenge of delineating normal age-related changes and onset of dementia. There is often not a clear line that separates the two. Sometimes symptoms creep up or pile on. Sometimes family members, co-workers, or neighbors notice a significant difference in an individual's behavior, mood, personality, problem solving or everyday functioning; and sometimes individuals themselves report significant subjective memory complaints (Mitchell, Beaumont, Ferguson, Yadegarfar, & Stubbs, 2014; Steinberg et al., 2013) that propel the individual and/or family to seek a formal diagnosis. It is also not uncommon for individuals and families to receive a diagnosis of "dementia" without understanding that dementia refers to a group of brain disorders—each with their own unique neurobiology.

PATHOPHYSIOLOGY OF DEMENTIA

What do we know about the underlying causes of dementia? First, it is important to understand that dementia is a general term for a group of brain disorders. It is not a specific disease in itself. Rather, dementia describes a group of symptoms affecting memory, thinking, and social abilities severely enough to interfere with daily functioning. There are often no clear indicators of the type of dementia until the condition progresses and further information on the causative factors can be identified based on available diagnostic data. If an etiology can be narrowed down, and this is not always possible, individuals may be given a diagnosis of a specific type of dementia. Although there are over 100 diseases that can cause dementia (Prince, Bryce, & Ferri, 2011), here we briefly describe the basic brain changes that occur in five of the most common forms of dementia: Alzheimer's disease, mixed dementia, vascular dementia, Lewy body dementia, and frontotemporal dementia (FTD). These are also summarized in Box 1-1.

Dementia is a syndrome with many potential underlying causes such as Alzheimer's Disease, Lewy Body Disease, vascular disease or a combination of these factors.

Alzheimer's Disease

Alzheimer's disease, the leading cause of dementia, is characterized by the presence in the brain of protein deposits called plaques, consisting predominately of the amyloid β peptide (Aβ or A-beta), and tangles, consisting primarily of neurofibrillary tangles of tau protein. Although plagues and tangles occur as part of normal aging, the higher concentrations of plaques and tangles in specific brain regions (such as the neocortex and hippocampus) and a clinical history of memory

> **Box 1-1**
> **Five Common Types of Dementia**
>
> - Alzheimer's Disease: Initial short-term memory loss followed by gradual loss of other cognitive and communication abilities; diagnosis often made retrospectively, slowly progressive over 5–12 years.
> - Mixed dementia: Alzheimer's disease and vascular dementia combined.
> - Vascular dementia: Abrupt onset, stepwise decline over 5 years, history of vascular risks, symptoms, and manifestations are dependent on the area of brain affected.
> - Lewy Body Dementia: Fluctuating levels of cognition, motor symptoms consistent with Parkinsonism, behavioral symptoms may include psychosis.
> - FTD (Pick's disease): Gradual onset between ages 45 and 65 years, progressive personality changes, behavioral disturbances, progressive decline in functioning.

problems are used to confirm the diagnosis of Alzheimer's disease (Hyman et al., 2012). The metabolic changes that result in plaques are considered the initiating events in Alzheimer's diseases, but these changes do not immediately affect memory or cognitive function. In other words, disease activity can be occurring for many years before cognitive symptoms appear. As a result, the concept of "preclinical Alzheimer's disease" has emerged as scientists seek to understand the early disease processes in the formation of plaques and tangles in order to develop treatments and facilitate timely diagnosis (Besson et al., 2015; Papp et al., 2015).

Mixed Dementia

While the $A\beta$ hypothesis is the most investigated and accepted over the past 20 years, the exact role of $A\beta$ in the onset of progression of Alzheimer's disease is not fully understood and continues to be debated. This debate has been fueled by the vascular hypotheses, as increasing research suggests that vascular disease also plays a key role in the onset and progression of a mixed form of dementia (Hayakawa et al., 2015; van Uden et al., 2015). Autopsy studies from individuals diagnosed with Alzheimer's disease suggest that a majority had a form of "mixed dementia," caused by both an Alzheimer's disease-related neurodegenerative processes and a vascular disease-related processes. More recent research suggests that mixed vascular-degenerative dementia is the most common cause of dementia in the elderly. In one study, approximately 40% of people who were thought to have Alzheimer's were found after autopsy to also have some form of cerebrovascular disease (Schneider, Arvanitakis, Leurgans, & Bennett, 2009). Given the clinical and biological complexity of Alzheimer's disease and mixed dementia, health care providers are often not forthcoming with information to help patients understand the disease process. Yet for patients diagnosed with Alzheimer's disease, the diagnosis is more frightening as receiving a cancer diagnosis and the need for information is great (Cahill, Pierce, Werner, Darley, & Boberbsky, 2015). Thus current research on "all-cause" dementia etiology is largely focused on the development and application of innovative approaches to analyze the complex interactions of multiple biological systems rather than on a single cause (Bergeron et al., 2015; DiMarco et al., 2015; Schott & Fox, 2016).

Vascular Dementia

Vascular dementia, the second most common form of dementia, results from injuries to the vessels supplying blood to the brain, often due to occlusions of blood vessels, hemorrhage in large or small blood vessels, or lacunar strokes of small cerebral blood vessels (Haffner, Malik, & Dichgans, 2016). The most prevalent is cerebral small vessel injury, or arteriolosclerosis, that supply deep nuclei and deep white matter areas in the brain. Symptoms of vascular dementia can begin suddenly and then either worsen or stabilize during an individual's lifetime based on the rates of these vascular injuries (Du et al., 2017). Similar to our understanding of Alzheimer's disease and mixed dementia, the particular pathways that lead to disease pathology remain poorly understood, leaving individuals and families often with more questions than answers regarding treatment decisions and prognosis (Helman & Murphy, 2016; Lopez-Haldes et al., 2016).

Lewy Body Dementia

Lewy body dementia—cited as one of the most common causes of dementia—is often one of the most frustrating to be accurately diagnosed because if it often misdiagnosed as a movement disorder of Alzheimer's diseases. Accurate diagnosis can take numerous diagnostic visits and tests before an accurate diagnosis is given (Zweig & Galvin, 2014). The pathology of Lewy body dementia involves protein aggregates (Lewy bodies) that are balloon-like structures inside nerve cells and the formation of Lewy neurites in the brain. Because these same pathologic changes also occur in persons with Parkinson's disease, Lewy body dementia and Parkinson's disease are considered part of a continuum of Lewy body diseases (Klein et al., 2010). The initial symptoms may vary, but over time individuals develop very similar cognitive, behavioral, physical, and sleep-related symptoms that include changes in alertness and attention, hallucinations, tremor, muscle stiffness, sleep problems, and memory loss.

Frontotemporal Dementia

Frontotemporal Dementia, or FTD, describes a group of neurodegenerative conditions associated with disorders of tau that result in atrophy in the frontal and temporal lobes of the brain and account for up to 10% of all dementia cases. FTD has been linked to five genetic markers, and 30%–50% of individuals with FTD have a family history of early onset dementias. Some forms of FTD are considered combinations of tau disease and vascular disease. To date, there is no specific abnormality associated with all cases of FTD. For example, in one type of FTD called Pick's disease, there are abnormal microscopic deposits called Pick bodies (Arvanitakis, 2010).

Does Etiology Matter?

In some respects, knowing the etiology of a dementia does not matter when considering lived experiences and daily consequences of dementia. The functional or daily consequences are very similar across all etiologies. Nevertheless, it can be helpful to know etiology for the purposes of understanding and planning. For example, as FTD is characterized by early onset and often extreme behavioral disturbances, understanding this particular disease can be very helpful to individuals and families. As Lewy body dementia has a strong movement component in advanced stages, receiving this as a diagnosis may help a family plan differently than if the dementia is due to another underlying disease.

At the very least, even when etiology cannot be determined, individuals with dementia are entitled to accurate, timely and sensitive disclosure of the diagnosis at the moment when they and their families express concerns and can benefit from advice, treatment, and support.

THE CHALLENGE OF DIAGNOSIS

Less than half of all individuals living with dementia are aware of their diagnosis. As many as 28 million of the world's 47 million people with dementia have yet to receive a diagnosis and therefore do not have access to treatment, information, and care (Prince et al., 2011). There are any number of factors that can explain this concerning fact. One is the very real stigma associated with dementia that often prevents open discussion about it (see Chapter 2: Lived Experiences of Individuals With Dementia). Despite the increasing prevalence of dementia in society, there is a lack of public recognition, awareness or discussion of dementia, and the benefits of early detection and diagnosis (Quaglio, Brand, & Dario, 2016). The second factor leading to low diagnosis awareness is a form of denial that memory problems are a normal part of getting older. This belief is often complicated by another false belief that "nothing can be done." Yet as we emphasize in this book, it is simply not true that there is "no point in a diagnosis" or that "nothing can be done."

Unfortunately, even for those who do seek assessment for memory changes, the process of obtaining a diagnosis is not straightforward, easy, or consistent. Obtaining a diagnosis can take a few months or a few years driven in part by a lack of clinician knowledge, time, and reimbursement structures to ensure a full assessment of cognitive impairment (Hinton et al., 2007). Disparities in diagnosis also exist by race/ethnic/cultural groups, with minority populations including African Americans and Latinos in the United States, receiving a diagnosis much later in the disease process if at all (Alzheimer's Association, 2014; Husaini et al., 2003). Social ecological forces appear to be at play and include a number of factors such as one's health literacy, access to resources, cultural beliefs, stigma, fear, and/or understanding of the need for a diagnosis (Chin, Negash, & Hamilton, 2011).

The Diagnosis Disclosure

Most people with dementia wish to be told of their diagnosis, but there is a concerning lack of practice guidelines to direct clinicians in interpreting diagnostic impressions and disclose the diagnosis (Borson et al., 2016). The tremendous focus in dementia research on characterizing the pathology of dementia has not been translated into routine clinical practice. There is no single definitive diagnostic test for dementia, and while clinicians may determine that a person has a dementia diagnosis, the exact cause is often difficult to confirm. For example, a diagnosis of Alzheimer's disease is often based on the clinician's judgment and may or may not be in concert with evidence-based guidelines from the Alzheimer's Association, the National Institute on Aging, and the US Preventative Task Force (Hyman et al., 2012).

At a minimum the essentials of any assessment for dementia includes a medical history, clinical examination, laboratory tests, and an imaging test (MRI or CT scan, if indicated) to rule out underlying medical conditions that may contribute to memory changes. This is followed by a comprehensive assessment of multiple cognitive domains to pinpoint the memory deficits and further refine the diagnostic impressions. Often a referral to a specialist based in a memory clinic is needed in order to access experts in diagnosing, treating, and advising people with dementia and their families.

Once diagnostic procedures have been completed, revealing test results and a diagnosis to individuals and their family members can be challenging for health providers. This is because clinicians often do not receive specialized training in how to effectively relay a diagnosis of such a profound and complex condition and are often unprepared to respond to questions concerning next steps and care planning.

Upon receiving a diagnosis of "dementia," most families may not fully understand that this is a general term for a group of brain disorders—each with their own unique neurobiology. Most persons newly diagnosed with dementia are left to grapple with the stigma of the disease, an uncertain treatment course and may be unclear as to the implications of the diagnosis for everyday life. Moreover, although dementia has immediate and long-term implications for daily living, individuals and families are typically left on their own to figure it out after receiving a diagnosis.

The response of individuals and families to the disclosure of a diagnosis of dementia may depend in part upon the manner in which the diagnosis is imparted. Some common issues reported, both from the perspectives of individuals and their families, include being unprepared for the bad news, having the diagnosis disclosed insensitively, or receiving inadequate information with no follow-up (Lecouturier et al., 2008). Sometimes a diagnosis is not shared with individuals themselves but rather only with the family who receive very little information about the condition, resources, education, and support. Except in unusual circumstances, physicians and the care team should disclose the diagnosis to the individual with Alzheimer's disease because of the individual's moral and legal right to know" (Alzheimer's Association, 2014).

Current evidence-based recommendations include eight key elements of good practice in delivering a dementia diagnosis—preparation; involving family members; exploring the individual's perspective; disclosing the diagnosis; responding to individual and family reactions; focusing on quality of life; future planning; and effective communication. This process has been termed "making the diagnosis well"

(Lecouturier et al., 2008). As with any diagnosis of a serious illness, the disclosure conversation is the first in many conversations about the impact of the disease on the individual and family. Five additional key concepts that should be used to guide ongoing conversations about the dementia diagnosis are summarized in Box 1-2. Evidence suggests that when individuals with dementia and their families are well prepared and supported, initial feelings of shock, anger, and grief are balanced by a sense of reassurance and empowerment (Milby, Murphy, & Winthrop, 2015).

Benefits of Early Diagnosis

There are clearly tangible benefits to earlier recognition of dementia (Jack et al., 2011). Population-based survey findings indicate that early disclosure of the diagnosis is preferred by most individuals (Blendon et al., 2012). Timely diagnosis could offer many potential benefits to individuals with dementia and families, especially the opportunity to obtain treatment to control symptoms, avoid medications that may worsen symptoms, and access to treatments that slow or lessen the disease process (Prince et al., 2011). Additional benefits of making a diagnosis include ending uncertainty about the cause of alarming or disturbing symptoms and behavior change, with a greater understanding of why they may be occurring; giving access to appropriate support; promoting positive coping strategies; and facilitating the planning and fulfillment of short-term goals. Early, accurate, and documented diagnosis of dementia has been shown to result in better outcomes for

---

Box 1-2

Five Goals of Dementia Disclosure

1. Provide individuals and caregivers with general information about dementia, and include the stage of disease and classification of disease.
2. Provide information on pharmacologic and nonpharmacologic treatment options.
3. Refer individuals and caregivers to resources in their community, such as the Alzheimer's Association.
4. Where no proxy or caregiver exists, encourage the individual to name a health care and a financial proxy.
5. Develop and document a plan of care in collaboration with the individual and caregiver.

> **Box 1-3**
> **Benefits of Timely Diagnosis of Dementia**
>
> - Maximizes treatment options that have potential to slow disease process
> - Accesses pathway of evidence-based treatments and support services
> - Facilitates advanced care planning
> - Eases uncertainty
> - Individuals "right to know"
> - Helps individual and family plan for the future

individuals and their caregivers (Cahill et al., 2015). Of importance is that an early diagnosis affords an important opportunity to gather information from individuals themselves about their future wishes for care and treatment (Box 1-3)

ROLE OF BIOMARKERS IN DIAGNOSIS

The need for additional information to improve the timeliness and accuracy of diagnosis has led to growing interest in the role of biomarkers. Biomarkers are characteristics of diseases that can be objectively measured and evaluated as an indicator of either a normal or pathogenic processes. Biomarkers for dementia fall into two categories: fluid biomarkers and imaging biomarkers.

Fluid Biomarkers

Fluid biomarkers for dementia are found in cerebrospinal fluid and include measures of inflammation, infection, and markers of amyloid protein metabolism. The most commonly studied fluid biomarkers are molecular pathology of amyloid proteins that are seen in Alzheimer's disease—Aβ peptides. Low levels of Aβ in cerebrospinal fluid are indicative of Alzheimer's disease (Dubois et al, 2016). The second category of fluid biomarker for dementia measures neuronal or brain cell injury. These biomarkers assess for the presence of tau—the primary component of the tangles seen in brains of persons with Alzheimer's diseases. The usefulness of fluid biomarkers in determining dementia diagnosis has been mostly limited to research applications focused on the accuracy of diagnosis of Alzheimer's disease in clinical trials. If both biomarkers are positive, the likelihood of an Alzheimer's disease pathology is very high. Having one of these two biomarkers would be interpreted as a moderate likelihood, and having neither of these biomarkers would be interpreted as a low likelihood for Alzheimer's disease. For example, low cerebrospinal fluid concentrations of the Aβ peptide, in combination with high total tau and phosphorylated tau, would be considered highly predictive of progression to Alzheimer's dementia in patients with mild cognitive impairment.

Worldwide standardization efforts and quality control programs include standard operating procedures for both preanalytical (e.g., lumbar puncture to obtain cerebrospinal fluid and sample handling) and analytical procedures are being designed to improve observed variations in laboratory values. Efforts are also ongoing to develop highly reproducible assays on fully automated instruments. These global standardization and harmonization measures will provide the basis for the generalized international application of biomarkers into more routine clinical diagnosis. Once successful, these approaches would allow clinicians to intervene earlier, identify people at risk, and initiate treatments much earlier to prevent or delay the progression of the disease.

Imaging Biomarkers

Structural brain imaging (e.g., CT scan or MRI) is currently recommended in all persons being evaluated for dementia, according to the UK, European, and US guidelines. Brain imaging can assess for vascular damage and brain signal changes with a wide range of causes. The pattern of regional brain loss that can be observed through brain imaging is currently being incorporated into diagnostic criteria for several dementia syndromes (Dubois et al., 2007). Functional imaging techniques such as positron emission tomography (PET) and single photon emission tomography allow for measurement of patterns of brain metabolism, which show characteristic patterns that differ in different dementia syndromes. For example, PET tracers that bind to brain proteins such as Aβ or tau can be used to assess Alzheimer's disease pathology.

These are just a few of the more common applications of biomarkers to early detection and study of dementia, and there are other techniques being explored as biomarkers. While the biomarkers discussed above are invasive, expensive, and difficult to obtain in most clinical settings, other newer diagnostic tests offer promise as noninvasive, inexpensive biomarkers of dementia. One test, the Olfactory Identification Test, is based on the premise that neurofibrillary tangles in the olfactory bulb are among the earliest pathologic features of Alzheimer's disease. Current research is exploring if odor identification impairment can be used as a useful tool to improve diagnostics (Devanand, 2016).

It is important to remember that while the specific biomarkers vary across different dementias and at present are focused on the diagnosis of Alzheimer's disease, there are common themes including their potential ability to allow for early or pre-symptomatic diagnosis, track disease progression by the sequence of changes in biomarkers, and reflect underlying pathology. Many of the biomarkers have shown to be useful at a group level, but if and how they can be applied on an individual level and in clinical practice requires further investigation. No one biomarker is diagnostic of any one condition in its own right, each has limitations, and interpretation should always be done in the appropriate clinical context.

Biomarkers are now making it possible to detect abnormal changes in the brain associated with Alzheimer's disease long before any symptoms of dementia emerge. As a result, expert groups have recommended new definitions when referring to Alzheimer's disease to reflect these discoveries. For example, the term "Alzheimer's disease pathology" is used to refer to the changes in the brain underlying Alzheimer's disease, irrespective of the stage or phase (i.e., with or without dementia) (Alzheimer Europe's Ethics Working Group, 2016). These new definitions expand the conceptualization of the Alzheimer's disease to encompass a continuum from very early ("preclinical") stage before symptoms are detectable, to mild cognitive impairment when memory symptoms emerge, and finally Alzheimer's disease (Dubois, Feldman, Jacova, & Cummings, 2010, 2014; Dubois et al., 2016).

THE TRAJECTORY OF DEMENTIA

Once a diagnosis is confirmed, the individual and family need education on the expected course or trajectory of dementia. Despite the variations in the type and severity of symptoms, most dementias typically involve a gradual onset, are progressive in nature, and are irreversible. The course of dementia is often characterized as occurring in three stages (Welsh, Butters, Hughes, Mohs, & Heyman, 1992) as shown in Fig. 1-1:

1. Mild or early-stage dementia: Deficits are evident in a number of areas such as memory and personal care, but the individual can still function with minimal assistance. In the early stage of disease, or the mild cognitive impairment stage of disease, the first symptom may be expressed as anxiety. The individual may notice some early memory changes particularly in the area of executive functioning or problem solving. Often small memory losses can be hidden from family members. Individuals may have difficulties initiating, organizing, planning or sustaining their attention and being engaged

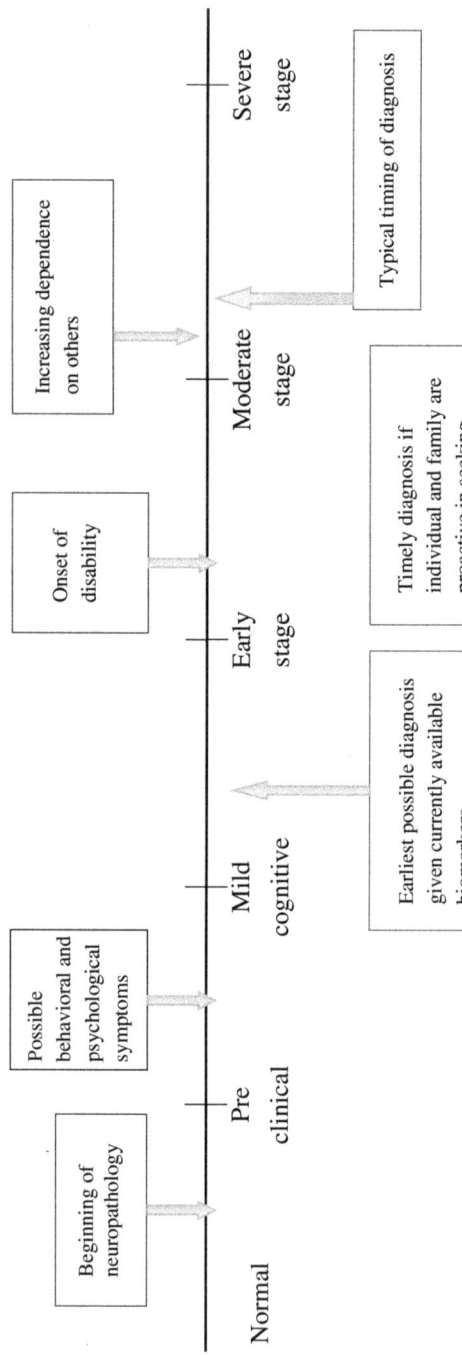

FIGURE 1.1 Brain-related changes and timing of diagnosis disclosure in the clinical trajectory of dementia.

in familiar activities or those they participated in before. In this stage, individuals begin to have more emotional distress, particularly as they begin to fear that they have a disease that is progressive and irreversible. At the same time, they face decisions about giving up aspects of independence and activities that they enjoy such as driving and work. Unless individuals and their families are proactive in seeking information about memory changes, most individuals do not receive a dementia diagnosis in the early stage of the disease.

2. Moderate or middle-stage dementia: Memory loss becomes more obvious and severe, and an increasing level of assistance is required to help the individual maintain daily functioning in the home and community. At the moderate stage of the disease, we see an increase in behavioral symptoms such as restlessness, anxiety, agitation, worry, irritability, and aggressiveness. These behavioral symptoms occur with greater frequency and severity and can cause distress to persons themselves as well as family caregivers. In the moderate stage, there is a dramatic decline in the individual's ability to be independent or even participate in any of the instrumental activities of daily living such as shopping or financial management or laundry and housekeeping. As this stage progresses, there is a decline in basic self-care such as brushing teeth or other aspects of grooming, bathing, and dressing. Home safety concerns become heightened because the person becomes at much greater risk of vulnerability to features in their home environment, of falling and taking medications appropriately. At the moderate disease stage, families report feeling the most distressed and burdened. It is in this stage too that persons may receive a confirmed diagnosis.

3. Severe or late-stage dementia: This stage is characterized by almost total dependence on care and the constant need for supervision by others. In the severe stage of dementia, the individual has lost the ability to communicate verbally with others and the ability to care for themselves and is dependent on others for their day-to-day needs. Quality of life issues become at the foremost of importance and includes maintaining dignity, promoting comfort, and providing opportunities to enjoy sensory experiences. This is also a time when caregivers can experience a great amount of anxiety and depression and also need respite and support.

CHANGING NEEDS

The needs of individuals living with dementia change over the disease trajectory. It is essential to remember that during all stages and in all types of dementia, the concerns of individuals and families vary tremendously due to personal histories, unique personality characteristics, coexisting conditions (e.g., depression and functional impairments), living conditions, access to diagnosis and care, and resources (e.g., informal and formal carers). As we will discuss in later chapters, the variations in each person's needs are in large part due to the widening gap between neurodegenerative processes, the declining cognitive and physical abilities, and increased vulnerabilities to physical and social environments. It is not possible to predict the amount of time for any one stage or movement through stages. These tremendous uncertainties have a profound effect on a person living with dementia and their family, often resulting in feelings of isolation, embarrassment, and intense frustration and confusion about what to expect next as the disease progresses.

> The current demographic imperative ensures that dementia will continue to be a significant clinical issue now and into the foreseeable future. Clinical guidelines are essential for providing a roadmap for how clinicians should approach the diagnosis of dementia to individuals and their family members from diverse backgrounds and cultures and intervene in ways that will help to maximize the individual's quality of life while helping families plan, prepare for, and cope with the symptoms of dementia.

The overall goals of dementia care are to achieve timely and accurate diagnosis, and to maximize individual's quality of life, promote decision-making and planning, maintain independence, delay institutionalization, and lessen the burden on caregivers. Management should first focus on optimizing both physical and mental health function. This involves treating coexisting diseases and cardiovascular risks of vascular and mixed dementia. Although the focus of this book is not on the diagnostic process itself, this is clearly an area for which there is great need for research and specifically for the development and testing of strategies to reduce disparities in access. Furthermore, there is a great need for the advancement of clinical guidelines for making a timely and accurate diagnosis and identification and evaluation of effective strategies for revealing it to individuals and families. Therefore, early diagnosis and early treatment and support can help with modest delays in progression of dementia, could bring major benefits, and should be a public health priority moving forward (Naylor et al., 2012). Some of the outstanding areas of research for enhancing timely diagnosis are outlined in Box 1-4. In the chapters to follow, we discuss in greater depth the research evidence for the nonpharmacologic options that are the cornerstone of dementia care.

> **Box 1-4**
> **Key Research Needs to Understand Disparities in Timely and Accurate Dementia Diagnosis**
>
> - Understand the lived experience of the diagnostic process for individuals and families.
> - Identify role of social determinants and cultural factors on diagnosis-seeking behavior.
> - Develop innovative approaches to support individuals with low health literacy and from different race, ethnic, and cultural groups to obtain diagnosis.

KEY POINTS

- The specific underlying cause of dementia may remain unknown early in the disease process; yet obtaining a diagnosis early on enables opportunities for planning and prompt referral to support services and information, leading to better outcomes for individuals and their family members.
- It is essential to clearly explain to individuals and their family members that dementia is a complex, degenerative, and terminal disorder with multiple potential causes due to a range of possible lifetime exposures including vascular, amyloid, and other risk factors.
- Clinicians need basic competencies in early detection of dementia and in disclosing a dementia diagnosis.
- Where possible, memory centers with specialists in dementia assessment should be established in health care systems to promote dementia awareness, confirm dementia diagnosis, and help individuals and families establish a plan of care.

> **What Actions Can be Taken Now**
>
> - Become familiar with existing diagnostic guidelines
> - Seek consultation with a specialist (geriatrician, geropsychiatrist, neurologist) for any subjective memory complaints or change in personality or abilities
> - If a family member, insist on meeting with a clinician (Nurse, geriatric social worker) who can explain the disease and help with care planning
> - Upon diagnosis, consult with vetted websites such as ADEAR, National Institute on Aging, Alzheimer's Association for more disease information

> **A Conversation with Dr. Ester Oh, MD, PhD**
>
> 1. *What are the implications of using biomarkers as a feature of diagnosing individuals?*
>   Biomarkers are rapidly becoming an integral part of diagnosing various types of dementias. Biomarkers are important in determining if the cognitive symptoms are due to a neurodegenerative disease. For patients and caregivers, this may bring relief if certain biomarkers indicate that the cognitive symptoms may not be due to a neurodegenerative disease. For clinicians, this would enable starting or stopping certain medications depending on the underlying etiology of cognitive symptoms. For researchers, this would enable a more targeted approach to developing new therapeutic agents.
> 2. *What do you recommend as the key messages when initially disclosing a diagnosis to a person and also his/her care partner or family member*
>   The key messages are that they are not alone, and that dementia is a very common condition that is often associated with aging. I would also encourage the patients to engage in physical exercise and social activities to optimize their condition. I would encourage the caregivers to join support groups and become more educated about the condition, and remember to take care of themselves.
> 3. *What research do you believe is needed to understand the diagnostic process and its impact for diverse individuals?*
>   One of the more important factors in patient/family discussion about diagnostic work-up or the disclosure of dementia diagnosis is not to make any assumptions based solely on their race, ethnicity, or religious backgrounds. While more research may be helpful in determining how dementia diagnosis is perceived in certain groups, each patient and his/her family members have different life experiences that may inform the extent of the diagnostic work up and how to proceed with the disclosure of dementia diagnosis.

References

Alzheimer's Association. (2014). *2014 Alzheimer's disease facts & figures*. Retrieved from https://www.alz.org/downloads/facts_figures_2014.pdf.

Alzheimer Europe's Ethics Working Group. (2016). *Ethical issues linked to the changing definitions/use of terms related to Alzheimer's disease*. Retrieved from http://www.alzheimer-europe.org.

Arvanitakis, Z. (2010). Update on frontotemporal dementia. *The Neurologist, 16*(1), 16–22. Available from https://doi.org/10.1097/NRL.0b013e3181b1d5c6.

REFERENCES

Bergeron, D., Beauregard, J.-M., Guimond, J., Fortin, M.-P., Houde, M., Poulin, S., & Laforce, R. (2015). Clinical impact of a second FDG-PET in atypical/unclear dementia syndromes. *Journal of Alzheimer's Disease, 49*(3), 695–705. Available from https://doi.org/10.3233/JAD-150302.

Besson, F. L., La Joie, R., Doeuvre, L., Gaubert, M., Mezenge, F., Egret, S., & Chetelat, G. (2015). Cognitive and brain profiles associated with current neuroimaging biomarkers of preclinical Alzheimer's disease. *Journal of Neuroscience, 35*(29), 10402–10411. Available from https://doi.org/10.1523/JNEUROSCI.0150-15.2015.

Blendon, R. J., Benson, J. M., Wikler, E. M., Weldon, K. J., Georges, J., Baumgart, M., & Kallmyer, B. A. (2012). The impact of experience with a family member with Alzheimer's disease on views about the disease across five countries. *International Journal of Alzheimer's Disease, 2012*, 1–9. Available from https://doi.org/10.1155/2012/903645.

Borson, S., Boustani, M. A., Buckwalter, K. C., Burgio, L. D., Chodosh, J., Fortinsky, R. H., & Geiger, A. (2016). Report on milestones for care and support under the U.S. National Plan to Address Alzheimer's disease. *Alzheimer's & Dementia, 12*(3), 334–369. Available from https://doi.org/10.1016/j.jalz.2016.01.005.

Cahill, S., Pierce, M., Werner, P., Darley, A., & Bobersky, A. (2015). A systematic review of the public's knowledge and understanding of Alzheimer's disease and dementia. *Alzheimer Disease & Associated Disorders, 29*(3), 255–275. Available from https://doi.org/10.1097/WAD.0000000000000102.

Chin, A. L., Negash, S., & Hamilton, R. (2011). Diversity and disparity in dementia. *Alzheimer Disease & Associated Disorders, 25*(3), 187–195. Available from https://doi.org/10.1097/WAD.0b013e318211c6c9.

Devanand, D. P. (2016). Olfactory identification deficits, cognitive decline, and dementia in older adults. *The American Journal of Geriatric Psychiatry, 24*(12), 1151–1157. Available from https://doi.org/10.1016/j.jagp.2016.08.010.

Di Marco, L. Y., Venneri, A., Farkas, E., Evans, P. C., Marzo, A., & Frangi, A. F. (2015). Vascular dysfunction in the pathogenesis of Alzheimer's disease—A review of endothelium-mediated mechanisms and ensuing vicious circles. *Neurobiology of Disease, 82*, 593–606. Available from https://doi.org/10.1016/j.nbd.2015.08.014.

Du, S.-Q., Wang, X.-R., Xiao, L.-Y., Tu, J.-F., Zhu, W., He, T., & Liu, C.-Z. (2017). Molecular mechanisms of vascular dementia: What can be learned from animal models of chronic cerebral hypoperfusion? *Molecular Neurobiology, 54*(5), 3670–3682. Available from https://doi.org/10.1007/s12035-016-9915-1.

Dubois, B., Feldman, H. H., Jacova, C., DeKosky, S. T., Barberger-Gateau, P., Cummings, J., & Scheltens, P. (2007). Research criteria for the diagnosis of Alzheimer's disease: Revising the NINCDS–ADRDA criteria. *The Lancet Neurology, 6*(8), 734–746. Available from https://doi.org/10.1016/S1474-4422(07)70178-3.

Dubois, B., Feldman, H., Jacova, C., Cummings, J., et al. (2010). Revising the definition of Alzheimer's disease: A new lexicon. *The Lancet Neurology, 9*(October), 1118–1127.

Dubois, B., et al. (2014). Advancing research diagnostic criteria for Alzheimer's disease: The IWG-2 criteria. *The Lancet Neurology, 13*(6), 614–629.

Dubois, B., Hampel, H., Feldman, H. H., Scheltens, P., Aisen, P., Andrieu, S., & Jack, C. R. (2016). Preclinical Alzheimer's disease: Definition, natural history, and diagnostic criteria. *Alzheimer's & Dementia, 12*(3), 292–323. Available from https://doi.org/10.1016/j.jalz.2016.02.002.

Haffner, C., Malik, R., & Dichgans, M. (2016). Genetic factors in cerebral small vessel disease and their impact on stroke and dementia. *Journal of Cerebral Blood Flow & Metabolism, 36*(1), 158–171. Available from https://doi.org/10.1038/jcbfm.2015.71.

Hayakawa, T., McGarrigle, C. A., Coen, R. F., Soraghan, C. J., Foran, T., Lawlor, B. A., & Kenny, R. A. (2015). Orthostatic blood pressure behavior in people with mild cognitive impairment predicts conversion to dementia. *Journal of the American Geriatrics Society, 63*(9), 1868−1873. Available from https://doi.org/10.1111/jgs.13596.

Helman, A. M., & Murphy, M. P. (2016). Vascular cognitive impairment: Modeling a critical neurologic disease in vitro and in vivo. *Biochimica et Biophysica Acta (BBA)— Molecular Basis of Disease, 1862*(5), 975−982. Available from https://doi.org/10.1016/j.bbadis.2015.12.009.

Hinton, L., Franz, C. E., Reddy, G., Flores, Y., Kravitz, R. L., & Barker, J. C. (2007). Practice constraints, behavioral problems, and dementia care: Primary care physicians' perspectives. *Journal of General Internal Medicine, 22*(11), 1487−1492. Available from https://doi.org/10.1007/s11606-007-0317-y.

Husaini, B. A., Sherkat, D. E., Moonis, M., Levine, R., Holzer, C., & Cain, V. A. (2003). Racial differences in the diagnosis of dementia and in its effects on the use and costs of health care services. *Psychiatric Services, 54*(1), 92−96. Available from https://doi.org/10.1176/appi.ps.54.1.92.

Hyman, B. T., Phelps, C. H., Beach, T. G., Bigio, E. H., Cairns, N. J., Carrillo, M. C., & Montine, T. J. (2012). National Institute on Aging−Alzheimer's Association guidelines for the neuropathologic assessment of Alzheimer's disease. *Alzheimer's & Dementia, 8*(1), 1−13. Available from https://doi.org/10.1016/j.jalz.2011.10.007.

Jack, C. R., Albert, M. S., Knopman, D. S., McKhann, G. M., Sperling, R. A., Carrillo, M. C., & Phelps, C. H. (2011). Introduction to the recommendations from the National Institute on Aging-Alzheimer's Association workgroups on diagnostic guidelines for Alzheimer's disease. *Alzheimer's & Dementia, 7*(3), 257−262. Available from https://doi.org/10.1016/j.jalz.2011.03.004.

Klein, J. C., Eggers, C., Kalbe, E., Weisenbach, S., Hohmann, C., Vollmar, S., & Hilker, R. (2010). Neurotransmitter changes in dementia with Lewy bodies and Parkinson disease dementia in vivo. *Neurology, 74*(11), 885−892. Available from https://doi.org/10.1212/WNL.0b013e3181d55f61.

Lecouturier, J., Bamford, C., Hughes, J. C., Francis, J. J., Foy, R., Johnston, M., & Eccles, M. P. (2008). Appropriate disclosure of a diagnosis of dementia: identifying the key behaviours of "best practice. *BMC Health Services Research, 8*(1), 95. Available from https://doi.org/10.1186/1472-6963-8-95.

Milby, E., Murphy, G., & Winthrop, A. (2015). Diagnosis disclosure in dementia: Understanding the experiences of clinicians and patients who have recently given or received a diagnosis. *Dementia.* Available from https://doi.org/10.1177/1471301215612676.

Mitchell, A. J., Beaumont, H., Ferguson, D., Yadegarfar, M., & Stubbs, B. (2014). Risk of dementia and mild cognitive impairment in older people with subjective memory complaints: Meta-analysis. *Acta Psychiatrica Scandinavica, 130*(6), 439−451. Available from https://doi.org/10.1111/acps.12336.

Naylor, M. D., Karlawish, J. H., Arnold, S. E., Khachaturian, A. S., Khachaturian, Z. S., Lee, V. M.-Y., & Trojanowski, J. Q. (2012). Advancing Alzheimer's disease diagnosis, treatment, and care: Recommendations from the Ware Invitational Summit. *Alzheimer's & Dementia, 8*(5), 445−452. Available from https://doi.org/10.1016/j.jalz.2012.08.001.

Papp, K., Rentz, D., Mormino, E., Amariglio, R., Burnham, S., Johnson, K., & Sperling, R. (2015). The neuropsychology of preclinical Alzheimer's disease: Differential sensitivity of component processes of memory performance on biomarker evidence of amyloidosis (S41.004). *Neurology, 84*, 14.

Prince, M., Bryce, R., & Ferri, C. (2011). *World Alzheimer Report 2011.* London, United Kingdom: Alzheimer's Disease International.

Quaglio, G., Brand, H., & Dario, C. (2016). Fighting dementia in Europe: The time to act is now. *The Lancet Neurology, 15*(5), 452−454. Available from https://doi.org/10.1016/S1474-4422(16)00079-X.

Schneider, J. A., Arvanitakis, Z., Leurgans, S. E., & Bennett, D. A. (2009). The neuropathology of probable Alzheimer disease and mild cognitive impairment. *Annals of Neurology*, *66*(2), 200–208. Available from https://doi.org/10.1002/ana.21706.

Schott, J. M., & Fox, N. C. (2016). Inflammatory changes in very early Alzheimer's disease: Friend, foe, or don't know? *Brain*, *139*(3), 647–650. Available from https://doi.org/10.1093/brain/awv405.

Steinberg, S. I., Negash, S., Sammel, M. D., Bogner, H., Harel, B. T., Livney, M. G., & Arnold, S. E. (2013). Subjective memory complaints, cognitive performance, and psychological factors in healthy older adults. *American Journal of Alzheimer's Disease & Other Dementias*, *28*(8), 776–783. Available from https://doi.org/10.1177/1533317513504817.

van Uden, I. W. M., van der Holst, H. M., Tuladhar, A. M., van Norden, A. G. W., de Laat, K. F., Rutten-Jacobs, L. C. A., & de Leeuw, F.-E. (2015). White matter and hippocampal volume predict the risk of dementia in patients with cerebral small vessel disease: The RUN DMC study. *Journal of Alzheimer's Disease*, *49*(3), 863–873. Available from https://doi.org/10.3233/JAD-150573.

Welsh, K. A., Butters, N., Hughes, J. P., Mohs, R. C., & Heyman, A. (1992). Detection and staging of dementia in Alzheimer's disease. Use of the neuropsychological measures developed for the Consortium to Establish a Registry for Alzheimer's disease. *Archives of Neurology*, *49*(5), 448–452.

Zweig, Y. R., & Galvin, J. E. (2014). Lewy body dementia: The impact on patients and caregivers. *Alzheimer's Research & Therapy*, *6*(2), 21. Available from https://doi.org/10.1186/alzrt251.

Further Reading

Kumar, A., Singh, A., & Ekavali. (2015). A review on Alzheimer's disease pathophysiology and its management: An update. *Pharmacological Reports*, *67*(2), 195–203. Available from https://doi.org/10.1016/j.pharep.2014.09.004.

López-Valdés, H. E., & Martínez-Coria, H. (2016). The role of neuroinflammation in age-related dementias. *Revista de Investigacion Clinica; Organo Del Hospital de Enfermedades de La Nutricion*, *68*(1), 40–48.

Vigliettta, V., O'Gorman, J., Williams, L., Tian, Y., Sandrock, A., Doody, R., & Sevigny, J. (2016). Randomized, double-blind, placebo-controlled studies to evaluate treatment with aducanumab (BIIB037) in patients with early Alzheimer's disease: Phase 3 study design (S1.003). *Neurology*, *86*(16).

CHAPTER 2

Lived Experiences of Individuals With Dementia

I am still a person **Title of poem by Judy Lauer, a caregiver for her 70-year-old husband.**

Things are at a slightly different stage. [my mom] has slowed down, with a little more confusion at times, more sleepiness, less balance, more use of the walker especially outside. She is still very sweet and has a smile and a nice word for everyone. Thank goodness for the Senior Center, where they talk about how remarkable [my mom] is, and how they all love her. Rarely is she agitated, but it happens. **Daughter caring for her mother with moderate dementia in an email exchange with a relative.**

As highlighted by these quotes, dementia impacts the fabric of daily life of individuals both positively and negatively, and in different ways. A range of factors as illuminated in our social ecological model (Fig. 2-1, Introduction) shape impact. For example, individual factors affecting the lived experience may include living situation (living alone or with others), stage of disease, race/ethnicity/cultural group and associated values, beliefs, and/or understandings. Social factors affecting the lived experience may include access to resources, social capital, neighborhood safety, and societal policies concerning reimbursement for care and services. Consider a person diagnosed with early stage dementia who lives alone, without social support or financial resources. This person will have a vastly different disease experience compared to a person living with a family member or who has access to a network of family members who can assist in daily life. Similarly, consider an individual living in a community which has become dementia friendly (see Chapter 9: Living in the Community); this person may not experience the same type or depth of stigma, social isolation, or anxiety to which an individual living in an unsupportive environment may be exposed.

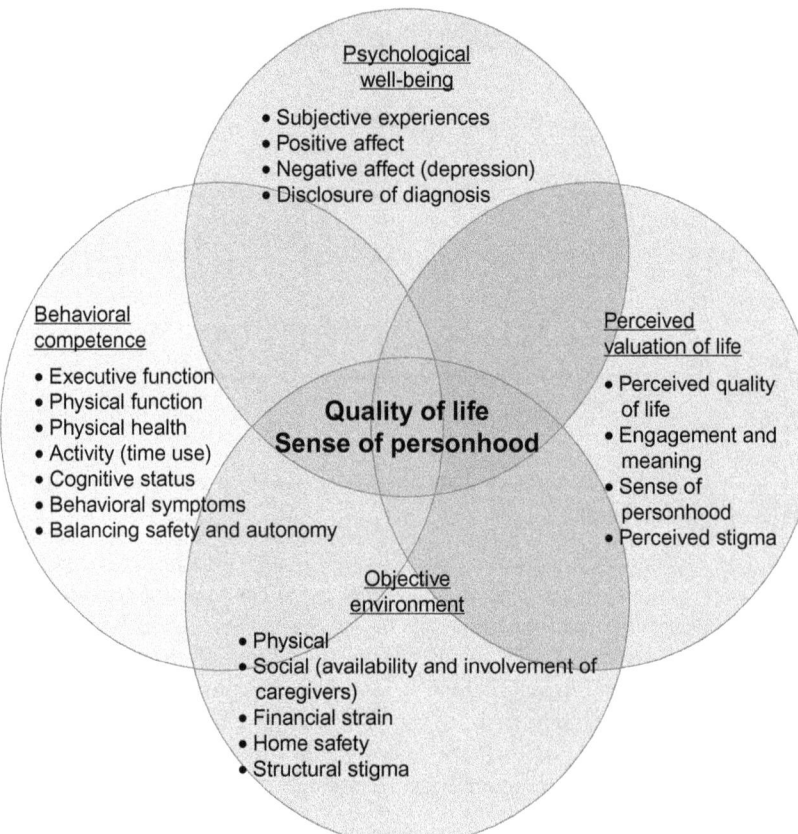

FIGURE 2-1   Sectors of quality of life.

Whereas in Chapter 1, How the Brain Is Affected, we discussed the pathophysiology and clinical features of dementia, here we consider the range of lived experiences of individuals regardless of etiology, and identify potential barriers to well-being and quality of life. Although family members are interwoven in the disease trajectory, in this chapter and in Chapter 3, Breaking the Cycle of Despair, we exclusively focus on persons themselves and then in Chapters 5 and 6, Family Member as Care Partner, and How We Can Support Families, respectively, we examine impacts on family caregivers. In this chapter, we show that the physical, social, and policy environments (identified in our socio-ecological model) play a considerable role in how dementia is experienced. We suggest that while at this point in time the pathophysiology or underlying neuronal disease processes are not well understood and appear immutable to treatments, we are able to make important changes to the life space or physical and social environments of individuals living with dementia that can mitigate their negative impacts as the disease progresses and improve the daily lived experience.

PRINCIPLES FOR UNDERSTANDING LIVED EXPERIENCES

Three key principles guide our discussion and which must be considered in any discussion of the impact of dementia on the daily lives of affected individuals. First is that we must recognize that our understanding of the experiences of living with dementia is limited. To date, our knowledge typically stems from the perspectives of others such as family members or clinicians and reflects research understandings generated from an outsider's perspective. As such, our understandings of dementia are not entirely grounded in the perceptions, viewpoints, and world views of individuals themselves who are living with a dementia.

Although individuals with mild cognitive impairment or early dementia have participated in research concerning their own perceived quality of life, experiences and needs, this body of research is small. Furthermore, individuals with language difficulties or at the moderate to severe stages of the disease may find existing measures and research protocols challenging and barriers to study participation. The lack of representation of individuals at all disease stages in our studies is due principally to the limitations of existing research methodologies and measures, and the pervasive misunderstanding and misguided orientation that individuals living with dementia are not capable of study participation or providing insights as to how the disease effects the sense of self and every day life. Consequently, our presentation of the impact on dementia is necessarily limited by the limitations of research to date. However, at the very least, we seek to provide emerging insights gained through direct observation and from reports by individuals themselves on key facets of their experiences and at each stage of the disease process.

Second, research has focused on the devastating and deleterious effects of the disease process. Yet, this is only one part of the story. We have a limited understanding of coping mechanisms and adaptive responses, how to support and build on preserved capabilities at each disease stage, and how to address enduring needs such as for engagement and purpose of affected individuals. As the dementias eat away at a sense of self-identity, the strategies used to maintain a sense of self at each stage and the impact of adaptive processes on behaviors are important aspects to study and which are part of the lived disease experience of individuals.

Third, our understanding of the dementia experience must extend beyond the biological and medical aspects (see Chapter 1: How the

Brain Is Affected) and include a holistic understanding of the person in their entirety.

THE GOOD LIFE MODEL

To understand the multiple aspects of the "self" of individuals living with dementia, we draw upon and adapt a multifactorial quality of life model. This model was initially developed by Lawton (1983), and previously referred to as the "Good Life." The model suggests that there are independent and joint effects of four interrelated sectors, quadrants, or components of what makes up a good life. We have adapted this model by adding to the factors to be considered in each quadrant. These quadrants or sectors and their respective factors include the following:

- Behavioral competencies—This refers to executive function, physical function, physical health, activity and time use, cognitive status, behavioral and psychological symptoms.
- Psychological well-being—This refers to subjective experiences, positive effect, negative effect and depression.
- Perceived valuation or appraisal of life—This refers to perceived quality of life, engagement and meaning, sense of personhood or person agency and connectedness.
- Objective environment—This includes physical and social characteristics such as caregiver availability and involvement, financial status/strain, home safety, home layouts, community resources/supports, and safety.

Fig. 2.1 graphically displays the four sectors or domains of the "good life" as applied to persons living with dementia and the categories within each.

The "Good Life" model has important implications for how we think about, transform, and create comprehensive dementia care. Comprehensive dementia care must include an assessment of each quadrant and their respective categories from which to design and execute an integrated and coordinated care plan that addresses identified areas of concerns and needs in each quadrant and disease stage. The following case snapshot illustrates the Good Life Model, its respective quadrants and factors, and its utility in understanding different areas of daily life affected by dementia for a given individual.

Case Snapshot Highlighting the Good Life Model

Mrs. B is an 85 year old African American with moderate dementia. A widow for 10 years, she had lived alone until it was evident that she was unsafe and unable to engage in self-care (bathing, dressing) or carry out instrumental activities of daily living such as shopping, medication taking and so forth (behavioral competence). She moved in with her daughter who lived in an apartment in another city (objective environment). The move was distressful and disorienting and Mrs. B became increasingly anxious in this unfamiliar environment; consequently she began shadowing her daughter and panicking when she left the room or was out of sight (psychological well-being). Mrs. B's daughter modified her apartment to create a more simplified and decluttered environment by removing objects that might be confusing to her mother including disabling the oven (objective environment). Mrs. B is worried about her mother's quality of life as she had nothing to do all day, appeared bored and disengaged (perceived value of life).

We continue in this chapter by examining the known needs of individuals with dementia and as they change with disease progression, referring to when appropriate the four sectors of the Good Life model. We focus on individuals living at home primarily. We then examine one of the most significant impacts of dementia—that of perceived stigma (affecting the valuation of life) and structural stigma (environmentally imposed discriminatory practices), as well as other core challenges individuals with dementia and their family members confront that are relevant to the Good Life Model. These include when and how to disclose a diagnosis (psychological well-being quadrant of the Good Life Model), balancing autonomy and safety (behavioral competence quadrant of the Good Life Model), and the imperative of preserving a sense of self and personhood (intersection of all quadrants of the model).

We conclude by suggesting that an important dynamic dominates the lived experience throughout the disease trajectory. This concerns the imperative of continuously making adjustments to obtain a "just right fit" or balance between safety and security (typically overarching goals of providers and family caregivers) with the enduring need for and desire of individuals living with dementia for meaningful participation, control, and agency in everyday life.

DIFFERENTIAL NEEDS OF PEOPLE LIVING WITH DEMENTIA

Obtaining the just right fit between changing cognitive abilities and environmental demands involves understanding the changing needs of people living with dementia. However, in this regard, only a few well-conducted studies have systematically examined needs with each study evaluating different aspects of well-being and for the most part without the benefit of employing a theoretical framework or overarching conceptual compass. Thus, of no surprise, our understanding of needs is necessarily piecemeal reflecting the whim of different research perspectives as to what constitutes well-being for persons living with dementia. Nevertheless, taken as a whole, various conclusions can be drawn from this limited but important body of research as summarized in Box 2-1. As indicated, needs appear to vary by various factors including disease stage and social determinants including race and ethnicity, as well as age of onset.

Needs by Disease Stage

It is helpful to understand how disease stage affects needs in order to inform effective care planning, organization of services, and policies. Research to date suggests that needs emerge immediately upon diagnosis and at the earliest disease stages and continue through disease progression. Some needs remain and endure across disease stages. For example, the need for a home environment that supports a person's daily functioning and affords safety and security; and the need for meaning and purposeful engagement are enduring, regardless of disease stage.

Box 2-1

Needs of People With Dementia: A Summary of the Research

- People with dementia are living at home with many unmet and significant needs
- Unmet needs are addressable
- Needs emerge in each of the four sectors of the Good Life and at each disease stage
- Needs in each sector of the Good Life Model vary widely based on a combination of factors including disease stage, personal characteristics (e.g., race, ethnicity, and culture), and age of onset
- Some needs are specific to disease stage (e.g., end of life care)
- Some needs persist throughout disease trajectory (e.g., safety)
- Needs appear to transcend disease etiology although there is the need for disease specific education
- Perceived needs differ: people with dementia are typically concerned about inclusion and meaningful engagement, whereas caregivers typically focus on safety

Other needs are stage-specific and reflect the variegated cognitive, functional, and behavioral profiles that emerge, such as the need for compensatory techniques to address memory impairment early on or for pain management at the end of life. There is very limited research as to whether needs differ by disease etiologies. Certainly, the needs of those with young onset who are still working and with young children will be quite different than individuals diagnosed with dementia at an advanced age. However, as needs reflect the outcomes of a degenerative brain disease process, we can surmise that most needs traverse specific etiologies, except of course the need of individuals and families to have access to disease-specific education. Fig. 2-2 maps the needs that have been identified in research to each disease stage.

As suggested by Fig. 2-2, we find that in the early disease stage, home safety (objective environment of the Good Life Model), and basic disease education (behavioral competence of the Good Life) initially emerge as of utmost importance to individuals (Gitlin & Corcoran, 2000; Hodgson, Black, Johnston, Lyketsos, & Samus, 2014). Living arrangement also becomes important with those living alone at significant greater risk for poor health, increased safety concerns, and more unmet needs than those who are living with others. As assistance with instrumental activities of living (shopping, finances, and meal preparation) becomes increasingly central to daily life followed by some beginning oversight of self-care (dressing, grooming, and bathing) and attention to accidental self-harm (Miranda-Castillo, Woods, & Orrell, 2010), those living alone may be at a distinct disadvantage.

In early disease stages, the loss of meaningful daytime activities (Behavioral Competence, Good Life Model) and the sense of purpose in day-to-day living (Perceived Quality of Life, Good Life Model) become perhaps one of the most profound consequences of the disease that is experienced. The desire and need for meaningful activities dominates with most individuals in surveys reporting boredom and little to do that is meaningful (Black et al., 2013; Millenaar et al., 2016). As individuals also report early on depression and anxiety (psychological well-being of the Good Life Model), we see that each sector of the Good Life is immediately impacted.

Concomitantly, ethical dilemmas begin to emerge immediately that are expressed in tensions between the perceived needs of individuals themselves for continued engagement (e.g., driving) and safety concerns of informal and formal caregivers. Although caregivers tend to focus on risk reduction and safety, individuals themselves tend to be more concerned about remaining meaningful engaged and maintaining a purposeful life (Millenaar et al., 2016; Lach & Chang, 2007).

Although some needs continue into the moderate disease stage, new needs also emerge. Individuals with moderate dementia, for example,

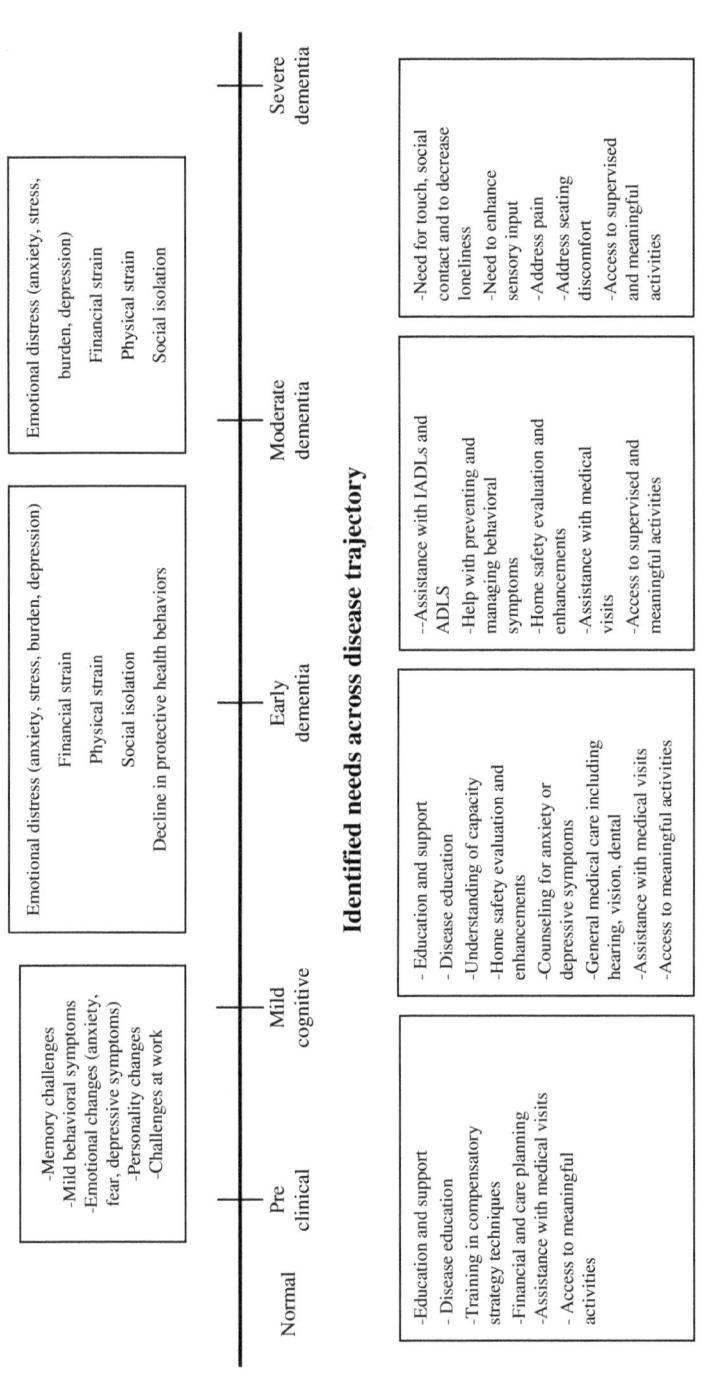

FIGURE 2-2 Clinical trajectory of dementia, identified needs and impacts.

tend to need increased supervision with daytime activities, attention to preventing and managing neuropsychiatric behaviors and psychological distress, as well as different levels of assistance—from supervision to cueing to physical support—with instrumental and basic activities of daily living. There is also the increased need for assistance with coordination of medication taking and medical care, disease education, and social engagement (Black et al., 2013; Hodgson et al., 2014; van der Roest et al., 2009).

A snapshot of other research studies uncover that people live with dementia with a wide array of unaddressed medical and safety issues. For example, a study of 88 families using both self-report and direct observation found that individuals with moderate dementia were living at home with an average of eight neuropsychiatric behaviors and six chronic health conditions. About 70.7% ($n = 58$) were observed as having a fall risk, 60.5% ($n = 52$) reported sleep problems one or more times weekly, and 42.5% ($n = 37$) reported daily pain (Gitlin, Hodgson, Piersol, Hess, & Hauck, 2014).

In a study of 265 persons with dementia living at home, 36% ($n = 96$) had clinical findings indicative of undetected but treatable illnesses. These included bacteriuria (15%), followed by hyperglycemia (6%), and anemia (5%). The behavioral symptom most often reported by caregivers was resisting or refusing care (66% vs 47% for those without detected illness). Also, individuals with detected illness had significantly lower functional status scores, lower cognitive status scores, and were more likely to be prescribed psychotropic medications for behavior (41% vs 26%, $w2 = 3.67$, $P < 0.05$) than those without illness (Hodgson, Gitlin, Winter, & Czekanski, 2011). These findings suggest that individuals with dementia may have atypical presentations of illness and also may not be effectively monitored by primary care offices; this in turn may affect everyday quality of life.

These and other studies suggest that comorbidities may be affected by and interact with dementia, further complicating disease management and the lived experience. For example, an individual with moderate dementia plus sensory impairments (hearing or vision loss) will have different daily challenges and needs than those without these types of comorbidities. Furthermore, unmanaged pain, sleep disturbances, and neuropsychiatric behaviors are all associated with poor quality of life (Hodgson et al., 2014).

Individuals with severe or end-stage disease may have the highest level of unmet needs in the area of emotional distress (Hodgson et al., 2014). Other commonly identified areas of concern include the need for appropriate social contact, overcoming boredom and sensory deprivation, and meaningful engagement—these all remain priorities of families across the disease trajectory and into the end stage of life. Discomfort, pain, and uncomfortable seating positions have also been noted as unmet needs with severe dementia (Cohen-Mansfield, Dakheel-Ali, Marx, Thein, & Regier, 2015).

The needs of individuals with dementia arise immediately with diagnosis and persist across the disease trajectory, regardless of etiologies. Dementia impacts every aspect including overall well-being, medical (co-morbidities), psychological (depression), and social profiles, and living environments. In considering needs, it is not just about neuropathology or medical issues; rather a holistic, transformative approach is required as suggested by the "Good Life" model, to identify needs in all sectors of well-being from which to derive integrative supportive solutions that encompass the psychological, social, medical and environmental, to support the whole person.

Race, Ethnicity, and Culture

Race, ethnicity, and culture are all factors as well that shape daily living with dementia and overlay disease stage. There is consistent and strong evidence of significant disparities with regard to detection, diagnosis, disease management, medication use, and access to supportive and care services according to an individual's race, ethnicity, and culture. Individuals from low-resourced countries, minority, and low-income groups, individuals living in remote areas and older adults often experience poor detection, delayed diagnosis, inadequate disease management, and inappropriate antipsychotic treatment use (Gilligan, Malone, Warholak, & Armstrong, 2012; Nielsen, Andersen, Kastrup, Phung, & Waldemar, 2011; Puyat, Law, Wong, Sutherland, & Morgan, 2012; Sivananthan, Lavergne, & McGrail, 2015; Zilkens, Duke, Horner, Semmens, & Bruce, 2014).

In contrast, in the United States and throughout the world, those with higher incomes, younger age, and who are white, have better odds of receiving a diagnosis, guideline treatments, and access to follow-up supportive services including referrals or counseling. Similarly, high-income and white populations have lower odds of being prescribed nonrecommended medications such as antipsychotics and antidepressants (Gilligan et al., 2012; Sivananthan et al., 2015). Correspondingly, in the United States, there are significant disparities in the rate of diagnosis, access to disease management, use of inappropriate medications, use of physical restraints, and cost among minority groups, with African Americans followed by Hispanics, having the poorest odds of receiving a timely diagnoses, adequate care and services, inappropriate medications, and having higher costs (Cassie & Cassie, 2013; Gilligan, Malone, Warholak, & Armstrong, 2013). These differences may be due to a combination of factors including implicit bias among health practitioners, financial constraints, and lack of knowledge and access by the populations involved.

Age of Onset

Another factor differentiating how individuals experience dementia is age of onset. Individuals with early onset (≤60 years of age) confront unique needs including access to companionship, meaningful occupation, or daytime activities, negotiating engagement in social and intimate relationships. Additional challenges for those with early onset include determining when and how and to whom to disclose the diagnosis, reconciling the need for employment and driving with decreasing abilities to participate in both, and managing the impact of the disease on children, other family members, and one's own care responsibilities. Furthermore, addressing psychological distress, medical needs, and providing disease information and care planning all become critical needs for those with young onset (Bakker et al., 2014; Levine, 2013; Millenaar et al., 2016). Those who receive a diagnosis at an older age also confront unique challenges, the most pressing being ageism and stigma (discussed below).

DAILY CHALLENGES

The specific daily challenges that individuals with dementia routinely confront are unlike those associated with other chronic conditions. Due to degeneration and that all areas of cognition, physical function, and behavior are affected, challenges are in many ways unique to this condition. The key challenges for individuals that we examine in this chapter are listed in Box 2-2 and include home safety, managing stigma, deciding when and how to disclose a diagnosis to family, friends, and employers, remaining engaged in meaningful activities, and maintaining a sense of purpose and control. Here we examine each of these in more detail.

Remaining Safe at Home

As most people with dementia live at home and for the duration of the disease, a universal and consistently documented need is in the area

> **Box 2-2**
> **5 Key Daily Challenges**
>
> - Remaining safe
> - Managing stigma
> - Disclosing diagnosis
> - Staying engaged
> - Maintaining purpose, control, and agency

of safety (see Fig. 2-2). This need transcends disease etiology and stage and is the most prominent documented unmet need across studies. Concerns for safety emerge almost immediately and persist, although specific safety concerns and unsafe conditions change with disease progression. For example, although in the early disease stage safety concerns may focus on driving, at the moderate−severe disease stage, safety concerns center on the persons' ability to remain alone at home or in a room with limited or no supervision. A study of 254 individuals with cognitive impairment who were interviewed and observed at home found that 90.6% had one or more home hazards. In a home-based observational study mentioned above, an average of eight home hazards were observed along with 51.7% of families reporting an unmet assistive device (e.g., grab bars, monitors) or ambulation (tripping hazards, walking aids) need for the person with dementia (Gitlin et al., 2014). Home safety concerns are considered in depth in Chapter 8, The Physical Home Environment: A Neglected Therapeutic Context.

Managing Stigma

> Dementia is often regarded as an embarrassing condition that should be hushed up and not spoken about. But I feel passionately that more needs to be done to raise awareness...
> Kevin Whately, British Actor.

Of the many negative emotional consequences of having a dementia diagnosis, stigma is perhaps one of the most pernicious and secondary to the experience of progressive cognitive and functional declines. Individuals living with dementia and their families often express feeling stigmatized by a dementia diagnosis. This may be due to various factors including poor awareness about the disease on the part of family members, friends, neighbors, and employers and society at-large, such as believing it is a "mental illness" which is highly stigmatizing in most countries. Awareness about dementia is typically quite low as shown in surveys worldwide leading to a wide variety of misperceptions and misinterpretations concerning the meaning and cause of dementia and its symptoms (Alzheimer's Disease International, 2012; Bamford, Holley-Moore, & Watson, 2014). This has resulted in the high prevalence of stigma in all countries (Borochowitz, 2011; McParland, Devine, Innes, & Gayle, 2012; Navab, Negarandeh, Peyrovi, & Navab, 2013; Piver et al., 2013; Zeng et al., 2015.

The specific aspects of dementia that are stigmatizing are not quite clear. One research study for example found that the label "Alzheimer's disease" was not associated with more stigmatizing reactions. Rather it was being told that symptoms would worsen which resulted in greater perceived structural discrimination and social distancing (Johnson, Harkins, Cary, Sankar, & Karlawish, 2015).

What Is Stigma?

There are many different definitions of stigma, a few of which are highlighted in Box 2-3. Regardless of definition, there are common themes suggesting consensus that stigma reflects inaccurate beliefs based on misinformation and disparages an individual or group of individuals; and that it has a negative impact on targeted individuals—in this case, people with dementia and their caregivers, involving both experienced or actual as well as perceived stigma. Regardless of definition, there is no doubt that stigma is a complex construct encompassing

---

Box 2-3

Examples of Definitions of Stigma

- "A mark of disgrace associated with a particular circumstance, quality, or person." Oxford English Dictionary
- "A set of negative and often unfair beliefs that a society or group of people have about something." Merriam-Webster dictionary
- "A strong lack of respect for a person or a group of people or a bad opinion of them because they had done something society does not approve of." Cambridge Dictionary
- "Stigma results from a process whereby certain individuals and groups are unjustifiably rendered shameful, excluded and discriminated against." World Psychiatric Association, World Health Organization, Reducing stigma and discrimination against older people with mental disorders, 2002.

different components and impacting individuals, family members, communities, and society in ways that affect every level—from the individual in terms of their daily life to the family and care decisions to societal level regarding health care policies.

Understandings about dementia vary widely by cultural groups with some believing dementia is a form of insanity, the work of the devil, a mental illness, a fault of the individual, or a natural part of aging (Adebiyi, Fagbola, Olakehinde, & Ogunniyi, 2016; Alzheimer's Disease International, 2012). The stigma associated with dementia is also intertwined with agism or the "...systematic stereotyping and discrimination against people because they are old" (Butler, 2005; Mazerolle et al., 2016). Additionally, some consider dementia a mental illness. As mental disorders have long been shown to be highly stigmatizing, people with dementia also experience stigma from being perceived as having a mental illness. (Blay & Peluso, 2010). Thus, all three forms of stigma subject individuals with dementia, and their families, to a triple jeopardy, the effects of which are malignant with real, immediate, and long-term negative consequences for both individuals and their families and society at large.

Effects of Stigma

Box 2-4 lists the most common and known perceived and experienced effects of stigma for individuals with dementia.

One of the most pernicious forms of experienced stigma is structural. This form is evident in the common belief among health and human service professionals that nothing can be done. It is also evident in the avoidance by physicians to disclose a diagnosis to an individual or their care partner, openly discuss the disease process, or help families with care planning, as expressed by a woman caring for her mother:

> ...I felt like the doctors were really not much help to me. They didn't know what to do...It seems that once a person has been diagnosed with dementia, many doctors just ignore them... *Markut, L. A., Crane A. Dementia Caregivers share their stories. Nashville, TN. Vanderbilt*

The lack of adequate training of health and human service professionals in dementia and care options, lack of needed services, and continuous under-resourcing of dementia research reflect different aspects of structural stigma (Benbow & Jolley, 2012). One consequence is that individuals with dementia and their family members may be denied needed support and services or be deterred from seeking such help (Phillipson, Magee, Jones, Reis, & Skaldzien, 2015). Thus, the view that "nothing can be done" and singular societal and research focus on a cure at the expense of care continues to perpetuate stigmatized practices with individuals with dementia.

Box 2-4
Effects of Stigma

- Perceived stigma
  - Fear of diagnosis
  - A sense of shame
  - Emotional consequences (frustration, boredom, anxiety, fear, upset)
  - Change in social standing, feelings of social rejection
- Experienced stigma
  - Lack of help-seeking for supportive services
  - Avoidance by others including health and human service professionals
  - Avoidance by friends/family/neighbors of persons with dementia
  - Social isolation
  - Being treated differently (infantilization)
  - Withdrawal from meaningful activities
  - Caregiver burden

The effects of stigma may be perceived and experienced even at the earliest stages of the disease. Burgener, Buckwalter, Perkhounkova, and Liu (2015) in a study of 50 persons with dementia and 47 family caregivers found that individuals experienced persistent perceived stigma across the early stages with some variation by age (older individuals reported less perceived stigma) and geographic location (persons in urban areas reported high levels of stigma than those in rural areas).

Stigma may also contribute to caregiver burden over and above other contributors. One consequence of perceived stigma among adult children is increased feelings of shame and decreased involvement. The latter is a known outcome of stigma in the care of family members with mental illness as well (Werner, Mittelman, Goldstein, & Heinik, 2012).

Research Needs

Despite the documented effects of stigma, it is still unclear as to the underlying factors that contribute to the stigma specifically experienced by individuals with dementia and their families as well as the underlying motivations and cultural nuances of stigma and its impacts. Also the different components of stigma (e.g., stereotypes, prejudice, and discrimination) require further refinement and measurement and an examination of their independent and joint effects on individuals and families (Blay & Peluso, 2010). Although there are some measures of stigma (see, for example, the Family Stigma in Alzheimer's Disease Scale; Werner, Goldstein, & Heinik, 2011), more work in this area is important in developing ways to systematically elicit the lived experience of dementia from individuals themselves (Swaffer, 2014). Furthermore, there may be differences in the experience of stigma based on an individual's gender, age, living arrangement, and/or relationship (Werner, Goldberg, Mandel, & Korczyn, 2013). Thus, there are clear research needs to more fully understand stigma in order to effectively minimize its presence and individual/family/societal impacts.

Strategies to Address Stigma

So what can be done about stigma? Addressing stigma is an important strategy for helping to improve the quality of life of individuals with dementia and their family members as it has a significant role in the experience of dementia. As Benbow and Jolley (2012, 170) argue: "To further combat stigma and provide for the future, person-centered care of people who develop a dementia will need concerted effort in four areas: policy, research, information and education and service design." Box 2-5 outlines key strategies that individuals, communities, and the public at-large can utilize.

Box 2-5
Strategies to Address Stigma

- Increase public awareness through education and media campaigns
- Build on preserved capabilities and establish a supportive environment in order to include people with dementia in everyday activities at home and community
- Help to promote/develop dementia-friendly communities
- Be aware of and change language to be more inclusive, jargon-free, clear, non-judgmental
- Focus on the person, not the disease
- Promote or develop dementia friendly communities
- Use published language guidelines[1]
- Include persons with dementia in decision-making, planning ("nothing about me without me")
- Enhance training of health and human service professionals

[1]*For language guides see, for example, http://www.alzheimer-europe.org/Ethics/ Ethical-issues-in-practice/The-ethicalissues-linked-to-the-perceptions-and-portrayal-of-dementia-and-people-withdementia/GuidelinesOr https://fightdementia.org.au/ sites/default/files/20090600_Nat_NP_4DemFriendLang.pdf.*

An effective approach to addressing stigma is directly involving people with dementia and those without dementia in meaningful joint ventures. Harris and Caporella (2014), for example, developed an intergenerational choir involving college students and individuals with dementia and their families. Although it was only a small study of 13 individuals, their results are promising. They showed that individuals with dementia/families reported a decrease in their social isolation while college students demonstrated a decrease in negative attitudes toward people with the disease.

Disclosing Diagnosis to Family/Friends/Employers

> "In most circumstances I have found that if I have disclosed that I have dementia, my thoughts, opinions, conversations are discounted and dismissed." (Individual in the United States, cited in Alzheimer's Disease International, 2012, p. 24)

An immediate dilemma that many individuals confront is whether to disclose their diagnosis or not to family, friends, neighbors, and/or employers. Reactions to a diagnosis can vary widely with some individuals fearful of doing so and others directly experiencing negative consequences. As the above quote reveals, individuals often perceive a sense of immediate exclusion and stigma. Fear and stigma is shared worldwide as revealed by this gentleman in China with dementia:

> "Neighbours, the village leaders do not know. People who know that I am suffering from dementia will not treat us well." (reported in Alzheimer's Disease International, 2012, p. 24).

Yet others proceed differently as explained by this individual with dementia living in the United States:

> "If you are asking why I don't hide the fact that I have dementia, it is simple. I have it. If others know it, they are more apt to accept and understand." (reported in Alzheimer's Disease International, 2012, p. 24).

Regardless of stance, determining how and when to disclose one's diagnosis becomes part of the experience and task of living with dementia. Disclosure has to be thought through carefully given the potential for perceived and structural negative consequences. This is particularly the case when informing employers for which there is the need to disclose and derive a plan as to whether one can continue in one's position and if so for how long and with what types of accommodations. Employers in turn are challenged by how to support an employee with cognitive impairment and make the determination with them as to what responsibilities are possible to continue with, particularly in the early disease stage, as well as crafting a plan for moving forward. The ability to continue in a position obviously depends upon work demands, expectations, and disease stage.

Of importance is that disclosure becomes a task that individuals with dementia (and their family members) need to think through and determine how, when, where, and what to say. Controlling the timing and nature of disclosure may help individuals prepare for and/or effectively manage any negative consequences that follow.

Remaining Engaged in Meaningful Activity

With changes in cognitive abilities, staying engaged in meaningful activities becomes increasingly challenging. Engagement in meaningful activity is one of the most persistent and critical unmet needs cited by both individuals and family caregivers. As such, most individuals—from early to late stages—spend most of their days doing little that holds meaning for them (Ice, 2002; von Kutzleben, Schmid, Halek, Holle, & Bartholomeyczick, 2012; Miranda-Castillo, Woods, & Orrell, 2013; Phinney, Chaudhury, & O'Connor, 2007). A study using a national representative sample, the National Health and Aging Trends Study (NHATS) involving 5264 individuals with no dementia, 893 with possible dementia, and 518 with probable dementia found that those with cognitive impairment were less likely to indicate they were engaged in valued activities compared to their cognitively intact counterparts. Additionally, poor health and transportation difficulties were reported as limiting access to select activities (Parisi, Roberts, Szanton, Hodgson, & Gitlin, 2015).

Lack of stimulation has significant negative sequelae including isolation, increased dependency, and decreased quality of life. Inactivity is also associated with behavioral and psychological symptoms such as aggression, agitation, depression, and apathy (Gitlin, Kales, & Lyketsos, 2012). Alternately, engagement in meaningful activities has been shown to improve quality of life and reduce behavioral occurrences (Aronstein, Olsen, & Schulman, 1996), increase positive emotions (Schreiner, Yamamoto, & Shiotani, 2005), and improve quality of life when utilized in the home (Gitlin et al., 2009), hospital (Gitlin et al., 2017), or nursing home (Brooker & Woolley, 2007; Fossey et al., 2006; Kolanowski, & Buettner, 2008; Orsulic-Jeras, Judge, & Camp, 2000), and will be discussed in greater detail in Chapter 4, Making Life Better for Individuals Living With Dementia.

Maintaining a Sense of Purpose, Control, and Agency

An important outcome of enabling regular engagement in meaningful activities is the preservation of a sense of purpose in life and control over one's immediate life space. Having a sense of purpose and some control over daily life events remains an enduring need throughout disease progression, is highly valued by people living with dementia, and remains a universal need (Boyle, Buchman, Barnes, & Bennett, 2010; Irving, Davis, & Collier, 2017; Mak, 2011).

Purpose in life is a psychological construct referring to the "tendency to derive meaning from life's experiences and possess a sense of intentionality and goal directedness that guides behavior," (Boyle et al., 2010, p. 1096), or having experiences that are meaningful. Having a sense of purpose (or meaning) in life has been shown in research to have a protective benefit against negative health outcomes. While the exact mechanisms or pathways by which this psychological construct intersects with and/or impacts physiological functioning is unclear, it has been associated with a range of positive outcomes including better overall well-being, better sleep quality, and reduced incident disability, risk of mortality, and Alzheimer disease (Boyle et al., 2010; Turner, Smith, & Ong, 2017). Importantly, research suggests that having a sense of purpose is not a "trait" but rather is amenable to or modified through intervention or improvement strategies—that is we can enhance a person's sense of purpose or attributions of meaning in life (Gitlin, Parisi, Huang, Winter, & Roth, 2018).

Having a sense of purpose can be understood within the context of the Motivational Theory of Life-Span Development (Heckhausen, Wrosch, & Schulz, 2010). Briefly, this theory suggests that having some control over behavior-event contingencies in daily life is important for psychosocial well-being. Involvement in activities, for example, may provide a sense of control, connectivity, and meaning in daily life; this in turn may reduce behavioral and mood disturbances (Gitlin et al., 2016).

Relevant to a discussion of purpose is the construct of "personhood" as it emphasizes the need to understand that people with dementia are people first. This construct has helped to shift focus from loss, despair, and inabilities to an emphasis on identifying and supporting what people can do or their remaining or preserved abilities (Bartlett & O'Connor, 2007; Murray & Boyd, 2009; Nowell, Thornton, & Simpson, 2013; Potts, 2012). Thus, based on this construct, treatment focuses on ways to support capabilities and assure quality of life at every disease stage. Tom Kitwood (1997), who adapted this construct to dementia, argued that how people with dementia were treated often led to deterioration over and above the disease process itself. He redefined personhood from its previous historical enlightenment roots which focused on consciousness, rationality, memory, and intentionality to include how individuals relate to each other and the importance of interpersonal relationships. This moves the focus from a strictly biomedical paradigm to understand how quality of life is not only related to the neuropathology of dementia but also the physical and social environment including how one is perceived, interacted with, and included.

Noteworthy is that since Kitwood's groundbreaking work, others have argued that the personhood construct does not go far enough to create a meaningful, integrative environment to enable people with dementia to flourish. Bartlett and O'Connor (2007) have suggested an alternative view for example. They argue that the personhood construct is limited by its sole focus on persons at the exclusion of the sociopolitical sphere and how that impacts daily life. As such, it does not consider or lead to a push for how social and housing policies could change dementia care practices. Secondly, they suggest that while the focus of personhood is on supporting the person with dementia, it does not deliberately recognize the role of the person themselves and their need for and ability to exert agency; that is, people with dementia are not viewed as social actors who can contribute to an exchange but rather are implicitly considered as passive recipients of personalized care. Finally, they critique the term as residing only in the realm of the psychosocial and spirituality and consideration of the broader political environment of dementia care. They propose an alternative term, "citizenship," to complement and extend the principles of personhood to include a view of individuals as full members of a community with equal rights. The concept of citizenship leads to social policies that affirm the rights of individuals with dementia and which seek to provide dementia-friendly supportive communities (see Chapter 8: The Physical Home Environment: A Neglected Therapeutic Context). Higgs and Gilleard (2016) have similarly argued that the construct of personhood is too vague when applied to people with dementia and does not facilitate advancing a standard of care; rather, they suggest focusing on people's existing capabilities and minimizing potential detrimental effects resulting from cognitive decline.

We agree. While the losses that accumulate with dementia are well documented, less so are the ways in which individuals adapt to changing abilities as well as their preserved abilities, that is, what people are able to do at each disease stage and how individuals actively construct or act upon their environment to try to create meaning and purpose tends to be ignored and is understudied. For example, as some have argued, it may be that some behavioral symptoms are attempts of individuals to make meaning or address a need not recognized or understood by others. Thus, research is needed to understand preserved

> **Box 2-6**
> **Key Research Gaps**
>
> - Understand and identify positive coping mechanisms used by people with dementia upon diagnosis and throughout disease trajectory.
> - Develop measures to assess for positive psychological processes (e.g., purpose in life) that can be used with individuals with communication challenges and at different disease stages.
> - Develop assessments to quickly and validly elicit preferences, perceptions of what makes a good life, preferred treatment goals from the individual and family perspective.
> - Develop efficient approaches to assess preserved capabilities (not just what a person cannot do).
> - Develop and test interventions to support capabilities throughout disease process and for different care settings.
> - Develop new measures for each quadrant of the Good Life that also reflect the preferences of persons living with dementia and their caregivers and for different etiologies and disease stages.

capabilities and assure a comprehensive supportive dementia care approach. Key research gaps are identified in Box 2-6 and range from descriptive to measurement to intervention development.

PRACTICAL IMPLICATIONS FOR DEMENTIA CARE

From this chapter a broad vision emerges as ways to transform dementia care at the individual level that will continue to be fleshed out in subsequent chapters. This involves first and foremost recognizing that quality of life is multifaceted and individuated, thus necessitating a comprehensive assessment of all aspects or sectors of our model, the Good Life (Fig. 2.1), as well as at each disease juncture, change in cognitive, functional, or behavioral status, or other life events including changes in comorbid status (Fig. 2.2). In this way, a dementia care plan will need to reflect a living document that changes with disease progression to address the factors in each of the four quadrants of the "good life" and as needs and living circumstances change.

KEY POINTS

Several conclusions can be drawn from the extant research on the needs of individuals with dementia.

- Individuals with dementia have multiple and different needs at each point along the disease trajectory.
- Abilities and needs change with disease progression.
- Abilities and needs are highly individualized and reflect the confluence of person-related factors (age, gender, race/ethnicity/culture, and cognitive status) and environmental-related factors (access to support, living arrangements, community, and societal policies).
- Individuals encounter key challenges including assuring their sense of security and safety at home (and outside the home), overcoming stigma, determining when and how to disclose a diagnosis and cope with the consequences of the label of dementia, maintaining engagement and a purposeful life.
- An understanding of varied impacts leads to a different way of thinking about and executing comprehensive dementia care; this would involve identifying opportunities for ongoing assessment and care planning and purposeful support in key areas such as helping individuals determine how to disclose, providing coping mechanisms to overcome or manage stigma, and facilitating activity engagement.
- Understanding the characteristics and impacts of stigma and effective messaging could address societal level misconceptions that impinge on a person's daily life and self-identity.

What Can Be Done Now

- Recognize that having a sense of purpose is an enduring need throughout disease progression.
- Understand that dementia and associated stigma impacts self-identity.
- Upon diagnosis, particularly early stage, provide to person: (1) referral numbers and link to Alzheimer's Association and other helpful websites; (2) counseling to discuss best ways of disclosing; (3) opportunity to discuss treatment preferences with disease progression.
- If early stage, consider preference for joining an advocacy group and early stage support groups.
- Ask for consultation with an occupational therapist trained in dementia care to help determine cognitive functional abilities,

home safety needs and modifications, and compensatory strategies to support engagement in daily activities.
- Identify strategies to support each sector of the "Good Life" model.
- Identify meaningful activities and ways to support the person's continued participation (consult with occupational therapist trained in dementia care).
- Encourage participation in physical exercises as possible.
- Manage comorbidities.
- Start conversations about power of attorney, end-of-life decisions, and finances.
- Develop a dementia care plan that is revisited with disease progression and which includes attention to oral, hearing and vision care and sleep patterns.
- Establish a daily predictable and structured routine.
- Provide opportunities for person living with dementia to process and discuss their lived experiences and ways they would like to be supported.

A Conversation with Dr. Jason Karlowish

1. *What aspects of living with dementia and/or having this diagnosis are stigmatizing?*
Stigma is the toxic chemistry catalyzed by a disease label. It's a distinctly human experience. In healthcare, the term describes how either a person's social identity or sense of self is harmed by being associated with a disease. The person becomes a member of a group associated with unwanted behaviors, disabilities, and negative experiences ascribed to the diagnosis. For a person diagnosed with dementia, the label "dementia" implies a set of undesired behaviors the person has and also is expected to develop and negative expectations about the person's future, such as prognosis and life expectancy (Scambler, 2009). Adding the "Alzheimer's" label only intensifies this stigma.
Public stigma describes how the public may carry negative or pejorative beliefs that cause them to act in discriminatory, exclusionary or patronizing ways towards persons who either have or are closely associated with persons with dementia. The beliefs include that persons with Alzheimer's are unkempt, dangerous, and out of control (Johnson et al., 2015; Stites et al., 2016). In the extreme, they are a living dead, or, in a word, zombies (Behuniak, 2011). Self-stigma describes a person

absorbing negative beliefs, attitudes, assumptions, and stereotypes related to the disease. These include feelings ashamed and inferior because of being closely linked to the disease (Corrigan, 2007). Among persons with dementia cause by Alzheimer's disease, self-stigma, also referred to as "felt" or "internalized" stigma, is associated with depression, avoidant coping, social avoidance, low self-esteem, hopelessness, relatively worse psychiatric symptoms, and decreased help-seeking behaviors (Mukadam & Livingston, 2012).

Persons caring for a person with dementia experience stigma as well. This "spillover stigma" affects individuals who share close social proximity to those who do have the disease, such family members and caregivers (Werner et al., 2011). It can also affect individuals who have a condition that while distinct is also related to dementia, such as Mild Cognitive Impairment (MCI; Beard, 2013). It is possible that the stigma experience of dementia caused by Alzheimer's disease could spillover to cognitively unimpaired persons who are diagnosed with Alzheimer's using biomarkers.

2. *Why is stigma one of the most critical issues in dementia care that must be addressed?* The symptoms of dementia are many and manifold, but they have a common theme, a chipping away at identity, privacy, authority, normality, and responsibility. In short, a chipping away at autonomy. Self and public stigmas both work to undermine each of these aspects of an adult's agency. Stigma is the suffering of dementia. Stigma affects patients' and caregivers' health and well-being, relationships, and financial well-being throughout most stages of disease. The stress of managing the psychosocial consequences of the disease can lead to development and exacerbation of existing symptoms (Jolley & Benbow, 2000). This is sometimes misconstrued by patients or their caregivers as evidence of decline, increasing the burden of morbidity, likelihood of social withdrawal, and risk of institutionalization (Aneshensel, Pearlin, & Schuler, 1993). It can also lend to relationship conflict and loss, particularly with family members. Stigma of Alzheimer's disease dementia can create financial difficulties, like being fired or forced into early retirement, or being unable to secure insurance to cover the cost of care (Francesca et al., 2011).

Patients often worry about conforming to stereotypes of the disease, embarrassing themselves, and how others might react to their diagnosis (Ballard, Boyle, Bowler, & Lindesay, 1996). When faced with the threat of feeling that they're at risk for conforming to a stereotype, some react by exhibiting signs that confirm that stereotype. This phenomenon, called stereotyped threat, has been found to affect individuals even before the onset of cognitive symptoms; persons who learned their genetic risk for developing Alzheimer's disease dementia performed much lower on memory tasks than others who are at-risk but uninformed (Lineweaver, Bondi, Galasko, & Salmon, 2014).

3. *What research is needed to fully understand stigma and its effects on the lived experience?*
There's an expression that keeps science true and honest, "No measurement, no science." Scales are available to measure stigma in persons with dementia and in the general public (see for example Werner et al., 2011). Cohort studies need to more routinely measure these so that we learn more about who experiences stigma, who's protected from it and why. We need to learn these things so that we can improve living with dementia. Talking about stigma can be, well, stigmatizing. We mustn't avoid the topic, but we can use a richer language. Messages about stigma should talk about what we're trying to preserve: identity, privacy, authority, normality, and responsibility. The more we understand the experience of stigma, the better we can intervene to reduce or even prevent it. Interventions need to include careful attention to our language, to the words, images and stories we use when we talk about dementia and Alzheimer's disease. Studies need to discover what messages create the intention to want to have a meaningful conversation with someone with dementia.

References

Adebiyi, A. O., Fagbola, M. A., Olakehinde, O., & Ogunniyi, A. (2016). Enacted and implied stigma for dementia in a community in south-west Nigeria. *Psychogeriatrics*, 16 (4), 268−273. Available from https://doi.org/10.1111/psyg.12156.

Aneshensel, C. S., Pearlin, L. I., & Schuler, R. H. (1993). Stress, role captivity, and the cessation of caregiving. *Journal of Health and Social Behavior*, 34(1), 54−70.

Alzheimer's Disease International. (2012). *World Alzheimer Report 2012: Overcoming the stigma of dementia*. London: Alzheimer's Disease International (ADI). Retrieved from https://www.alz.co.uk/research/WorldAlzheimerReport2012.pdf.

Aronstein, Z., Olsen, R., & Schulman, E. (1996). The nursing assistant's use of recreational interventions for behavioral management of residents with Alzheimer's disease. *American Journal of Alzheimer's Disease*, 11(3), 26−31. Available from https://doi.org/10.1177/153331759601100304.

Bakker, C., de Vugt, M. E., van Vliet, D., Verhey, F., Pijnenburg, Y. A., Vernooij-Dassen, M. J. F. J., & Koopmans, R. T. C. M. (2014). Unmet needs and health-related quality of life in young-onset dementia. *The American Journal of Geriatric Psychiatry*, 22(11), 1121−1130. Available from https://doi.org/10.1016/j.jagp.2013.02.006.

Ballard, C., Boyle, A., Bowler, C., & Lindesay, J. (1996). Anxiety disorders in dementia sufferers. *International Journal of Geriatric Psychiatry, 11*(11), 987–990.

Bamford, S. M., Holley-Moore, G., & Watson, J. (2014). *New perspectives and approaches to understanding dementia and stigma*. International Longevity Centre United Kingdom.

Bartlett, R., & O'Connor, D. (2007). From personhood to citizenship: Broadening the lens for dementia practice and research. *Journal of Aging Studies, 21*(2), 107–118. Available from https://doi.org/10.1016/j.jaging.2006.09.002.

Beard, R. L., & Neary, T. M. (2013). Making sense of nonsense: Experiences of mild cognitive impairment. *Sociology of Health & Illness, 35*(1), 130–146. Available from https://doi.org/10.1111/j.1467-9566.2012.01481.x.

Behuniak, S. M. (2011). The living dead? The construction of people with Alzheimer's disease as zombies. *Ageing and Society, 31*(1), 70–92. Available from https://doi.org/10.1017/S0144686X10000693.

Benbow, S. M., & Jolley, D. (2012). Dementia: Stigma and its effects. *Neurodegenerative Disease Management, 2*(2), 165–172. Available from https://doi.org/10.2217/nmt.12.7.

Black, B. S., Johnston, D., Rabins, P. V., Morrison, A., Lyketsos, C., & Samus, Q. M. (2013). Unmet needs of community-residing persons with dementia and their informal caregivers: Findings from the Maximizing Independence at Home Study. *Journal of the American Geriatrics Society, 61*(12), 2087–2095. Available from https://doi.org/10.1111/jgs.12549.

Blay, S. L., & Peluso, É. T. P. (2010). Public stigma: The community's tolerance of Alzheimer disease. *The American Journal of Geriatric Psychiatry, 18*(2), 163–171. Available from https://doi.org/10.1097/JGP.0b013e3181bea900.

Borochowitz, K. (2011). Dementia: The stigma and the challenges: Conference paper. *ESR Review: Economic and Social Rights in South Africa, 12*(1), 32–33.

Boyle, P. A., Buchman, A. S., Barnes, L. L., & Bennett, D. A. (2010). Effect of a purpose in life on risk of incident Alzheimer disease and mild cognitive impairment in community-dwelling older persons. *Archives of General Psychiatry, 67*(3), 304. Available from https://doi.org/10.1001/archgenpsychiatry.2009.208.

Brooker, D. J., & Woolley, R. J. (2007). Enriching opportunities for people living with dementia: The development of a blueprint for a sustainable activity-based model. *Aging & Mental Health, 11*(4), 371–383. Available from https://doi.org/10.1080/13607860600963687.

Burgener, S. C., Buckwalter, K., Perkhounkova, Y., & Liu, M. F. (2015). The effects of perceived stigma on quality of life outcomes in persons with early-stage dementia: Longitudinal findings: Part 2. *Dementia, 14*(5), 609–632. Available from https://doi.org/10.1177/1471301213504202.

Butler, R. N. (2005). Ageism: Looking back over my shoulder. *Generations, 29*(3), 84–86.

Cassie, K. M., & Cassie, W. (2013). Racial disparities in the use of physical restraints in U. S. nursing homes. *Health & Social Work, 38*(4), 207–213. Available from https://doi.org/10.1093/hsw/hlt020.

Cohen-Mansfield, J., Dakheel-Ali, M., Marx, M. S., Thein, K., & Regier, N. G. (2015). Which unmet needs contribute to behavior problems in persons with advanced dementia? *Psychiatry Research, 228*(1), 59–64. Available from https://doi.org/10.1016/j.psychres.2015.03.043.

Corrigan, P. W. (2007). How clinical diagnosis might exacerbate the stigma of mental illness. *Social Work, 52*(1), 31–39. Available from https://doi.org/10.1093/sw/52.1.31.

Francesca, C., Ana, L.-N., Jérôme, M., & Frits, T. (2011). *OECD health policy studies help wanted? Providing and paying for long-term care: Providing and paying for long-term care.* OECD Publishing.

Fossey, J., Ballard, C., Juszczak, E., James, I., Alder, N., Jacoby, R., & Howard, R. (2006). Effect of enhanced psychosocial care on antipsychotic use in nursing home residents with severe dementia: Cluster randomised trial. *British Medical Journal, 332*(7544), 756−761. Available from https://doi.org/10.1136/bmj.38782.575868.7C.

Gilligan, A. M., Malone, D. C., Warholak, T. L., & Armstrong, E. P. (2012). Racial and ethnic disparities in Alzheimer's disease pharmacotherapy exposure: An analysis across four state Medicaid populations. *The American Journal of Geriatric Pharmacotherapy, 10*(5), 303−312. Available from https://doi.org/10.1016/j.amjopharm.2012.09.002.

Gilligan, A. M., Malone, D. C., Warholak, T. L., & Armstrong, E. P. (2013). Health disparities in cost of care in patients with Alzheimer's disease. *American Journal of Alzheimer's Disease & Other Dementias, 28*(1), 84−92. Available from https://doi.org/10.1177/1533317512467679.

Gitlin, L. N., & Corcoran, M. (2000). Making homes safer: Environmental adaptations for people with dementia. *Alzheimer's Care Quarterly, 1*(1), 50−58.

Gitlin, L. N., Hodgson, N., Piersol, C. V., Hess, E., & Hauck, W. W. (2014). Correlates of quality of life for individuals with dementia living at home: The role of home environment, caregiver, and patient-related characteristics. *The American Journal of Geriatric Psychiatry, 22*(6), 587−597. Available from https://doi.org/10.1016/j.jagp.2012.11.005.

Gitlin, L. N., Kales, H. C., & Lyketsos, C. G. (2012). Nonpharmacologic management of behavioral symptoms in dementia. *Journal of the American Medical Association, 308*(19), 2020. Available from https://doi.org/10.1001/jama.2012.36918.

Gitlin, L. N., Marx, K. A., Alonzi, D., Kvedar, T., Moody, J., Trahan, M., & Van Haitsma, K. (2017). Feasibility of the Tailored Activity Program for Hospitalized (TAP-H) patients with behavioral symptoms. *The Gerontologist, 57*(3), 575−584. Available from https://doi.org/10.1093/geront/gnw052.

Gitlin, L. N., Piersol, C. V., Hodgson, N., Marx, K., Roth, D. L., Johnston, D., ... Lyketsos, C. G. (2016). Reducing neuropsychiatric symptoms in persons with dementia and associated burden in family caregivers using tailored activities: Design and methods of a randomized clinical trial. *Contemporary Clinical Trials, 49*, 92−102. Available from https://doi.org/10.1016/j.cct.2016.06.006.

Gitlin, L. N., Parisi, J. M., Huang, J., Winter, L., & Roth, D. L. (2018). Valuation of Life as outcome and mediator of a depression intervention for older African Americans: The Get Busy Get Better Trial. *International Journal of Geriatric Psychiatry, 33*(1), e31−e39. Available from https://doi.org/10.1002/gps.4710.

Gitlin, L. N., Winter, L., Vause Earland, T., Adel Herge, E., Chernett, N. L., Piersol, C. V., & Burke, J. P. (2009). The Tailored Activity Program to reduce behavioral symptoms in individuals with dementia: Feasibility, acceptability, and replication potential. *The Gerontologist, 49*(3), 428−439. Available from https://doi.org/10.1093/geront/gnp087.

Harris, P. B., & Caporella, C. A. (2014). An intergenerational choir formed to lessen Alzheimer's disease stigma in college students and decrease the social isolation of people with Alzheimer's disease and their family members. *American Journal of Alzheimer's Disease & Other Dementias, 29*(3), 270−281. Available from https://doi.org/10.1177/1533317513517044.

Heckhausen, J., Wrosch, C., & Schulz, R. (2010). A motivational theory of life-span development. *Psychological Review, 117*(1), 32−60. Available from https://doi.org/10.1037/a0017668.

Higgs, P., & Gilleard, C. (2016). Interrogating personhood and dementia. *Aging & Mental Health, 20*(8), 773−780. Available from https://doi.org/10.1080/13607863.2015.1118012.

Hodgson, N. A., Black, B. S., Johnston, D., Lyketsos, C., & Samus, Q. M. (2014). Comparison of unmet care needs across the dementia trajectory: Findings from the maximizing independence at home study. *Journal of Geriatrics and Palliative Care, 2*(2), 5.

Hodgson, N. A., Gitlin, L. N., Winter, L., & Czekanski, K. (2011). Undiagnosed illness and neuropsychiatric behaviors in community residing older adults with dementia.

Alzheimer Disease & Associated Disorders, 25(2), 109–115. Available from https://doi.org/10.1097/WAD.0b013e3181f8520a.

Ice, G. H. (2002). Daily life in a nursing home. *Journal of Aging Studies, 16*(4), 345–359. Available from https://doi.org/10.1016/S0890-4065(02)00069-5.

Irving, J., Davis, S., & Collier, A. (2017). Aging with purpose. *The International Journal of Aging and Human Development, 85*(4), 403–437. Available from https://doi.org/10.1177/0091415017702908.

Johnson, R., Harkins, K., Cary, M., Sankar, P., & Karlawish, J. (2015). The relative contributions of disease label and disease prognosis to Alzheimer's stigma: A vignette-based experiment. *Social Science & Medicine, 143,* 117–127. Available from https://doi.org/10.1016/j.socscimed.2015.08.031.

Jolley, D. J., & Benbow, S. M. (2000). Stigma and Alzheimer's disease: Causes, consequences and a constructive approach. *International Journal of Clinical Practice, 54*(2), 117–119.

Kitwood, T. (1997). *Dementia reconsidered: The person comes first.* Buckingham: Open University Press.

Kolanowski, A., & Buettner, L. (2008). Prescribing activities that engage passive residents. *Journal of Gerontological Nursing, 34*(1), 13–18. Available from https://doi.org/10.3928/00989134-20080101-08.

Lach, H. W., & Chang, Y.-P. (2007). Caregiver perspectives on safety in home dementia care. *Western Journal of Nursing Research, 29*(8), 993–1014. Available from https://doi.org/10.1177/0193945907303098.

Lawton, M. P. (1983). Environment and other determinants of well-being in older people. *The Gerontologist, 23*(4), 349–357. Available from https://doi.org/10.1093/geront/23.4.349.

Levine, D. A. (2013). Young-onset dementia. *Journal of the American Medical Association Internal Medicine, 173*(17), 1619. Available from https://doi.org/10.1001/jamainternmed.2013.8090.

Lineweaver, T. T., Bondi, M. W., Galasko, D., & Salmon, D. P. (2014). Effect of knowledge of APOE genotype on subjective and objective memory performance in healthy older adults. *American Journal of Psychiatry, 171*(2), 201–208. Available from https://doi.org/10.1176/appi.ajp.2013.12121590.

Mak, W. (2011). Self-reported goal pursuit and purpose in life among people with dementia. *The Journals of Gerontology Series B: Psychological Sciences and Social Sciences, 66B*(2), 177–184. Available from https://doi.org/10.1093/geronb/gbq092.

Mazerolle, M., Régner, I., Barber, S. J., Paccalin, M., Miazola, A.-C., Huguet, P., & Rigalleau, F. (2016). Negative aging stereotypes impair performance on brief cognitive tests used to screen for predementia. *The Journals of Gerontology Series B: Psychological Sciences and Social Sciences, 72*(6), 932–936. Available from https://doi.org/10.1093/geronb/gbw083.

McParland, P., Devine, P., Innes, A., & Gayle, V. (2012). Dementia knowledge and attitudes of the general public in Northern Ireland: An analysis of national survey data. *International Psychogeriatrics, 24*(10), 1600–1613. Available from https://doi.org/10.1017/S1041610212000658.

Millenaar, J. K., Bakker, C., Koopmans, R. T. C. M., Verhey, F. R. J., Kurz, A., & de Vugt, M. E. (2016). The care needs and experiences with the use of services of people with young-onset dementia and their caregivers: A systematic review. *International Journal of Geriatric Psychiatry, 31*(12), 1261–1276. Available from https://doi.org/10.1002/gps.4502.

Miranda-Castillo, C., Woods, B., & Orrell, M. (2010). People with dementia living alone: What are their needs and what kind of support are they receiving? *International Psychogeriatrics, 22*(4), 607–617. Available from https://doi.org/10.1017/S104161021000013X.

Miranda-Castillo, C., Woods, B., & Orrell, M. (2013). The needs of people with dementia living at home from user, caregiver and professional perspectives: A cross-sectional survey. *BMC Health Services Research*, *13*(1), 43. Available from https://doi.org/10.1186/1472-6963-13-43.

Mukadam, N., & Livingston, G. (2012). Reducing the stigma associated with dementia: Approaches and goals. *Aging Health*, *8*(4), 377–386. Available from https://doi.org/10.2217/ahe.12.42.

Murray, L. M., & Boyd, S. (2009). Protecting personhood and achieving quality of life for older adults with dementia in the U.S. health care system. *Journal of Aging and Health*, *21*(2), 350–373. Available from https://doi.org/10.1177/0898264308329017.

Navab, E., Negarandeh, R., Peyrovi, H., & Navab, P. (2013). Stigma among Iranian family caregivers of patients with Alzheimer's disease: A hermeneutic study. *Nursing & Health Sciences*, *15*(2), 201–206. Available from https://doi.org/10.1111/nhs.12017.

Nielsen, T. R., Andersen, B. B., Kastrup, M., Phung, T. K. T., & Waldemar, G. (2011). Quality of dementia diagnostic evaluation for ethnic minority patients: A nationwide study. *Dementia and Geriatric Cognitive Disorders*, *31*(5), 388–396. Available from https://doi.org/10.1159/000327362.

Nowell, Z. C., Thornton, A., & Simpson, J. (2013). The subjective experience of personhood in dementia care settings. *Dementia*, *12*(4), 394–409. Available from https://doi.org/10.1177/1471301211430648.

Orsulic-Jeras, S., Judge, K., & Camp, C. (2000). Montessori-based activities for long-term care residents with advanced dementia: Effects on engagement and affect. *The Gerontologist*, *40*(1), 107–111. Available from https://doi.org/10.1093/geront/40.1.107.

Parisi, J. M., Roberts, L., Szanton, S. L., Hodgson, N. A., & Gitlin, L. N. (2015). Valued activities among individuals with and without cognitive impairments: Findings from the National Health and Aging Trends Study. *The Gerontologist*, *57*(2), 309–318. Available from https://doi.org/10.1093/geront/gnv144.

Phillipson, L., Magee, C., Jones, S., Reis, S., & Skaldzien, E. (2015). Dementia attitudes and help-seeking intentions: An investigation of responses to two scenarios of an experience of the early signs of dementia. *Aging & Mental Health*, *19*(11), 968–977. Available from https://doi.org/10.1080/13607863.2014.995588.

Phinney, A., Chaudhury, H., & O'Connor, D. L. (2007). Doing as much as I can do: The meaning of activity for people with dementia. *Aging & Mental Health*, *11*(4), 384–393. Available from https://doi.org/10.1080/13607860601086470.

Piver, L. C., Nubukpo, P., Faure, A., Dumoitier, N., Couratier, P., & Clément, J.-P. (2013). Describing perceived stigma against Alzheimer's disease in a general population in France: The STIG-MA survey. *International Journal of Geriatric Psychiatry*, *28*(9), 933–938. Available from https://doi.org/10.1002/gps.3903.

Potts, D. C. (2012). The art of preserving personhood. *Neurology*, *78*(11), 836–837. Available from https://doi.org/10.1212/WNL.0b013e318249f789.

Puyat, J. H., Law, M. R., Wong, S. T., Sutherland, J. M., & Morgan, S. G. (2012). The essential and potentially inappropriate use of antipsychotics across income groups: An analysis of linked administrative data. *The Canadian Journal of Psychiatry*, *57*(8), 488–495. Available from https://doi.org/10.1177/070674371205700807.

Scambler, G. (2009). Health-related stigma. *Sociology of Health & Illness*, *31*(3), 441–455. Available from https://doi.org/10.1111/j.1467-9566.2009.01161.x.

Schreiner, A. S., Yamamoto, E., & Shiotani, H. (2005). Positive affect among nursing home residents with Alzheimer's dementia: The effect of recreational activity. *Aging & Mental Health*, *9*(2), 129–134. Available from https://doi.org/10.1080/13607860412331336841.

Sivananthan, S. N., Lavergne, M. R., & McGrail, K. M. (2015). Caring for dementia: A population-based study examining variations in guideline-consistent medical care.

Alzheimer's & Dementia, 11(8), 906–916. Available from https://doi.org/10.1016/j.jalz.2015.02.008.

Stites, S. D., Johnson, R., Harkins, K., Sankar, P., Xie, D., & Karlawish, J. (2016). Identifiable characteristics and potentially malleable beliefs predict stigmatizing attributions toward persons with Alzheimer's disease dementia: Results of a survey of the U.S. general public. *Health Communication, 33*(3), 264–273, 10.1080/10410236.2016.1255847.

Swaffer, K. (2014). Dementia: Stigma, language, and dementia-friendly. *Dementia, 13*(6), 709–716. Available from https://doi.org/10.1177/1471301214548143.

Turner, A. D., Smith, C. E., & Ong, J. C. (2017). Is purpose in life associated with less sleep disturbance in older adults? *Sleep Science and Practice, 1*(1), 14. Available from https://doi.org/10.1186/s41606-017-0015-6.

van der Roest, H. G., Meiland, F. J. M., Comijs, H. C., Derksen, E., Jansen, A. P. D., van Hout, H. P. J., … Dröes, R.-M. (2009). What do community-dwelling people with dementia need? A survey of those who are known to care and welfare services. *International Psychogeriatrics, 21*(5), 949. Available from https://doi.org/10.1017/S1041610209990147.

von Kutzleben, M., Schmid, W., Halek, M., Holle, B., & Bartholomeyczik, S. (2012). Community-dwelling persons with dementia: What do they need? What do they demand? What do they do? A systematic review on the subjective experiences of persons with dementia. *Aging & Mental Health, 16*(3), 378–390. Available from https://doi.org/10.1080/13607863.2011.614594.

Werner, P., Goldstein, D., & Heinik, J. (2011). Development and validity of the Family Stigma in Alzheimer's Disease Scale (FS-ADS). *Alzheimer Disease & Associated Disorders, 25*(1), 42–48. Available from https://doi.org/10.1097/WAD.0b013e3181f32594.

Werner, P., Mittelman, M. S., Goldstein, D., & Heinik, J. (2012). Family stigma and caregiver burden in Alzheimer's disease. *The Gerontologist, 52*(1), 89–97. Available from https://doi.org/10.1093/geront/gnr117.

Werner, P., Goldberg, S., Mandel, S., & Korczyn, A. D. (2013). Gender differences in lay persons' beliefs and knowledge about Alzheimer's disease (AD): A national representative study of Israeli adults. *Archives of Gerontology and Geriatrics, 56*(2), 400–404. Available from https://doi.org/10.1016/j.archger.2012.11.001.

Zeng, F., Xie, W. T., Wang, Y. J., Luo, H. B., Shi, X. Q., Zou, H. Q., … … … Lian, Y. (2015). General public perceptions and attitudes toward Alzheimer's disease from five cities in China. *Journal of Alzheimer's Disease, 43*(2), 511–518. Available from https://doi.org/10.3233/JAD-141371.

Zilkens, R. R., Duke, J., Horner, B., Semmens, J. B., & Bruce, D. G. (2014). Australian population trends and disparities in cholinesterase inhibitor use, 2003 to 2010. *Alzheimer's & Dementia, 10*(3), 310–318. Available from https://doi.org/10.1016/j.jalz.2013.04.001.

Further Reading

Colombo, F., Llena-Nozal, A., Mercier, J., & Tjadens, F. (2011). *Help wanted? Providing and paying for long-term care*. Paris: OECD Publishing. Available from https://doi.org/10.1787/9789264097759-en.

Hodgson, N., Gitlin, L. N., & Huang, J. (2014). The influence of sleep disruption and pain perception on indicators of quality of life in individuals living with dementia at home. *Geriatric Nursing, 35*(5), 394–398. Available from https://doi.org/10.1016/j.gerinurse.2014.08.005.

World Health Organization. (2002). *Reducing stigma and discrimination against older people with mental disorders*. Geneva: World Health Organization.

CHAPTER 3

Breaking the Cycle of Despair

While no one can change the outcome of dementia or Alzheimer's, with the right support you can change the journey. **Tara Reed from A Practical Guide to Dealing with a Dementia or Alzheimer's Diagnosis in the Family.**

Those with dementia are still people and they still have stories and they still have character and they're all individuals and they're all unique. And they just need to be interacted with on a human level. **Carey Mulligan, British actress.**

Over the past 20 years, tremendous progress has been made concerning our understanding of the underlying pathophysiology of the dementias (see Chapter 1: How the Brain Is Affected). Nevertheless, we have a long way to go to fully comprehend, prevent, cure, and/or manage this extremely complex condition. As of the writing of this chapter, Eli Lilly announced that one of their most promising Alzheimer's drug, solanezumab, failed in a late stage Phase III trial. Earlier trials with this drug had shown a signal that people living with mild cognitive impairment may have a slowing of disease progression. However, in this most recent definitive trial, those receiving the drug fared no better those in the placebo group, leaving the field without much hope for an immediate potential disease-modifying treatment. Another drug company, Pfizer, also recently (2018) announced termination of their dementia drug discovery program.

Nevertheless, there are other ways—other treatments (e.g., non-drug) we should be seriously investing in developing and evaluating that may modify disease trajectory, reduce excess disabilities, or possibly compress morbidity and disease burdens. The consideration of other treatments requires adopting a different orientation towards dementia than what is currently endorsed. It involves viewing, understanding, and acting upon disease processes in their totality including the biological, social, psychological, and environmental context in which the disease occurs and transpires.

To begin to understand what is possible in comprehensive dementia care, we first describe in this chapter three primary buckets of research currently underway on dementia: these are prevention, cure (and an iteration of cure which refers to a search to slow disease progression with drug therapeutics) and slowing disease progression, and care and services. We then explore the consequences of the singular focus on preventive–curative research that dominates policy discourse and resource allocation. We argue that this singular focus creates a "cycle of despair" and perpetuates continuance of barriers to developing and accessing effective care and services and that even further, providing effective care and services may slow disease progression.

To move forward with effective care and services, we need to construct a different paradigm. We suggest that fundamental to a new paradigm in dementia are eight basic assumptions. Our intent here is to offer a way to begin to think differently about dementia care. In Chapter 4, Making Life Better for Individuals Living With Dementia, we build upon these basic assumptions and examine specific actions that can be taken at this moment in time to assure quality of life for people living with dementia.

THREE BUCKETS OF RESEARCH

Current research on dementia can be categorized into three broad areas or "buckets" as shown in Fig. 3-1: prevention, cure, and care and services. These three areas have been identified in most national plans on dementia as important for knowledge development and action (see Chapter 10: Services and Settings of Care).

Prevention is a relatively new research pathway in response to the consistent finding that the pathophysiology of the dementias begins many years prior to its clinical manifestations. Identifying strategies for preventing cognitive impairment is methodologically challenging given the complexities in manipulating lifestyle changes identified as possibly lowering dementia risk and the need to evaluate prevention at the population level over a long time frame. Nevertheless, some initial headway in this area has been made and there is a growing corpus of research signaling in particular four areas as possibly thwarting dementia and/or lowering its risk. These involve attending regular physical activity (Global Council on Brain Health, 2016), diet, social engagement and cognitive stimulation, and treating cardiovascular disease (Livingston et al., 2017). Specifications for each of these preventive actions such as how much and what type of exercise is most beneficial are still lacking and need to be fully investigated as well as the mechanisms of action and extent of risk reduction possible.

It remains unclear how early in one's life one must adopt healthy lifestyle choices to maximize benefit and if all areas must be simultaneously

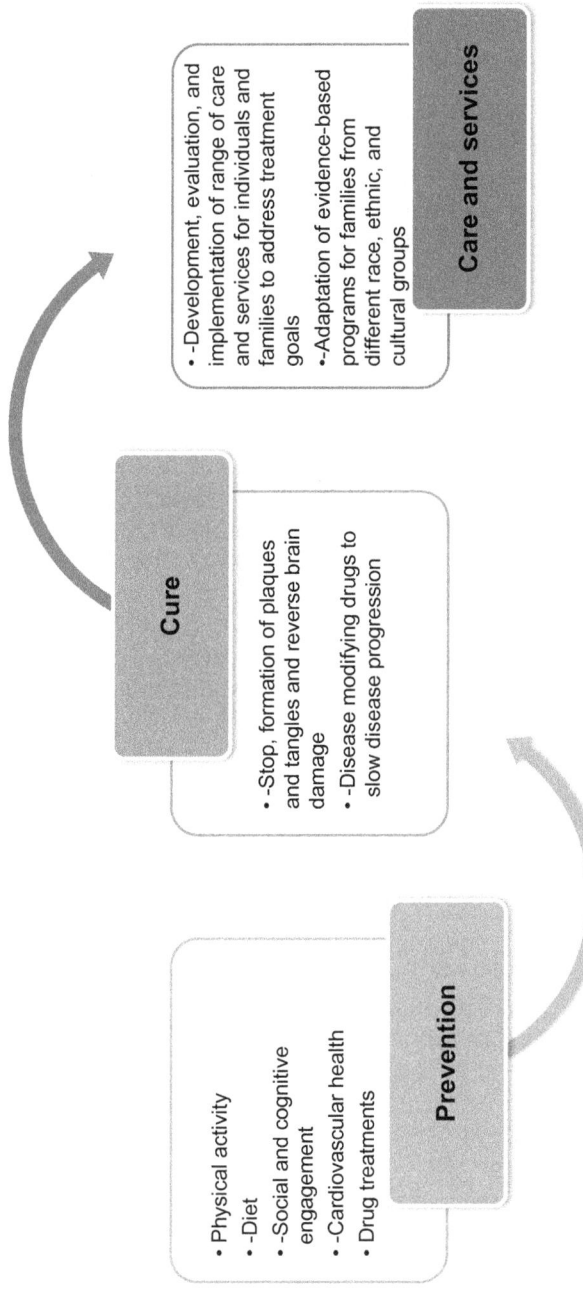

FIGURE 3-1 Three buckets of research and most promising topics within each area.

pursued in order to significantly reduce risks. However, these strategies remain the most promising actions that may prevent or lower dementia risk that require more research attention. Other potential candidates for lowering dementia risk include bilingualism, higher education, and addressing depression early on (Langa et al., 2017). These areas also warrant more research investment and have significant implications for health and social policies (e.g., assuring quality education, and access to language learning). For example, a recent study in the United States using data from the Health and Retirement Survey, a nationally representative, population-based longitudinal survey of individuals 65 years or older, compared the prevalence of dementia among participants from two study waves, 2000 ($n = 10,546$) and 2012 ($n = 10,511$). They found a significant decline in dementia prevalence over the 12 years from 11.6% in 2000 to 8.8% in 2012. The researchers found that an increase in educational attainment and better control of cardiovascular risk factors (such as diabetes) was associated with some of the decline, although other social, behavioral, and medical factors may also have contributed as well (Langa et al., 2017). Similar trends have been reported in Western Europe (Wu et al., 2016) and Scandinavia (Christensen, Davidsen, Kjoller, & Juel, 2014; Schrijvers et al., 2012). If findings are confirmed, results have dramatic implications for population health and national educational policies. Additionally, it is unclear as to the role of other social determinants such as financial strain, and what aspects of low education and socioeconomic status or other social determinants impact risk.

As to *cure*, this has dominated the focus and allocations of research dollars particularly in the United States. Nevertheless, as we have previously discussed, drug trials have failed to find promising treatments to date, and no therapies are on the horizon that are designed to totally reverse brain damage caused by a dementia. Consequently, attention has begun to shift and to an enhanced focus on ways to slow disease progression. This has involved identifying therapies such as immunotherapies, targeting individuals with early or mild dementia to try to slow disease progression so that individuals may live better and longer with dementia as a chronic disease (Davtyan et al., 2016). Such therapies would have the effect of compressing morbidity and possibly reducing caregiver burden or the time needed for care. This shift from prevention or the reversal of brain damage reflects the realization of the extreme complexities of dementia and that a single methodology/treatment/strategy is not possible.

A focus on research on *care and services* is slowly gaining recognition as an important strategy. This is the case for several reasons. First, strategies for slowing disease progression have yet to be developed and shown to work. Yet, even if there should be a pharmacological treatment that can slow disease progression, people living with dementia and their caregivers would still require care and supportive services. That is, the need for care and services will not go away even if we are able to slow disease progression. In fact, the need will only increase with individuals being diagnosed more and earlier on in the disease process. As a "cure" is decades away and not in sight, and disease modifying therapies may only slow disease progression but not address all disease symptoms and impacts, we must refocus and extend our energies to assuring appropriate care and services. Importantly, as stated above, a critical empirical question is whether providing evidence-informed care and services can modify disease course or slow its progression. There is some evidence to suggest for example, that effectively reducing risk for and/or managing behavioral and psychological behaviors can reduce the rate of decline. This is a critical area for investigation.

> Even if there is a "cure" and/or drug treatment that slows disease progression and it becomes available in the very near future, there would still be a significant need to advance comprehensive, evidence-informed and evidence-based care and supportive strategies; that is, care and services are essential now and will continue to be in the near and far future for those with a dementia and their caregivers, as well for those who would benefit from a future disease modifying treatment. This is the case even if there was some miracle breakthrough drug.

PARADIGM OF DESPAIR

An unfortunate consequence of the singular but also understandable focus on uncovering a cure has been the creation of a cycle of despair. Fig. 3.2 illustrates the psychology of this cycle. Specifically, the messaging in health care and among health providers and societies at-large has been as follows:

- There is no cure
- Therefore, nothing can be done
- As nothing can be done, nothing is provided families including basic education or referrals for support
- Nothing being done leads to hopelessness, resulting in poor quality of life

This "no cure—nothing can be done" mindset in turn underlies and perpetuates various factors that in turn inhibit or serve as barriers to access to and provision of adequate care and support. We have identified six key barriers to treatment planning and effective interventions shown in Fig. 3.3. These barriers in particular characterize the US context in which the despair cycle is reinforced by payment structures that reward curative therapies versus disease management and coordination

58   3. BREAKING THE CYCLE OF DESPAIR

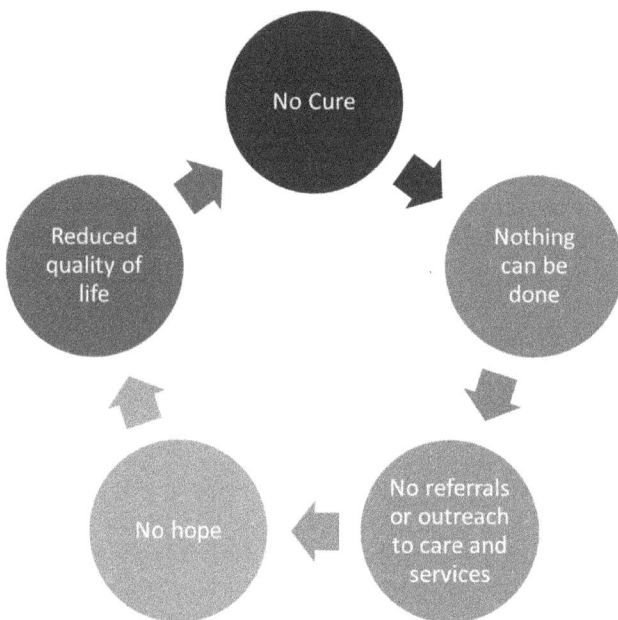

FIGURE 3-2 Cycle of despair imposed by the "no cure" paradigm.

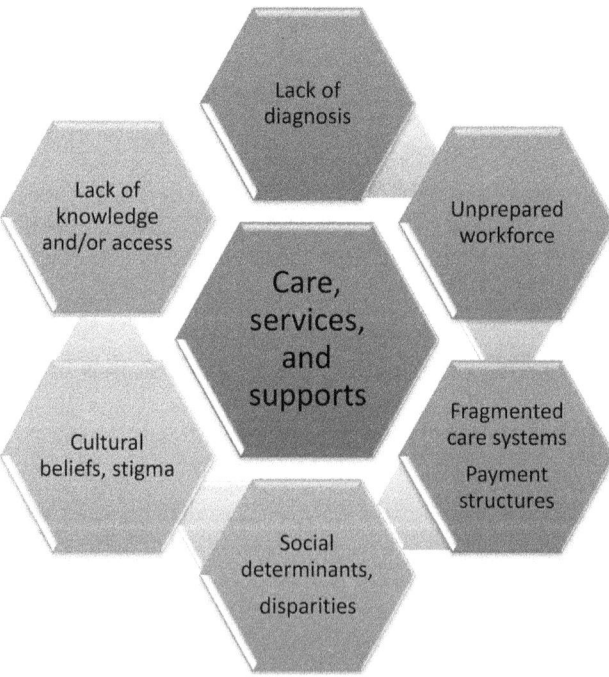

FIGURE 3-3 Key factors that must be addressed to enhance care that supports the "good life."

approaches, an inadequately prepared workforce in dementia care, structural and perceptual stigma (see also Chapter 2: Lived Experiences of Individuals With Dementia), and lack of access to diagnosticians and dementia care specialists for treatment planning and services. In turn, social determinants and health disparities in turn contribute to uneven and unequal access to and receipt of needed education and assistance.

To reiterate, these barriers conspire to make it almost impossible for people living with dementia and their families do obtain even the basic information, knowledge, skills, and resources to help them better manage disease progression and its complexities at home. It may be shocking to know that families usually do not receive even simple referrals to existing local, national, and/or global resources or websites such as the Alzheimer's Association or other associations (e.g., Lewy Body Dementia Association) and encouragement to access local care and services such as Adult Day Services or other strategies for respite, or when and how to access lawyers specializing in elder care to assist with financial and advanced care planning.

Individuals with dementia and their caregivers are basically left on their own to figure things out with the parting words from health professionals often being, "there is nothing that can be done." With little to no knowledge about the disease and potential resources and effective care strategies (albeit they are typically limited), families along with their health providers often experience a sense of hopelessness.

> There is no question that more evidence must be generated and there are huge gaps in ways to provide effective care. For example, we have no proven protocols for reducing fall risk, enhancing mobility, nor managing co-morbidities and sensory impairments. However, there are approaches that can be used now and from which we can build comprehensive dementia care for individuals and their caregivers with resultant improvements in quality of life.

This cycle of despair and the barriers it creates dominates the approach to dementia care, particularly in the United States. This is illustrated in the case snapshot of Mr. and Mrs. Smith.

Case Snapshot of Mr. and Mrs. Smith

Mr. Smith, an 82 year old African American cares for his wife at home in an urban area, who was diagnosed with dementia 4 years ago. Upon diagnosis, Mrs. Smith's doctor prescribed Aricept but indicated "nothing else can be done – there is nothing to do." As the medication caused side effects and seemed ineffective, it was shortly stopped. Mr. Smith only learned of the Alzheimer's Association by chance from a neighbor and he received some helpful information from their website, but he was not interested in attending their support groups. After about a year, Mr. Smith had to stop working to care for his wife full time as she could not be left alone at home safely. He began to feel isolated, overwhelmed and depressed. He could not afford paying for assistance at home and he was experiencing difficulty managing Mrs. Smith's increasing physical dependencies in self-care and behavioral symptoms including her periodic crying, pacing, and rejection of needed care. His two grown children have full time employment and their own families and do not live nearby. Mr. Smith is also very worried about his wife's quality of life, and he feels despair over their finances and future. He, in turn, is aging with diabetes and high blood pressure and has no time for himself or to keep his own doctor's appointments.

Mr. and Mrs. Smith are on their own to figure things out. However, we can design a model of dementia care to address their multiple needs. In the chapters that follow, we will begin to outline what dementia care should look like. We need to ask ourselves: What can we do for this family now?

Although disease progression and the lived experience of dementia as well as family dynamics and situations are highly unique and individualized, this case snapshot represents the experiences of most families. Families confront common challenges in understanding dementia and identifying and addressing the wide range and changing needs and challenges they experience. The case also illustrates the necessity of rapidly advancing research on care and services. Rigorous and systematic attention in this area is as important to pursue as research on prevention and cure.

So how can we support Mr. and Mrs. Smith? What are the principles that should underlie care and services and what are specific and obtainable treatment goals? How can we assure Mr. and Mrs. Smith are not in this alone? We tackle these next.

ASSUMPTIONS FOR DEVELOPING A SYSTEM FOR CARE AND SUPPORTIVE SERVICES

When it comes to the third "bucket"—research on care and services—there is a strong message of hope—we can make a positive difference in the quality of life of individuals with dementia and their family members and address many of the common stressors, unmet needs and challenges of families as illustrated by Mr. and Mrs. Smith.

Given the complexities of dementia and its on-going and differential impact on all aspects of daily life, we must carefully craft an approach for developing an effective system of care and supportive services. To begin to reimagine dementia care, we have identified eight assumptions that we believe must underlie or ground any new systems of care and services. These assumptions, listed in Box 3-1, are based on what we know about dementia and are in contrast with present-day approaches, assumptions, and actions in health care systems.

Box 3-1

Assumptions for Developing a System of Care and Services

- There is not a single solution or magic bullet or one point in time intervention.
- One treatment, care strategy, or clinical intervention in itself will not be able to address all unmet needs and over the disease trajectory.
- Given the multiple care and supportive service needs, care coordination and integration of social and medical approaches are an imperative.
- To be effective, strategies need to be identified through a systematic process that involves assessment, generation of a treatment plan, implementation of specific care strategies tailored to persons and environmental conditions, and evaluation of what works and what does not, followed by continuous opportunities for modification of treatment plans.
- A strategy or approach that works for one individual, family, and home, may or may not be effective for another even with the same treatment goals and disease etiology and stage; individuation; and tailoring in treatment planning and implementation is critical.
- All health and human service professionals have a role in dementia care; there is not one professional group who can be the sole point of contact or provider or who "owns" dementia care.
- Given the interprofessional team needed in dementia care, careful coordination across clinical encounters, care settings, professionals, and over the disease trajectory is critical.
- Involvement of persons with dementia and their caregivers in all aspects of care planning is essential.

CONCLUSION

To derive new understandings of dementia, it is critical that we devote equivalent efforts and resources to each of the three areas outlined earlier in this chapter—prevention, cure, care and services—as only then will we be able to derive health and social policies that fully support persons with dementia and their families. Each of these three research directions must be pursued simultaneously and worldwide to impact disease burden. In doing so, we may find that the understandings and knowledge emerging from one bucket (e.g., prevention) may provide important insights and advance another bucket (e.g., cure and care). Specifically, this tri-directional approach involves giving comparable attention and resources to prevention, cure, and care.

In this chapter we have argued for the following. As funding for dementia has been and continues to be limited relative to commitments to other diseases and conditions (cancer, heart disease, and stroke), we must balance all of our efforts to traverse three buckets: prevention, cure, and care. As we evolve a new and comprehensive approach to dementia care, it must be based on eight fundamental principles or assumptions. There is not now nor will there be one solution, one treatment, one approach, and only one point in time that a treatment/program/strategy will work for all families living with dementia. Dementia is a dynamic condition that defies simple solutions or our traditional medical models of care, and new ways of thinking about and addressing dementia must emerge. This includes identifying the outcomes of most importance to people living with dementia and their caregivers for specific etiologies and disease stages, and then the treatments, strategies, and approaches within etiology and disease stage that work.

What Can Be Done Now

- Seek opportunities to learn about the experience of having dementia from the perspective of individuals themselves.
- Derive a treatment plan responsive to individual preferences, etiologies, disease stage, and living contexts.
- Help individuals become linked community resources.
- Help individuals living with dementia remain engaged in activities they value and which have meaning to them.
- Reassess needs, preferences, capabilities with disease progression, etiologies, and living contexts.

References

Christensen, A. I., Davidsen, M., Kjoller, M., & Juel, K. (2014). What characterizes persons with poor mental health? A nationwide study in Denmark. *Scandinavian Journal of Public Health*, 42(5), 446–455. Available from https://doi.org/10.1177/1403494814532877.

Davtyan, H., Zagorski, K., Rajapaksha, H., Hovakimyan, A., Davtyan, A., Petrushina, I., & Ghochikyan, A. (2016). Alzheimer's disease AdvaxCpG—Adjuvanted MultiTEP-based dual and single vaccines induce high-titer antibodies against various forms of tau and Aβ pathological molecules. *Scientific Reports*, 6(July), 28912. Available from https://doi.org/10.1038/srep28912.

Global Council on Brain Health. (2016). *The brain–body connection: GCBH recommendations on physical activity and brain health*. Retrieved from http://www.GlobalCouncilOnBrainHealth.org.

Langa, K. M., Larson, E. B., Crimmins, E. M., Faul, J. D., Levine, D. A., Kabeto, M. U., & Weir, D. R. (2017). A comparison of the prevalence of dementia in the United States in 2000 and 2012. *JAMA Internal Medicine*, 177(1), 51. Available from https://doi.org/10.1001/jamainternmed.2016.6807.

Livingston, G., Sommerlad, A., Orgeta, V., Costafreda, S. G., Huntley, J., Ames, D., & Mukadam, N. (2017). Dementia prevention, intervention, and care. *The Lancet*, 390 (10113), 2673–2734. Available from https://doi.org/10.1016/S0140-6736(17)31363-6.

Schrijvers, E. M. C., Verhaaren, B. F. J., Koudstaal, P. J., Hofman, A., Ikram, M. A., & Breteler, M. M. B. (2012). Is dementia incidence declining? Trends in dementia incidence since 1990 in the Rotterdam Study. *Neurology*, 78(19), 1456–1463. Available from https://doi.org/10.1212/WNL.0b013e3182553be6.

Wu, Y.-T., Fratiglioni, L., Matthews, F. E., Lobo, A., Breteler, M. M. B., Skoog, I., & Brayne, C. (2016). Dementia in Western Europe: Epidemiological evidence and implications for policy making. *The Lancet Neurology*, 15(1), 116–124. Available from https://doi.org/10.1016/S1474-4422(15)00092-7.

CHAPTER 4

Making Life Better for Individuals Living With Dementia

Nothing about us without us

Case Snapshots

Mrs. S is an 85 year old African American who cares for her husband who is 88 and is in the moderate stage of dementia. They have had a close, loving 60 years long marriage. With dementia, Mr. S has become very irritable, easily upset, and angry. In turn, Mrs. Smith is becoming overwhelmed as his physical care needs increase and his behaviors become more challenging to manage. In the morning, Mr. S needs help with dressing and grooming and knowing what to do next. Then throughout the day, Mrs. S is not sure what to do—he seems bored, and disengaged, and he sometimes tries to walk out of the home. She has been leaving him alone to run errands but is not sure if that is the right thing to do as he sometimes makes himself tea and has left the stove on such that the kettle has burnt. Their two sons live in other cities and are unable to help out on a daily basis. Also, they don't seem to understand their father's disease and believe their mother is exaggerating his needs. Furthermore, Mrs. S has hypertension and is pre-diabetic and has to be careful with her nutrition and care for her own self-care needs.

Mrs. L, 78 years old, is a white, Italian immigrant to the United States who became a widow about 8 years ago. After her husband died, she noticed that she was having significant difficulties remembering doctor appointments, where she left her keys, and finding words in English. Her subjective memory complaints and getting lost in a familiar place prompted her to seek physician's input. She was diagnosed with early stage dementia. Her children do not live close by and she has limited financial resources. Planning for her future has been difficult and overwhelming to her. She also has arthritis and a heart condition for which she has to take various medications at prescribed times during the day.

These two snapshots reflect a small segment of the lives of two different families living with dementia in the United States. Taken together they highlight some of the nuances and individuated contexts in which dementia is experienced and the disease unfolds. Mrs. L in an early disease stage lives alone and has limited resources. She represents a growing number of individuals that will need external supports from their community to manage the disease. Alternately, Mr. S lives with his wife and is in the moderate to moderate–severe stage of the disease. His care needs are more extensive at this point than in the case of Mrs. L. Although he has more social capital and resources than her, Mr. S confronts other challenges such as managing comorbidities and his wife, the caregiver, has significant medical conditions which presents as a concern to the family unit—both in terms of her ability to provide on-going care to Mr. S as well as how dementia progression may exacerbate her own medical conditions. Each case illustrates just a few of the many factors affecting disease course such as living arrangement, disease stage, access to resources, care context, gender, and age—all of which and more need to be considered in treatment planning. We also witness in these two snapshots how women are differentially affected by dementia: they are overwhelmingly affected by dementia compared to men either as the person diagnosed with the condition or as the family caregiver (in this case spouse) tasked with providing long-term care to the affected family member.

In this chapter we examine two fundamental questions:

- What can and should be the treatment goals for Mrs. L and Mr. S?
- What does research suggest that we can offer Mrs. L and Mr. S to help support a "good" life?

TREATMENT GOALS

As we have discussed in Chapter 2, Lived Experiences of Individuals With Dementia, what matters most to individuals themselves may vary by life space including culture, living environment, resources as well as disease stage, and the presence of other medical conditions. While what matters most to individuals living with dementia is not well understood, we do know that it often differs between the perspectives of caregivers and providers. Whereas most individuals seek "living well" and opportunities for continued meaningful engagement and connectivity, caregivers and providers typically focus on treatments for "getting better." These are important differences warranting careful reflection as they affect how we evolve care services. These differences also stress the importance of identifying care preferences of persons themselves and suggest that caregivers/providers may need support to cognitively reframe their concerns. An important area for research is identifying strategies for eliciting care preferences at each disease stage.

One way to understand multifaceted treatment goals, preferences, and actions is with the Good Life model as we presented in Chapter 2, Lived Experiences of Individuals With Dementia. The Good Life model serves as a broad framework from which to identify key outcomes of importance to individuals and families in each of four quadrants. Consideration of these quadrants in turn can lead to advancing a range of strategies that are tailored to particular quadrants and life/environmental conditions.

Most approaches to specifying treatment goals have not been based on a conceptual underpinning as we suggest with the Good Life model. Furthermore, only a few attempts have been made to identify measurable treatment goals for people with dementia for use in care settings, and these have primarily reflected a medical perspective. That is, while items (e.g., assess for cognitive decline) are important to individuals and families, such measures have not encapsulated the full range of considerations for making life better across disease stages. Nevertheless, these measures for guiding treatment in medical encounters are important stepping stones. For example, in 2012, the American Academy of Neurology along with other medical organizations derived 10 measurements for use by physicians primarily in primary care practices to guide treatment of their patients with dementia (assess for and manage stage of disease, cognitive status, functional status, neuropsychiatric symptoms, depressive symptoms, provide counseling for safety concerns, counsel concerning risks of driving, provide palliative care counseling and advance care planning, and provide caregiver education and support). These were subsequently published in 2014 (Odenheimer et al., 2014) and revised in May 2017 (https://www.psychiatry.org/psychiatrists/practice/quality-improvement/quality-measures-for-mips-quality-category/dementia-updates). Unfortunately, neither versions have been widely implemented in primary care in the United States. More recently, the International Consortium for Health Outcomes (ICHOM) has developed a set of measures with consultation from a panel of international experts that also included people living with dementia and caregivers.

These measures, which can be found at http://www.ichom.org/medical-conditions/dementia/ (International Consortium for Health Outcomes Measurement's Standard Set for Dementia, 2016), reflect a wider swath of considerations and address both medical and social aspects of dementia that need to be assessed, managed, and/or treated. Although these measures are being adapted for use in a few health systems in Europe, they have not been widely embraced and employed worldwide yet, nor are they being considered at this point in time in the United States. This may be due to a number of factors including the need for workforce preparation and training in the use of these measurements, unavailability of a dementia-ready workforce, care systems that do not facilitate systematic assessment, and treatment of nonmedical considerations such as care coordination, education of family caregivers, and transition planning. As such, these measurement sets may be too cumbersome to adopt.

Nevertheless, these efforts along with other relevant publications and the evidence to date (Callahan et al., 2014) serve as guideposts for identifying viable and important treatment goals that can be accomplished now. Based on a review of the evidence and published recommendations and practice-based measures, we offer 15 potential treatment goals shown in Box 4-1. Each of these goals reflects different quadrants of the Good Life Model and is achievable with the evidence we have at hand. Taken as a whole, these goals encapsulate what is important to different stakeholders ranging from the individual living with dementia to societal and policy perspectives, and these goals can serve as a pillar on which we base comprehensive dementia care.

These 15 treatment goals are not listed in any particular order or priority in Box 4-1. Rather, they represent goals that we argue are relevant to and should be addressed from the time that a diagnosis is received to the end of an individual's life. No doubt more and on-going research is necessary to delineate more precisely and specify the specific actions needed for achieving each goal. While goals remain the same across disease progression, specific actions will differ based on stage and other life conditions. This list represents a starting point for redesigning dementia care and can be used by providers to reflect upon how to organize their care and services to meet treatment goals.

We further categorize these 15 treatment goals into three large groupings: symptom management that includes six specific treatment goals, care planning with four treatment goals, and quality of life involving five treatment goals. Noteworthy is the complexity of dementia care: first, there is not just one treatment goal but rather all 15 are necessary for supporting a "good life"; second, treatment goals cannot be addressed by a singular health or human service professional but rather an interdisciplinary team and coordinated effort will be required; and third, the way in which each treatment goal is met will differ based on

> **Box 4-1**
> **15 Feasible and Interrelated Treatment Goals to Support Quality of Life**
>
> **Symptom Management**
> 1. Obtain a formal diagnosis
> 2. Ongoing assessment of cognition, executive functioning, disease stage, and capabilities
> 3. Consider cognitive enhancing drugs and regularly assess side effects
> 4. Assess for and manage comorbidities including pain and depression
> 5. Assess for and prevent, reduce/minimize, behavioral and psychological symptoms
> 6. Assess for and maintain/support daily physical function
>
> **Care Planning**
> 7. Provide ongoing care coordination/care management, referrals and linkages
> 8. Identify and discuss care goals and tracking outcomes
> 9. Palliative care counseling and advance care planning
> 10. Ongoing identification of and addressing unmet needs
>
> **Quality of Life**
> 11. Support personhood, dignity, agency, control
> 12. Enable engagement in meaningful activities and provide opportunities to maintain a sense of purpose and self-identify
> 13. Screen for and act upon safety hazards including fall risk, smoking, driving, vulnerability to scams, wandering or exiting home
> 14. Identify needs of and provide education and support for family caregivers
> 15. Promote aging in place at home and in the community if preference of individual/family and staying in place supports quality of life

various factors including disease stage, life conditions, values, preferences, and access to resource and needs, adding to the nuances that systems of care will need to address.

WHAT CAN WE DO NOW?

To understand what can be done now, we outline specific actions for each treatment goal based on the evidence to date as shown on Table 4-1. Table 4-1 also identifies key research needs to improve the

TABLE 4-1 15 Treatment Goals, Description and Possible Plan of Action, and Research Needed

Treatment goal (primary responsible parties)	Plan of action informed by evidence and best practice	Research needed to improve treatment
I. Symptom Management		
Obtain a formal diagnosis (Dementia specialists—neurologists, gero-psychiatrists)	• Use standard guidelines and neurological and other tests to confirm dementia diagnosis. A diagnosis is important to enable care planning and appropriate symptom monitoring (see Chapter 1: How the Brain Is Affected) • Seek diagnosis from a memory clinic, geriatric psychiatrist, neurologist and insist on disclosure to family members	• Develop biomarkers for more precise and rapid disease detection • Develop standardized scales that capture subjective memory complaints and neuropsychiatric symptoms predictive of dementia risk or diagnosis that can be used clinically
Ongoing assessment of cognition, executive functioning, disease stage, and capabilities (primary care, occupational therapist for capabilities)	• Use standardized tools to assess cognitive status (MOCA, MSSE, SLUMS, CDR) and executive function and inform families how best to support the person living with dementia • Establish a baseline to monitor change over time • Assess for preserved capabilities to identify what the person is able to do and from which to design a plan to support their daily functioning	• Develop new brief measures to identify cognitive, physical abilities of persons at each disease stage and specific types of cueing and other supports needed
Consider cognitive enhancing drugs and regularly assess side effects (primary care physicians)	• Determine if an anticholinesterase medication is appropriate, if so closely monitor for side effects and identify when to cease medication	• Ongoing drug discovery research to slow disease progression and manage cognitive symptoms
Assess for and prevent, reduce/minimize, behavioral and psychological symptoms (all health providers, caregivers)	• Assess for the presence of behaviors using standardized measures • Assess for known risk factors for behavioral symptoms • Use DICE approach to develop treatment plan that addresses triggers and which rules out underlying medical issues that may be contributing behaviors • Provide caregiver education • Assist with establishing daily and predictable routines • Introduce strategies including simplification of activities, simplification of caregiver communications and the physical environment	• Develop standardized measures for (1) assessing risk for behavioral symptoms and (2) systematically identifying context in which behaviors occur • Develop measures that do not only rely on proxy report

Assess for and manage comorbidities including pain and depression (primary care physicians)	• At routine medical visits, review medications, check for any underlying blood, urine abnormalities • Monitor conditions • Evaluate and address sensory changes (hearing, sight) • Help identify strategies for medication management • At routine medical visits, ask persons with dementia and their caregivers about any pain and engage in on-going monitoring for pain • Educate caregivers as to how to determine if person with dementia has pain	• Develop protocols and clinical guidelines for managing complex conditions such as sensory impairments and chronic conditions • Develop measurement approaches for eliciting self-report from persons with cognitive impairment or ways of detecting pain
Assess for and maintain/support daily physical function (occupational and physical therapists)	• Assess for different aspects of daily functioning including (1) underlying impairment; (2) level of dependence, and (3) extent of family involvement (time spent and to which family caregivers • Assure home safety • Identify assistive devices that may be useful (e.g., grab bars) • Provide education and strategies to caregivers to reduce excess disability • Assure proper body mechanics in helping a person dress, transfer and get into and out of bed/toilet/shower	• Advance interventions to address functional disability and ways to prevent and minimize functional impairments
II. Care Planning		
Provide ongoing care coordination/care management, referrals and linkages (Social agency; any health and human service provider, care manager)	• Use a proven care management program and needs assessment • Provide professional assistance with coordinating care including addressing unmet needs, and coordinating transitions across care settings, • Help address coordination and integration of medical and social services	• Implementation and disseminate studies of proven care management models connecting social-medical care services • Conduct cost and cost benefit analyses of care coordination models to improve efficiencies and understand societal commitment

(Continued)

TABLE 4-1 (Continued)

Treatment goal (primary responsible parties)	Plan of action informed by evidence and best practice	Research needed to improve treatment
Identify and discuss goals of care of individuals and families including tracking outcomes over time (health and human service professionals)	• Use published needs assessments and preference tools to elicit needs	• Develop measures for use across disease continuum to elicit preferences, treatment goals • Identify best ways of involving families with diverse values and cultures in treatment planning
Palliative care counseling and advance care planning (nurse)	• Have on-going discussions with individuals and families concerning advance care planning including health, financial, and end of life considerations • Use developed tools such as "Five Wishes" and others available on web adapted for use in individuals with dementia and family caregivers	• Determine best approaches to engaging families and ways to tailor approaches to values, cultural preferences
Ongoing identification of and addressing unmet needs	• Identify unmet needs as cognitive and functional changes occur to derive a treatment plan to address them • Conduct comprehensive assessment of needs at each disease stage (assessing all four sectors of the Good Life (see Chapter 2: Lived Experiences of Individuals With Dementia).	• Understand specific needs of persons with different types of dementia • Understand specific needs of persons from different race, ethnicities, cultures, and resources • Develop standardized assessments to address needs
III. Quality of Life		
Support personhood, dignity, agency, and control	• Establish predictable daily routines	
Enable engagement in meaningful activities and provide opportunities to maintain a sense of purpose and self-identify	• Provide activities as part of daily care that are tailored to the person's preserved abilities, functional capacity, and interests	• Understand underlying mechanisms as to how activity has its positive effects (e.g., what are the pathways) • Determine what activities work best by disease stage and time of day

Screen for and act upon safety hazards including fall risk, smoking, driving, vulnerability to scans, wandering or exiting home (occupational therapist, physical therapist)	• People with dementia are at high risk for falls (reasons for which remain unclear). • Use standardized assessment to determine balance, strength and fall risk (e.g., Timed Up and Go or Berg Balance Scales). • Introduce simple exercises including walking if possible • Declutter home, clearing pathways, and removing tripping hazards • Assure the home is safe for a person with dementia at each stage of the disease • Conduct a comprehensive home environmental assessment considering as well placement of dangerous objects (weapons), medications, and poisonous substances (e.g., cleaning fluids)	• Develop easy-to-use online home safety checklists and tools • Develop fall prevention strategies specific to persons living with dementia
Identify needs of and provide education and support for family caregivers	• Assess for capability, own needs and readiness to use different strategies • Evaluate availability and social support network • Determine employment and supports • Provide ongoing education and support	
Promote aging in place at home and in the community	• Provide a supportive network, opportunities for engagement, respite, connectivity of individuals and families • Provide home repair and other home-based services to enable families to continue to care at home	• Determine strategies for scaling up and disseminating proven caregiver support programs • Adapt programs for families from diverse cultural and race/ethnic backgrounds • Adapt evidence for delivery via different settings and through technologies • Identify models to reduce fragmentation in care and relationship between social and medical services

evidence for delivering better clinical, care and supportive services. Except for obtaining a timely diagnosis, each of the other 14 treatment goals and specific actions should be empirically aligned with a disease stage or etiology and other life situations, creating a matrix of care strategies and guideposts for delivery—this is an immediate research need.

Here we describe a few significant pharmacological and nonpharmacological care approaches for addressing the three core clinical features characterizing any type of dementia: cognitive changes, behavioral and psychological symptoms, and functional disability.

Pharmacological Treatment Options

Unfortunately, there are very few pharmacologic treatments for any of the core features of dementia. It should be appreciated that as a whole, pharmacologic treatments to date are not cures for dementia. However, these medications do have some role to play and should be considered, although not necessarily always prescribed, to treat someone with dementia.

The first category of medications is those that have been studied and approved for the treatment of memory loss. Medications in this category include cholinesterase inhibitors that act by increasing the level of acetylcholine in the brain. Acetylcholine—a chemical that is important to the functioning of memory—is lost early in Alzheimer's disease. Cholinesterase inhibitors boost, albeit temporarily, the amounts of acetylcholine in the brain. In the United States, the three marketed medicines in this category (rivastigmine, galantamine, and donepezil) go under the trademark names of Aricept, Exelon, or Razadyne and are considered as equivalent with regard to whether they are likely to help or harm. These therapeutics are typically applied early in the disease course and by the moderate stage are withdrawn.

One category of medications that has shown some evidence for slowing cognitive decline is known as NMDA antagonists. This category of medications works by limiting toxicity of a brain chemical called glutamate. Namenda, as it is marketed in the United States, or Ebixa, as it is marketed in many other parts of the world, is an example of this medicine. This medication is indicated in moderate or more severe stages of dementia for people with Alzheimer's disease because of its limited benefit in earlier stage dementia.

Another category of medications for the treatment of cognitive symptoms are anti-amyloid-β therapies, such as amyloid-β immunotherapy, which act to reduce the plaque burden or prevent the development of amyloid plaques. Despite early enthusiasm, recent trials of disease-modifying drugs for Alzheimer's disease have all failed to show any treatment benefit (e.g., LMTM, TauRx Therapeutics, Ltd.). One exception is a very recent Phase III trial of Aducanumab—a human IgG1 monoclonal antibody that has shown safety and efficacy in persons with early Alzheimer's disease (Viglietta et al., 2016). However, it is still in trial and the benefits versus risks are not clear.

The recent enthusiasm generated by antibody-based immunotherapies (e.g., Aducanumab) in slowing cognitive decline in early stage Alzheimer's disease is welcomed. However, this should not diminish our need to address the needs of the 47 million people living in the world with dementia. Even with drug therapeutics that treat, manage, or slow disease progression, individuals and their families will still be in need of supportive care and management strategies.

While these drugs may decelerate the progression of the disease, they do so only for a limited time, with many persons experiencing side effects and needing to discontinue treatments. These medications only provide symptomatic relief and for a few and fail to slow disease progression over time or achieve a cure (Kumar, Singh, & Ekavali, 2015).

The treatment of behavioral and psychological symptoms common in dementia with pharmaceutical agents is challenging. Medications referred to as atypical antipsychotics, such as risperidone, olanzapine, or quetiapine, may have limited usefulness with certain types of severe behavioral and psychological symptoms such as agitation, delusions, and hallucinations. However, the decision to use these agents must be balanced with the high risk of catastrophic side effects, including strokes, heart attacks, and death. On balance, therefore, antipsychotics should be used very uncommonly, after other medical problems as causes of behavioral and psychological symptoms have been clearly ruled out and after non-medication therapies have been tried first.

In summary, there is no agreed-upon pharmacologic approaches that are consistently applied for dementia. Medications may be useful for some symptoms and for some individuals but only on a time limited basis. Monitoring of their on-going use and decision-making as to their initiation and stoppage must be done in consultation with family members and physicians.

Nonpharmacological Options

In contrast to drug therapists, there is a wide range of nonpharmacological approaches, interventions, programs, or strategies that have been evaluated in randomized clinical trials and shown to result in benefits for outcomes important to persons living with dementia (better quality of life), families (improved sense of mastery and wellbeing), and society (reduced unnecessary hospitalizations and nursing home placements). While there is no doubt that more research is critically needed to advance care and supportive strategies, it is important to know that there are approaches that can be used right now to alleviate many of the concerns and stressors described above in the snapshot cases of Mr. S. and Mrs. L.

Over the past 30 years, there has been a plethora of studies such that there are now numerous Cochrane reports, systematic reviews, and meta-analyses which synthesize the empirical evidence. Despite inconsistencies in study designs, measures, and results, various systematic reviews and meta-analyses conclude that there is sufficient foundational evidence for advancing effective care and services in select areas and there is strong evidence and signals of approaches warranting continued investigation (Cohen-Mansfield, 2001; Gitlin & Hodgson, 2016; Gitlin, Hodgson, Choi, & Marx, in press; Gitlin, Marx, Stanley, & Hodgson, 2015; Gitlin, Kales, & Lyketsos, 2012; O'Neil et al., 2011).

The level and type of evidence for care strategies does vary by setting (home versus assisted living versus nursing home) and possibly etiology (Frontotemporal dementia versus Alzheimer's versus Lewy Bodies). For example, a recent review of nonpharmacological interventions in assisted living and nursing homes to address agitation and aggression found very poor evidence for a range of approaches due to limitations in study designs, measures, and small sample sizes to name a few (Jutkowitz et al., 2016).

In the home and community, however, the evidence is strong with many possibilities for positively intervening. In addition to the approaches gleaned from this literature that are listed in Table 4.1, here we list several emerging approaches that warrant consideration, replication, and implementation.

- Care coordination to reduce health care utilization and link families to needed medical and social resources (Frank, Feldman, & Schulz, 2011).
- Comprehensive needs assessment, provision of strategies for unmet needs, and enhancing home safety to help keep people living at home longer (Samus et al., 2014).
- Use of activities that are matched to interests and preserved capabilities as part of daily care to reduce behavioral symptoms and functional dependence (Gitlin et al., 2009; Gitlin et al., 2016; Gitlin et al., 2017).
- Caregiver education and support to help understand the disease process and reduce and manage behavioral symptoms (Belle et al., 2006; Brodaty & Arasaratnam, 2012).
- On-going support, counseling, and skills to delay nursing home placement (Gitlin, Reever, Dennis, Mathieu, & Hauck, 2006; Mittelman et al., 1993, 2006).
- Home environmental modifications, monitor health conditions, and provide caregivers specific skills to reduce functional dependence (Graff et al., 2006; Gitlin, Winter, Dennis, Hodgson, & Hauck, 2010).

We continue here to review a few significant approaches for addressing key clinical symptoms of dementia that are disturbing to persons living with the condition and their families. This does not reflect a comprehensive review of the existing evidence but rather is meant to provide insight as to the evidence that can be used to innovate and move forward with comprehensive dementia care.

Cognitive Decline

Various nonpharmacological cognitive approaches have been developed and evaluated to address cognitive declines. The field has generated inconsistent results and terms such as cognitive stimulation, cognitive training, and cognitive rehabilitation are often used interchangeably but have different meanings and involve distinct approaches. Cognitive Stimulation Therapy (CST) refers to a group activity approach, the goal of which is to stimulate cognitive and social functioning. CST has become of increasing interest particularly in Europe as a potential approach to improve cognition and slow down disease progression in persons at the mild to moderate disease stage. It is evidence-based and has its roots in several previous therapies including reality orientation that involves the presentation and repetition of information to orient individuals to "reality" such as repeated reminders as to the day, date, and weather. CST typically occurs in small group activities to heighten socialization experiences. A Cochrane review of 15 trials involving a total of 718 participants concluded that cognitive stimulation has a beneficial effect on memory and thinking tests (Woods, Aguirre, Spector, & Orrell, 2012). Other studies have shown that CST improves quality of life and cognitions (Spector et al., 2003), communications, and interactions. Further studies have shown that weekly booster sessions can extend or maintain cognitive outcomes (Orrell, Spector, Thorgrimsen, & Woods, 2005). As studies are conducted in congregate settings, its role in home care is not clear, although one study showed some memory benefits when caregivers at home provided specified cognitive activities (Orrell et al., 2017). Furthermore, there is no evidence of improvements in mood, behavioral and psychological symptoms, daily function, or objective memory performance. CST is currently the only nonpharmacological therapy recommended in guidelines by the National Institute for Health and Clinical Excellence in England.

Cognitive training refers to providing a series of guided tasks with the goal of improving attention, memory, and/or problem-solving. While there is some evidence of benefit in the areas targeted, there is no evidence that skills learned transfer over to everyday life tasks. Thus, the ecological validity of cognitive training has not been shown. Similarly, cognitive rehabilitation focuses on improving everyday life by introducing memory tasks and memory-enhancing strategies. Both of these approaches have limited efficacy compared to cognitive stimulation (Bahar-Fuchs, Clare, & Woods, 2013; Huntley, Gould, Liu, Smith, & Howard, 2015). Even cognitive stimulation results in small effect sizes and appears to benefit individuals early on in the disease process and for a short period of time. CST in particular has not been examined in combination with other approaches such as exercise or pharmacology (Mavros et al., 2017).

Functional Decline

Functional decline is a core characteristic of dementia which is associated with negative consequences including nursing home placement, hospitalization, frailty, need for assistance, and distress among family caregivers. Functional decline is not well understood but may be a consequence of neurodegeneration plus the interaction with factors that are potentially modifiable. These factors can be considered as intrinsic to the person such as pain, medication complications, poor balance, or extrinsic such as a cluttered environment, poor lighting, ineffective communication patterns, or tasks that are too complex (Gitlin et al., in press).

There are different strategies for addressing physical decline that have found to be modestly effective. These include for example engaging individuals in physical activity as part of care interactions, referred to as Function Focused Care (Galik, Resnick, Hammersla, & Brightwater, 2014; Resnick & Galik, 2013), other forms of exercise including aquatic (Henwood, Neville, Baguley, Clifton, & Beattie, 2015); Yoga (McCaffrey, Park, Newman, & Hagen, 2014); walking programs or other physical activity programs (Hauer et al., 2012; Potter, Ellard, Rees, & Thorogood, 2011; Vreugdenhil, Cannell, Davies, & Razay, 2012). Additionally, in-home caregiver skill building and environmental modification programs have also found to result in slower declines in functional dependence (Graff et al., 2006; Gitlin, Winter, Dennis et al., 2010). Similarly, an activity program, discussed in more detail below also has been found to result in slowing functional decline (Gitlin et al., 2017).

In a summary of 24 home-based trials seeking to improve functional outcomes for persons with dementia, most involved caregiver education about the disease and instruction in behavioral management strategies. A third included home environmental modifications and providing caregivers with care management and coping strategies. Another quarter or less of interventions involved other strategies such as cognitive training, activity engagement, or medical evaluations. Most studies targeted extrinsic versus intrinsic factors and as such focused on reducing the gap between what a person can do and what they do, or what has been referred to as excess disability (Gitlin et al., in press).

These interventions are promising and more research examining the combination of their strategies and also in pharmacological management may be a fruitful approach.

Behavioral and Psychological Symptoms

Behavioral and psychological symptoms are ubiquitous and occur across disease etiologies and stages (Gitlin et al., 2012). One important approach for identifying and managing behavioral symptoms in any care setting is a six-step process, the heart of which is the DICE approach. Fig. 4-1 graphically describes this process. The first step is to have on-going assessments of behavioral occurrences (their frequency and severity) along with the identification of risk factors for symptoms. There are approximately 45 standardized scales for assessing behavioral occurrences with the 13-item Neuropsychiatric Inventory (NPI) and its various forms (NPI-Q, NPI-C) the most widely used (Cummings, 1997; de Medeiros et al., 2010; Gitlin, Marx, Stanley, Hansen, & Van Haitsma, 2014). There is some research that has identified risk factors for behaviors (Kolanowski et al., 2017). These range from, for example, not having a daily routine to having an overwhelmed caregiver to having a history of a psychiatric condition. Unfortunately, to date, there is not a standardized measure to systematically assess risk factors, and thus health and human

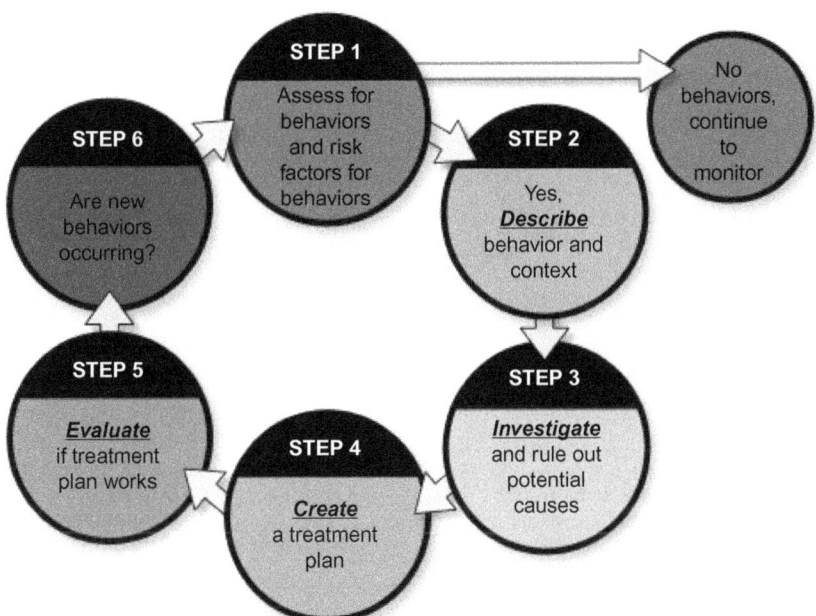

FIGURE 4-1 Steps involved in identifying and managing behavioral symptoms.

service professionals have to explore factors gleaned from the literature. If behaviors occur, then the DICE approach (Describe, Investigate, Create, and Evaluate) can be used (Kales, Gitlin, & Lyketsos, 2014). This approach provides a systematic strategy for *describing* the characteristics of a behavioral occurrence, *investigating* underlying contributors including ruling out medical and safety concerns, *creating* specific strategies to address underlying modifiable contributors, and *evaluating* whether strategies worked. The entire approach involves ongoing assessment and evaluation as shown in the sixth step of the process model.

In terms of creating a treatment plan, strategies for addressing behavioral symptoms may include drug options such as prescribing medications to control pain and/or nonpharmacological such as introducing good sleep hygiene, or ways to simplify communications, activities, or the environment. In creating a treatment plan, three "buckets" or areas need to be considered as shown in Fig. 4-2. Each bucket is composed of, modifiable factors related to the person living with dementia, the caregiver, and the physical environment.

DICE is currently being evaluated in different service contexts. It also has been operationalized into an interactive online platform, the WeCareAdvisor that guides families through a series of questions from which a WeCareAdvisor Prescription detailing strategies that may help to reduce and/or manage the targeted behaviors are provided

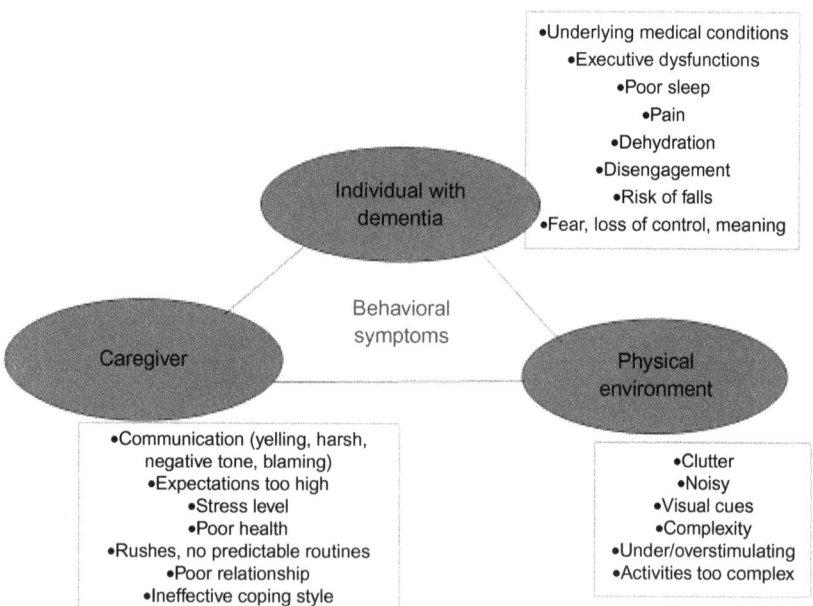

FIGURE 4-2 Targets for addressing behavioral symptoms.

(Gitlin, Kales, Marx, Stanislawski, & Lyketsos, 2017; Kales et al., 2017). Preliminary analyses of a randomized trial to evaluate feasibility, acceptability, and effectiveness have been promising, with family caregivers reporting reduced upset with behaviors and improved confidence managing behaviors (Kales et al., submitted).

Activity as a Therapeutic Agent

> "Although I've had to give up my job, stop driving and need help with many day-to-day things, I like to concentrate on what I can do rather than what I can't. I can still run with the help of guide runners, I get a lot of enjoyment from my music collection and have found a new talent in painting. I also like to keep up with the news, discuss current affairs and put the world to rights." Paul, 53 with Posterior Cortical Atrophy, in Callahan et al., 2014, p. 13

We highlight here one particular treatment approach that is extremely promising and has been shown to result in positive gains including reducing disability and maintaining physical function, preventing behavioral and psychological symptoms and reducing their frequency/severity of occurrence. Additionally, as the quote above suggests, remaining involved in activities can enhance enjoyment and quality of life.

Studies using various methodologies all signal the value of activity and in different settings including the home, adult-day services, and nursing homes. For example, a study evaluating a home recreational therapy intervention in which 29 individuals with dementia served as their own controls found reductions in passivity and agitation (Fitzsimmons & Buettner, 2002). In a clinical trial with 72 dyads, Teri Logsdon, Uomoto, and McCurry (1997) reported that two different interventions, instructing caregivers in problem solving and using pleasant events with persons with dementia, both resulted in reductions in depressive symptoms in individuals with dementia. In another randomized trial with 153 individuals with dementia, Teri et al. (2003) found that exercise plus caregiver training in behavioral management also resulted in better physical health and reduced depression in individuals with dementia.

Given the growing evidence base that activity participation can help to reduce agitation and may in turn decrease the inappropriate use of pharmacological or other restraints (Kolanowski, Buettner, & Fgsa-Faghe, 2008; Rovner, Steele, Shmuely, & Folstein, 1996), some governments such as the United Kingdom have begun to mandate the use of activity as part of standard treatment for individuals with dementia (United Kingdom's National Collaborating Centre for Mental Health, 2007).

To optimally engage individuals with dementia in activities requires a thoughtful and purposeful approach that accounts and compensates for differential impairments that occur throughout the disease process. Specifically, individuals may experience a range of cognitive impairments including difficulties with executive functioning (e.g., initiating, planning, organizing, and sequencing), and deficits in memory, language, and spatial recognition—all of which present unique challenges for engagement and participating in a desired activity (Trahan, Kuo, Carlson, & Gitlin, 2014).

The good news is that there are specific effective approaches and techniques such as simplifying the activity, providing cueing, drawing upon previously valued roles and activities, and using objects or tools that are familiar and which tap into the existing or preserved capabilities of the individual. Whereas an individual with mild dementia may find meaning participating in a cognitively demanding activity such as word puzzles, participating in a book or news club, with moderate to severe dementia, activities involving more repetitive type motions (washing windows, sorting objects of interest) may be more appropriate and of interest. Fig. 4-3 outlines a three-step approach for identifying and modifying activities based on disease stage.

Why is activity/engagement/participation important? It has been suggested that activity may fill a void, help a person to feel connected and maintain social roles, enable positive expressions, reduce frustrations, and enhance continuity of self-identity and purposefulness (Gitlin, Piersol, Hodgson, Marx, Roth, Johnston et al., 2016; Cohen-Mansfield, Parpura-Gill, & Golander, 2006; Kolanowski, Buettner, Costa, & Litaker, 2001; Phinney, Chaudhury, & O'Connor, 2007). Of importance is to recognize that the goal of an activity is to foster meaningful engagement versus seeking new learning, or enhancements in memory and cognitive functioning. While the latter is not the goal, the impact of participating in meaningful activity on cognition has yet to be evaluated in individuals with dementia with anecdotal evidence and case examples suggesting there may be some unexpected cognitive benefit. It is important to note that appropriate and meaningful activities can be developed for individuals at any level of cognitive status, from mild to severe, except perhaps at the end of life in which different sensory-based strategies (e.g., music, massage) would be more appropriate to make the person comfortable. Using activities as a therapeutic agent should follow various principles as outlined in Box 4-2.

First, an activity must have some intrinsic value or interest to a person. Thus, learning about previous roles, habits, occupations, and any recent or current interests can help guide activity selection. Second, it is

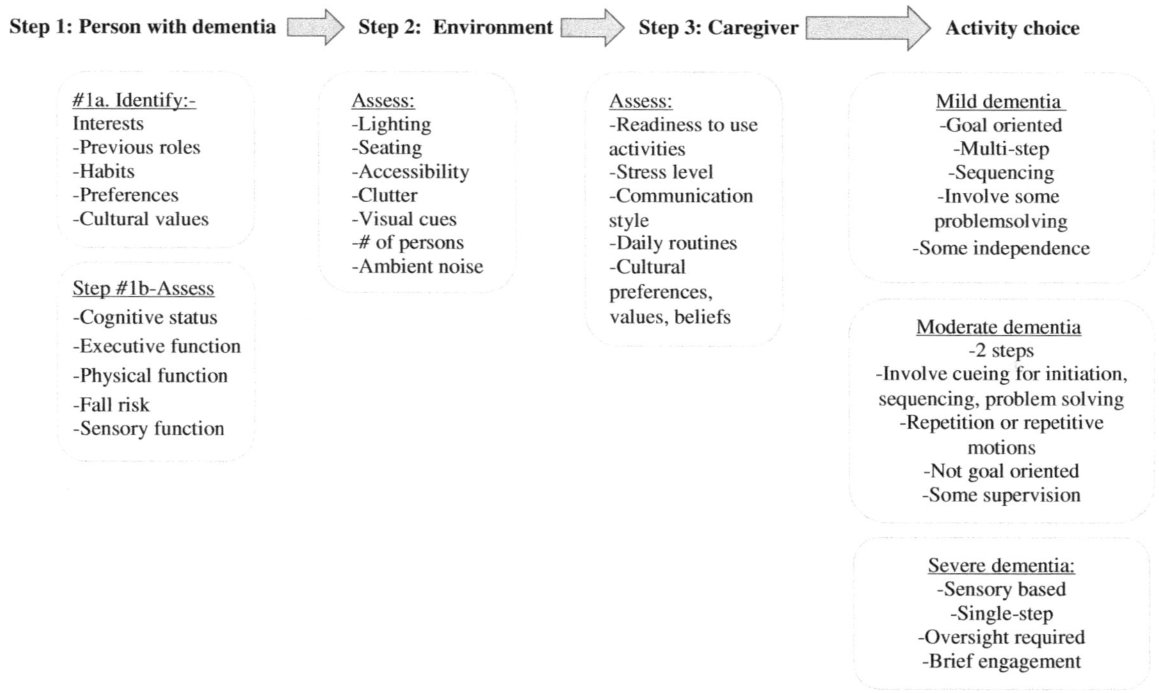

Step 1: Person with dementia ⇨ **Step 2: Environment** ⇨ **Step 3: Caregiver** ⇨ **Activity choice**

#1a. Identify:
- Interests
- Previous roles
- Habits
- Preferences
- Cultural values

Step #1b-Assess:
- Cognitive status
- Executive function
- Physical function
- Fall risk
- Sensory function

Assess:
- Lighting
- Seating
- Accessibility
- Clutter
- Visual cues
- # of persons
- Ambient noise

Assess:
- Readiness to use activities
- Stress level
- Communication style
- Daily routines
- Cultural preferences, values, beliefs

Mild dementia
- Goal oriented
- Multi-step
- Sequencing
- Involve some problemsolving
- Some independence

Moderate dementia
- 2 steps
- Involve cueing for initiation, sequencing, problem solving
- Repetition or repetitive motions
- Not goal oriented
- Some supervision

Severe dementia:
- Sensory based
- Single-step
- Oversight required
- Brief engagement

FIGURE 4-3 Three-step approach to activity selection.

> **Box 4-2**
> **Principles for Using Activity**
>
> - Consider previous and current roles, occupations, and interests to identify possibly meaningful activities
> - Assess a person's physical and cognitive functioning, sensory impairments, social comportment level, and fall risk from which to design the activity
> - With disease progression, activities will need to be simplified
> - Time engaged in an activity will decrease with disease progression
> - Consider time of day such that more cognitively demanding activities are introduced in late morning and relaxing type activities are used in the evening
> - Consider willingness and availability of caregiver(s) to set up, supervise, or use cues for an activity
> - Consider factors in the physical environment that support the activity including lighting, seating, and elimination of possible distractions (noise, clutter)

necessary to design an activity to fit a person's abilities and this includes their cognitive functioning, the extent to which they are social or follow social norms of interaction, their fall risk, and whether sensory impairments must be considered (e.g., hearing or vision loss). For example, an individual who enjoys gardening but is a fall risk would be safer engaging in table top gardening in which they can be seated or flower arranging, versus weeding or walking through uneven grounds in a garden. Third, it is important to understand that with disease progression, individuals will require that chosen activities be simplified. Take a multistep activity such as stringing beads following a pattern; this may need to be simplified to a one- to two-step activity such as sorting beads or moving beads from one container to another or working with stringing one bead color. Also with disease progression, auditory and tactile cueing to support initiation and sequencing of the steps in an activity will become necessary. Fourth, similarly, the time engaged in an activity will decrease, although at any stage, the quality of the engagement is the goal and not the length of time spent. Fifth, when introducing an activity, the time of day should be considered. More demanding types of activities should be introduced in the morning or early afternoon versus the evening. Sixth, with disease progression there will be greater reliance on caregivers to introduce activities. Thus, understanding caregivers' readiness to set up, help initiative, supervise, and provide cues is critical. Finally, the physical environment can either support or detract from engaging in an activity. For any activity, the physical features need to be considered to determine the best supportive setup. Specifically, lighting, seating, comfort, noise, and clutter are all considerations.

ETHICAL DILEMMAS PROVIDING CARE AND SUPPORTS

In providing care and services, there are common ethical dilemmas that individuals and their caregivers (family and others) typically confront. These are listed in Box 4-3 and illustrated in the case scenarios below.

Case Scenarios of Common Challenges

#1: Mr. J, now with moderate dementia, stays at home alone while his wife goes to work daily. Mrs. J prepares a sandwich and light snacks for Mr. J and calls him at lunch time to remind him to eat. Also, Mrs. J wants him to call her every few hours to check in with her. While this arrangement worked well in the past when Mr. J was first diagnosed 3 years ago, Mr. J is now forgetting to call and appears anxious, confused and agitated throughout the day. Initially, Mrs. J purchased a telephone with large numbers and set an alarm to remind her husband to call her. She thought that perhaps he could not see the numbers to dial correctly. However, one day she came home to find the oven burner on under an empty tea kettle which was beginning to smoke. She slowly came to realize that the issue was not Mr. J's eyesight but his cognitive decline. Although she must continue to work to support her family, she realizes Mr. J is unsafe to be home alone. Mrs. J is essentially on her own to figure out how to balance the safety of her husband with their financial situation and her employment responsibilities.

Box 4-3
Ethical Challenges Providing Care and Services

- Assure an individual's safety is not comprised by the need to fulfill other family obligations
- Balance safety of a person living with dementia with the person's need for asserting autonomy and control
- Attain just right fit between expectations of others and an individual's capacity or ability to carry out everyday activities and participate in daily life

This real-life vignette provides insight into a common dilemma. Employed caregivers represent a growing number of family members caring for persons with dementia and who are challenged by balancing work and care demands with the safety of persons with dementia (Schulz & Eden, 2016). Mrs. J would benefit from access to care coordination, a comprehensive needs assessment, home safety evaluation, and possible home modifications such as disabling the oven, knowledge of local resources, financial counseling and planning, and support from her employer to periodically take time off to solve care challenges. Additionally, these strategies may also be helpful to her:

- Enroll Mr. J into adult day services
- Identify volunteers who could serve as companions for Mr. J
- Consult with an elder care lawyer for financial and legal planning now and for the future
- Identify if there are employer-sponsored supportive care programs
- Have Mr. J assessed by an occupational therapist trained in dementia care to determine his level of cognitive functioning, home safety
- Develop a plan and backup plan for assuring Mr. J is not alone if Mrs. J has to leave the home for work and/or errands

#2: Mr. M was formerly a policeman for 35 years and consequently very facile with guns. He also enjoyed practicing at shooting ranges and he always kept a few guns in his home. Even with moderate dementia, he continues to keep one gun loaded under his mattress as he did in the past. His wife has become increasingly concerned about gun safety at home as she recognizes that he forgets how to do common everyday things he used to and he also doesn't always recognize neighbors and family who come to visit. He sometimes mistakes them for intruders. She is torn between wanting to remove the guns from their home and maintaining his autonomy and sense of self. As the use of guns was so much a part of his life, she feels she would be compromising his identity and taking one more thing away from him.

This true case is emblematic of the essential challenge families confront—balancing a person's safety with their ability to exert autonomy and maintain a sense of control over their daily lives. This issue arises in small and big ways and throughout the day. It may concern big decisions such as having to inform an individual that he/she can no longer drive, stay home alone, babysit for a grandchild by themselves, or venture to the supermarket alone. Or it may involve seemingly small matters, such as dressing the person versus having the person choose their clothing themselves or preparing a meal without offering a choice or selection. With disease progression, autonomy shrinks to maximize safety. However, providing safe opportunities to be in control throughout disease progression is essential. This may be one of the important functions of activity; engaging in an action/activity may provide individuals living with dementia a sense of control over their immediate environment.

#3: Mr. K was a brilliant mathematician but now with mild dementia, he was struggling to get through the day. He had to quit his position as a researcher and Professor. Given his intellectual capacity, he could often "fool" people in thinking that he was functioning at a higher level than in fact he was capable of performing. Consequently, his family often related to him using complex communications and expected him to engage in high level tasks (e.g., balancing check books and paying bills). Unfortunately, this created a gap between what Mr, K could understand and do and the expectations of his family such that it results in him "shutting down" completely, entering what appeared to be a catatonic state or conversely, becoming extremely angry, agitated and aggressive.

This mismatch between a person's capabilities and the expectations imposed by family members and formal providers is very common. Without careful assessment and reassessment as to the person's capabilities, it is quite challenging to obtain the just right fit between the person's abilities and care approaches. Most caregivers (family and others) assume the person can function at a higher level than they can. An occupational therapist trained in dementia care can be a valuable service to identify the person's best functioning and how communications and daily activities should occur to support them.

WHY INDIVIDUALS LIVING WITH DEMENTIA DO NOT RECEIVE EVIDENCE-BASED CARE, SERVICES AND SUPPORTS

We have shown in this chapter that there are strategies that can support 15 key treatment goals for individuals living with dementia. Yet, few individuals and their families have access to such approaches. Why this is the case is a complicated question and there is no easy answer or single solution. Although substantial progress has been made in identifying ways to support a "good life" with dementia, there are multiple challenges to infusing health and human services with evidence-derived practices and a person and family-centric care. These include the challenge of messaging or getting the word out to various stakeholders that there are positive, evidence-based, and evidence-informed approaches that can be introduced; preparing the workforce in dementia care; overcoming stigmata associated with dementia, having an effective dissemination and scaling plan; and adapting evidence-based practices for different social and medical contexts and race, ethnic, and cultural groups, so that all individuals with dementia and families have uniform access to appropriate and effective care throughout the disease trajectory when and where they need support. It is unclear as to the most effective approaches to addressing these challenges although public—private partnerships, moving to value-based care, realigning reimbursement to address dementia care needs, and linking community and medical services have all been cited as important in this regard (Samus et al., 2018).

KEY POINTS

This chapter suggests good news and that the glass is half full so to speak, as there is a growing evidentiary base that can inform how we effectively support individuals to make their life better now. Yet, we also balance or temper this good news with discussion of some of the shortcomings of the evidence and critical gaps in research and policy that prevent us from fully achieving quality care and services.

In this chapter we have argued that there is much hope in providing effective care and services that can make a difference in the lives of individuals with dementia, and in Chapter 5, Family Member as Care Partner, we will discuss the evidence for positively impacting family caregivers.

A Conversation with Dr. Helen Kales

1. *What is DICE and why is it a novel approach for addressing behavioral symptoms?* The DICE Approach stands for DESCRIBE-INVESTIGATE-CREATE-EVALUATE. It is an algorithmic approach to assist in the assessment and management of behavioral and psychological symptoms of dementia (BPSD) including depression, agitation, aggression and sleep problems. It is novel for two main reasons: 1) it systematizes and structures the way expert clinicians approach BPSD including the identification of possible underlying causes and etiologies; and 2) it combines pharmacological and non-pharmacological strategies.
2. *How do you use DICE in your clinical practice?*: First, we need to work with family caregivers and other members of the dementia care team to fully DESCRIBE the underlying behavior. As there are often several behaviors occurring, we strategize with caregivers to select the currently most problematic behavior. A full description includes "playing the behavior back" like one is fully relating the plot of a movie- we need the "who, when, what and where". That description then suggests the INVESTIGATION that needs to occur, and typically this includes

examining possible causes associated with the person living with dementia (e.g. medical problems, pain, medications, etc.), caregiver (communication issues, mismatch of abilities and expectations, etc.) and environment (clutter; over/understimulation; lack of activity, etc.). The investigation will then lead to the team to CREATE first line treatment options; non-pharmacologic strategies as well as treatment of underlying causes (e.g. urinary tract infection, pain, constipation) are prioritized. First-line psychotropic use is recommended for three situations only: 1) major depression with or without suicidality; 2) aggression with risk of harm to self/others; and 3) psychosis with risk of harm to self/others. Finally, we EVALUATE the impact of the strategies attempted and then make changes to the treatment plan based upon that feedback.
3. *What are some of the challenges in implementing DICE in a clinical setting?*: The main challenge is time. The DICE approach competes with the current paradigm of stakeholders, whether caregivers, providers, or health systems, expecting a "quick fix". Clearly it is easier and faster to write a prescription rather than undertake a thorough assessment and management of a symptom.
4. *What research do you believe is needed to address behavioral symptoms?*: More research is needed on how we can improve the dissemination and implementation of approaches like DICE given the current healthcare climate of time pressures.

References

Bahar-Fuchs, A., Clare, L., & Woods, B. (2013). Cognitive training and cognitive rehabilitation for mild to moderate Alzheimer's disease and vascular dementia. In A. Bahar-Fuchs (Ed.), *Cochrane database of systematic reviews*. Chichester, United Kingdom: John Wiley & Sons, Ltd. Available from https://doi.org/10.1002/14651858.CD003260.pub2.

Belle, S. H., Burgio, L., Burns, R., Coon, D., Czaja, S. J., Gallagher-Thompson, D., & Zhang, S. (2006). Enhancing the quality of life of dementia caregivers from different ethnic or racial groups: A randomized, controlled trial. *Annals of Internal Medicine, 145*(10), 727−738.

Brodaty, H., & Arasaratnam, C. (2012). Meta-analysis of nonpharmacological interventions for neuropsychiatric symptoms of dementia. *American Journal of Psychiatry, 169*(9), 946−953. Available from https://doi.org/10.1176/appi.ajp.2012.11101529.

Callahan, C. M., Sachs, G. A., LaMantia, M. A., Unroe, K. T., Arling, G., & Boustani, M. A. (2014). Redesigning systems of care for older adults with Alzheimer's disease. *Health Affairs, 33*(4), 626−632. Available from https://doi.org/10.1377/hlthaff.2013.1260.

Cohen-Mansfield, J. (2001). Nonpharmacologic interventions for inappropriate behaviors in dementia: A review, summary, and critique. *The American Journal of Geriatric Psychiatry: Official Journal of the American Association for Geriatric Psychiatry, 9*(4), 361−381. Retrieved from http://www.ncbi.nlm.nih.gov/pubmed/11739063.

Cohen-Mansfield, J., Parpura-Gill, A., & Golander, H. (2006). Utilization of self-identity roles for designing interventions for persons with dementia. *The Journal of Gerontology: Psychological Sciences and Social Sciences, 61B*(4), P202–P212. Available from https://doi.org/10.1093/geronb/61.4.P202.

Cummings, J. L. (1997). The Neuropsychiatric Inventory: Assessing psychopathology in dementia patients. *Neurology, 48*(5 Suppl 6), S10–S16.

de Medeiros, K., Robert, P., Gauthier, S., Stella, F., Politis, A., Leoutsakos, J., & Lyketsos, C. (2010). The Neuropsychiatric Inventory-Clinician rating scale (NPI-C): Reliability and validity of a revised assessment of neuropsychiatric symptoms in dementia. *International Psychogeriatrics, 22*(6), 984–994. Available from https://doi.org/10.1017/S1041610210000876.

National Collaborating Centre for Mental Health. (2007). *Dementia: A NICE-SCIE guideline on supporting people with dementia and their carers in health and social care* (1st ed.). Leicester: United Kingdom's National Collaborating Centre for Mental Health.

Dementia | ICHOM – International consortium for health outcomes measurement. (2016). *Ichom.org*. Retrieved from http://www.ichom.org/medical-conditions/dementia/ Accessed 19 February 2017

Fitzsimmons, S., & Buettner, L. L. (2002). Therapeutic recreation interventions for need-driven dementia-compromised. *American Journal of Alzheimer's Disease & Other Dementias, 17*(6), 367–381. Available from https://doi.org/10.1177/153331750201700603.

Frank, C., Feldman, S., & Schulz, M. (2011). Resources for people with dementia: The Alzheimer Society and beyond. *Canadian Family Physician Médecin de Famille Canadien, 57*(12), 1387–1391, e460-4. Retrieved from /pmc/articles/PMC3237510/?report = abstract.

Galik, E., Resnick, B., Hammersla, M., & Brightwater, J. (2014). Optimizing function and physical activity among nursing home residents with dementia: Testing the impact of function-focused care. *The Gerontologist, 54*(6), 930–943. Available from https://doi.org/10.1093/geront/gnt108.

Gitlin, L.N., Hodgson, N., Choi, S. & Marx, K. (in press). Interventions to address functional decline in persons with dementia: Closing the gap between what a person "does do" and what they "can do" In R. Park, et al., (Eds). *Neuropsychology of Alzheimer's disease and other dementias* (2nd ed.). Oxford University Press.

Gitlin, L. N., Arthur, P., Piersol, C., Hessels, V., Wu, S., Dai, Y., & Mann, W. (2017). Targeting behavioral symptoms and functional decline in dementia: A randomized clinical trial. *Journal of the American Geriatrics Society.* Available from https://doi.org/10.1111/jgs.15194.

Gitlin, L. N., & Hodgson, N. A. (2016). Who should assess the needs of and care for a dementia patient's caregiver? *The AMA Journal of Ethic, 18*(12), 1171–1181. Available from https://doi.org/10.1001/journalofethics.2016.18.12.ecas1-1612.

Gitlin, L. N., Kales, H. C., & Lyketsos, C. G. (2012). Nonpharmacologic management of behavioral symptoms in dementia. *JAMA, 308*(19), 2020. Available from https://doi.org/10.1001/jama.2012.36918.

Gitlin, L. N., Kales, H. C., Marx, K., Stanislawski, B., & Lyketsos, C. (2017). A randomized trial of a web-based platform to help families manage dementia-related behavioral symptoms: The WeCareAdvisor™. *Contemporary Clinical Trials, 62*, 27–36. Available from https://doi.org/10.1016/j.cct.2017.08.001.

Gitlin, L. N., Marx, K. A., Stanley, I. H., Hansen, B. R., & Van Haitsma, K. S. (2014). Assessing neuropsychiatric symptoms in people with dementia: A systematic review of measures. *International Psychogeriatrics, 26*(11), 1805–1848. Available from https://doi.org/10.1017/S1041610214001537.

Gitlin, L. N., Marx, K., Stanley, I. H., & Hodgson, N. (2015). Translating evidence-based dementia caregiving interventions into practice: State-of-the-science and next steps. *Gerontologist, 55*(2), 210–226. Available from https://doi.org/10.1093/geront/gnu123.

REFERENCES

Gitlin, L. N., Piersol, C. V., Hodgson, N., Marx, K., Roth, D. L., Johnston, D., & Lyketsos, C. G. (2016). Reducing neuropsychiatric symptoms in persons with dementia and associated burden in family caregivers using tailored activities: Design and methods of a randomized clinical trial. *Contemporary Clinical Trials, 49*, 92–102. Available from https://doi.org/10.1016/j.cct.2016.06.006.

Gitlin, L. N., Reever, K., Dennis, M. P., Mathieu, E., & Hauck, W. W. (2006). Enhancing quality of life of families who use adult day services: Short and long-term effects of the Adult Day Services Plus program. *The Gerontologist, 46*(5), 630–639. Available from https://doi.org/10.1093/geront/46.5.630.

Gitlin, L. N., Winter, L., Dennis, M. P., Hodgson, N., & Hauck, W. W. (2010). A biobehavioral home-based intervention and the well-being of patients with dementia and their caregivers. *JAMA, 304*(9), 983. Available from https://doi.org/10.1001/jama.2010.1253.

Gitlin, L. N., Winter, L., Vause Earland, T., Adel Herge, E., Chernett, N. L., Piersol, C. V., & Burke, J. P. (2009). The Tailored Activity Program to reduce behavioral symptoms in individuals with dementia: Feasibility, acceptability, and replication potential. *The Gerontologist, 49*(3), 428–439. Available from https://doi.org/10.1093/geront/gnp087.

Graff, M. J. L., Vernooij-Dassen, M. J. M., Thijssen, M., Dekker, J., Hoefnagels, W. H. L., & Rikkert, M. G. M. O. (2006). Community based occupational therapy for patients with dementia and their care givers: Randomised controlled trial. *BMJ, 333*(7580). Available from https://doi.org/10.1136/bmj.39001.688843.BE, 1196–1196.

Hauer, K., Schwenk, M., Zieschang, T., Essig, M., Becker, C., & Oster, P. (2012). Physical training improves motor performance in people with dementia: A randomized controlled trial. *Journal of the American Geriatrics Society, 60*(1), 8–15. Available from https://doi.org/10.1111/j.1532-5415.2011.03778.x.

Henwood, T., Neville, C., Baguley, C., Clifton, K., & Beattie, E. (2015). Physical and functional implications of aquatic exercise for nursing home residents with dementia. *Geriatric Nursing, 36*(1), 35–39. Available from https://doi.org/10.1016/j.gerinurse.2014.10.009.

Huntley, J. D., Gould, R. L., Liu, K., Smith, M., & Howard, R. J. (2015). Do cognitive interventions improve general cognition in dementia? A meta-analysis and meta-regression. *BMJ Open, 5*(4). Available from https://doi.org/10.1136/bmjopen-2014-005247, e005247–e005247.

Jutkowitz, E., Brasure, M., Fuchs, E., Shippee, T., Kane, R. A., Fink, H. A., & Kane, R. L. (2016). Care-delivery interventions to manage agitation and aggression in dementia nursing home and assisted living residents: A systematic review and meta-analysis. *Journal of the American Geriatrics Society, 64*(3), 477–488. Available from https://doi.org/10.1111/jgs.13936.

Kales, H. C., Gitlin, L. N., & Lyketsos, C. G. (2014). Management of neuropsychiatric symptoms of dementia in clinical settings: Recommendations from a multidisciplinary expert panel. *Journal of the American Geriatrics Society, 62*(4), 762–769. Available from https://doi.org/10.1111/jgs.12730.

Kales, H. C., Gitlin, L. N., Stanislawski, B., Marx, K., Turnwald, M., Watkins, D. C., & Lyketsos, C. G. (2017). WeCareAdvisor™: The development of a caregiver-focused, web-based program to assess and manage behavioral and psychological symptoms of dementia. *Alzheimer Disease and Associated Disorders, 31*(3), 263–270. Available from https://doi.org/10.1097/WAD.0000000000000177.

Kolanowski, A. M., Buettner, L., Costa, P. T., & Litaker, M. S. (2001). Capturing interests: Therapeutic recreation activities for persons with dementia. *Therapeutic Recreation Journal, 35*(3), 220–235.

Kolanowski, A., Buettner, L., & Fgsa-Faghe. (2008). Prescribing activities that engage passive residents. *Journal of Gerontological Nursing, 34*(1), 13–18. Available from https://doi.org/10.3928/00989134-20080101-08.

Kolanowski, A., Boltz, M., Galik, E., Gitlin, L. N., Kales, H. C., Resnick, B., & Scerpella, D. (2017). Determinants of behavioral and psychological symptoms of dementia: A scoping review of the evidence. *Nursing Outlook*. Available from https://doi.org/10.1016/j.outlook.2017.06.006.

Kumar, A., Singh, A., & Ekavali. (2015). A review on Alzheimer's disease pathophysiology and its management: An update. *Pharmacological Reports*, 67(2), 195–203. Available from https://doi.org/10.1016/j.pharep.2014.09.004.

Mavros, Y., Gates, N., Wilson, G. C., Jain, N., Meiklejohn, J., Brodaty, H., & Fiatarone Singh, M. A. (2017). Mediation of cognitive function improvements by strength gains after resistance training in older adults with mild cognitive impairment: Outcomes of the study of mental and resistance training. *Journal of the American Geriatrics Society*, 65(3), 550–559. Available from https://doi.org/10.1111/jgs.14542.

McCaffrey, R., Park, J., Newman, D., & Hagen, D. (2014). The effect of chair yoga in older adults with moderate and severe Alzheimer's disease. *Research in Gerontological Nursing*, 7(4), 171–177. Available from https://doi.org/10.3928/19404921-20140218-01.

Mittelman, M. S., Haley, W. E., Clay, O. J., & Roth, D. L. (2006). Improving caregiver well-being delays nursing home placement of patients with Alzheimer disease. *Neurology*, 67(9), 1592–1599. Available from https://doi.org/10.1212/01.wnl.0000242727.81172.91.

Mittelman, M. S., Ferris, S. H., Steinberg, G., Shulman, E., Mackell, J. A., Ambinder, A., & Cohen, J. (1993). An intervention that delays institutionalization of Alzheimer's disease patients: Treatment of spouse-caregivers. *The Gerontologist*, 33(6), 730–740. Available from https://doi.org/10.1093/geront/33.6.730.

Odenheimer, G., Borson, S., Sanders, A. E., Swain-Eng, R. J., Kyomen, H. H., Tierney, S., & Johnson, J. (2014). Quality improvement in neurology: Dementia management quality measures. *Journal of the American Geriatrics Society*, 62(3), 558–561. Available from https://doi.org/10.1111/jgs.12630.

O'Neil, M.E., Freeman, M., Christensen, V., Telerant, R., Addleman, A., & Kansagara, D. (2011). A systematic evidence review of non-pharmacological interventions for behavioral symptoms of dementia. VA-ESP Project #05-225.

Orrell, M., Spector, A., Thorgrimsen, L., & Woods, B. (2005). A pilot study examining the effectiveness of maintenance Cognitive Stimulation Therapy (MCST) for people with dementia. *International Journal of Geriatric Psychiatry*, 20(5), 446–451. Available from https://doi.org/10.1002/gps.1304.

Orrell, M., Yates, L., Leung, P., Kang, S., Hoare, Z., Whitaker, C., & Pearson, S. (2017). The impact of individual Cognitive Stimulation Therapy (iCST) on cognition, quality of life, caregiver health, and family relationships in dementia: A randomised controlled trial. *PLoS Medicine*, 14(3), e1002269.

Phinney, A., Chaudhury, H., & O'Connor, D. L. (2007). Doing as much as I can do: The meaning of activity for people with dementia. *Aging & Mental Health*, 11(4), 384–393. Available from https://doi.org/10.1080/13607860601086470.

Potter, R., Ellard, D., Rees, K., & Thorogood, M. (2011). A systematic review of the effects of physical activity on physical functioning, quality of life and depression in older people with dementia. *International Journal of Geriatric Psychiatry*, 26(10), 1000–1011. Available from https://doi.org/10.1002/gps.2641.

Resnick, B., & Galik, E. (2013). Using function-focused care to increase physical activity among older adults. *Annual Review of Nursing Research*, 31(1), 175–208. Available from https://doi.org/10.1891/0739-6686.31.175.

Rovner, B. W., Steele, C. D., Shmuely, Y., & Folstein, M. F. (1996). A randomized trial of dementia care in nursing homes. *Journal of the American Geriatrics Society*, 44(1), 7–13. Available from https://doi.org/10.1111/j.1532-5415.1996.tb05631.x.

Samus, Q. M., Johnston, D., Black, B. S., Hess, E., Lyman, C., Vavilikolanu, A., & Lyketsos, C. G. (2014). A multidimensional home-based care coordination intervention for elders with memory disorders: The Maximizing Independence at Home (MIND) pilot randomized trial. *The American Journal of Geriatric Psychiatry, 22*(4), 398–414. Available from https://doi.org/10.1016/j.jagp.2013.12.175.

Samus, Q., Black, B., Bovenkamp, D., Buckley, M., Callahan, C., Davis, K., Lyketsos, C. G., et al. (2018). Home is where the future is: The Bright Focus Foundation consensus panel on dementia care. *Alzheimer's & Dementia, 14*(1), 104–114. Available from http://dx.doi.org/10.1016/j.jalz.2017.10.006.

Schulz, R., & Eden, J. (Eds.), (2016). *Families caring for an aging America*. Washington, DC: National Academies Press. Available from https://doi.org/10.17226/23606.

Spector, A., Thorgrimsen, L., Woods, B., Royan, L., Davies, S., Butterworth, M., & Orrell, M. (2003). Efficacy of an evidence-based cognitive stimulation therapy programme for people with dementia: Randomised controlled trial. *The British Journal of Psychiatry, 183* (3), 248–254. Available from https://doi.org/10.1192/bjp.183.3.248.

Teri, L., Logsdon, R. G., Uomoto, J., & McCurry, S. M. (1997). Behavioral treatment of depression in dementia patients: A controlled clinical trial. *The Journals of Gerontology Series B: Psychological Sciences and Social Sciences, 52B*(4), P159–P166. Available from https://doi.org/10.1093/geronb/52B.4.P159.

Teri, L., Gibbons, L. E., McCurry, S. M., Logsdon, R. G., Buchner, D. M., Barlow, W. E., & Larson, E. B. (2003). Exercise plus behavioral management in patients with Alzheimer disease. *JAMA, 290*(15), 2015. Available from https://doi.org/10.1001/jama.290.15.2015.

Trahan, M. A., Kuo, J., Carlson, M. C., & Gitlin, L. N. (2014). A systematic review of strategies to foster activity engagement in persons with dementia. *Health Education & Behavior, 41*(1_suppl), 70S–83S. Available from https://doi.org/10.1177/1090198114531782.

Viglietta, V., O'Gorman, J., Williams, L., Tian, Y., Sandrock, A., Doody, R., & Sevigny, J. (2016). Randomized, double-blind, placebo-controlled studies to evaluate treatment with aducanumab (BIIB037) in patients with early Alzheimer's disease: Phase 3 study design (S1.003). *Neurology, 86*(16).

Vreugdenhil, A., Cannell, J., Davies, A., & Razay, G. (2012). A community-based exercise programme to improve functional ability in people with Alzheimer's disease: A randomized controlled trial. *Scandinavian Journal of Caring Sciences, 26*(1), 12–19. Available from https://doi.org/10.1111/j.1471-6712.2011.00895.x.

Woods, B., Aguirre, E., Spector, A. E., & Orrell, M. (2012). Cognitive stimulation to improve cognitive functioning in people with dementia. In B. Woods (Ed.), *Cochrane Database of Systematic Reviews*. Chichester, United Kingdom: John Wiley & Sons, Ltd. Available from https://doi.org/10.1002/14651858.CD005562.pub2.

PART II

ABOUT THE CAREGIVER

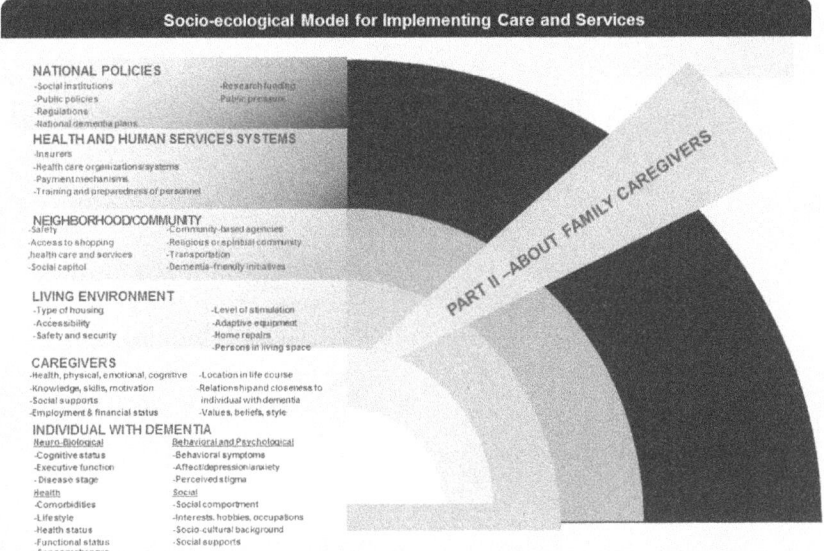

In Part II, we expand our lens to include the impact of dementia on family members. We first examine the characteristics of family members and who becomes care partners (see Chapter 5: Family Member as Care Partner). We explore the emotional, physical, financial, and social implications of being a care partner, and consider some of the characteristics of the disease that pose the most challenge as well. Furthermore, we examine how the caregiving experience differs by when it occurs in a person's life course and the role of social determinants. Then in Chapter 6, How We Can Support Families, we examine ways to support families. Here we find there is substantial evidence to move forward with evidence-based clinically meaningful approaches to providing caregivers education, support, skills, counseling, and respite opportunities. Finally, in Chapter 7, Formal Caregivers: The Role of the Interprofessional Team, we focus on the formal provider and show that they confront similar challenges as families—they are unprepared and poorly trained in dementia care, confront multiple stressors in working with persons with dementia, and are not given the time and support to provide adequate dementia care.

CHAPTER 5

Family Member as Care Partner

> *I learned to be a caregiver by doing it, because I had to do it; it was there to do.* **Arthur Kleinman, MD, Professor of Medical Anthropology and Sociology, Harvard.**
>
> *I believe it's helpful to acknowledge and to accept that no one ever asks or desires to become a dementia sufferer and that none of it, the onset of disease and the ongoing outcomes, is the fault of your loved one.* **Loretta Anne Woodward Veney, "Becoming My Mom's Mom" Infinity, 2013.**

In this chapter, we broaden our lens from focusing on the person living with dementia to the family caregiver. We consider the term "family caregiver" in its broadest sense to include one or more individuals who are related, fictive kin, or friends/neighbors who have a personal involvement with the person with dementia. We examine the multiple and evolving roles of the family caregiver and the impact of assuming these roles on the caregiver's health and well-being across the trajectory of dementia. We answer three key questions: "Who are the family caregivers of persons living with dementia?"; "What are the core tasks they are responsible for with disease progression?"; and "What are the consequences of caregiving for the family caregiver?"

We begin by considering the role of family caregivers through the "Good Life" model (Lawton, 1983). As reviewed in Chapter 2, Lived Experiences of Individuals With Dementia, the model proposes four interrelated components of what contributes to a good life. These include (1) behavioral and functional competencies; (2) psychological well-being; (3) perceived valuation of life; and (4) the objective environment. The following case snapshot illustrates the Good Life Model, its respective quadrants, and its utility in understanding the dynamic relationship between family caregivers and persons with dementia.

Case Snapshot
Suzanne and the Good Life Model

Suzanne expertly guides her mother to sit at the kitchen table, her hand gently supporting her mother's lower back as she helps to ease her into the chair. Placing the fork in her mother's hand, she cues her mother to show her the motion of moving the fork to her mouth (behavioral competence). Her mom eats heartily. Suzanne sits across from her mother and considers her plans for the day. As part of their daily routine there will be a short walk outside to show her mom the new flowers in the garden, then they will look through old postcards from her mother's many travels (objective environment). While her mom naps in the afternoon, Susanne will prepare their evening meal. Later in the afternoon, she will have her mom "help" in folding the laundry while she plays her familiar music. She says that this routine "just works" and that her mom seems comfortable and happy (psychological well-being). "No one taught me how to be a caregiver in the three years since her diagnosis- I just learned by doing it," Suzanne says proudly (perceived value of life).

WHO ARE FAMILY CAREGIVERS?

Suzanne is currently one of over 15 million family members providing care to persons living with dementia in the United States (Alzheimer's Association, 2016). Since most individuals living with dementia are residing in their own long-term residences or homes or that of a family member (see Chapter 8: The Physical Home Environment: A Neglected Therapeutic Context), 90% of care is provided by their family (O'Shaughnessy, 2014). We use the term "family" in its broadest sense. Family members may live with, nearby, or far away from, the person receiving care (Metlife Mature Market Institute, 2011). In the United States for example, 1.4–2.3 million caregivers of people with dementias are long-distance caregivers (Alzheimer's Association, 2012). As a result, a growing number of caregivers do not have a family kinship or legally defined relationship with the individual with dementia but rather are neighbors, partners, or friends. In some cases, although the prevalence is not known, even a divorced spouse may move in with the other upon a dementia diagnosis. Families often do not prepare for who becomes the main or caregiver and what supporting roles other family members will play. Caregiving may start

TABLE 5-1 Characteristics of Dementia Caregivers Internationally

Characteristic	% /Median	Source
Gender	% Female: 59%	Chow, Pio, and Rockwood (2011)
Age	Range: 28–78, and Median: 58	Chow, Pio, and Rockwood (2011)
Employment	% Employed: 27%	Joling et al. (2016)
Relationship	% Spouse: 59%	Joling et al. (2016)
Years Caregiving	Mean: 3.7, Range: 0.5–18 years	Gallego-Alberto, Losada, Márquez-González, Romero-Moreno, and Vara (2017)

when the sibling who lives nearby or has a close relationship to the parent helps out with small things or assumes that the nearest daughter will take care of emotional or physical care needs.

Regardless, family caregivers are defined as such as their involvement is primarily due to the personal relationship rather than by financial remuneration. Because of this personal relationship and commitment, many individuals providing care to persons with dementia do not even consider themselves "caregivers" because it is something they feel is their responsibility and simply part of being a member of a family. Different terms are used to refer to caregivers by researchers and health and human professionals and include: "key informant, proxy informant," "visit companion," "care partner," and "decision maker" to name a few.

The typical characteristics of dementia caregivers in the United States are summarized in Table 5-1. Like Suzanne, most family caregivers are women (60%), in their late 40s, employed, and caring for children and/or others in the home (National Alliance for Caregiving & AARP, 2015). As they are also providing 80% of the long-term care for persons living with dementia, they have been referred to as the "woman in the middle" (Brody, 1981) or the sandwich generation (Alzheimer's Association, 2016).

While traditionally caregiving has been mostly provided by women across all cultures, the number of male caregivers is increasing, especially for older males (Baker, Robertson, & Connelly, 2010) and spousal caregivers (Brown, Chen, Mitchell, & Province, 2007). Rapid population aging coupled with a higher proportion of women affected by dementia compared with men means that the number of male family caregivers of persons with dementia is anticipated to increase. With this shift in caregiving trends, male family caregivers of persons with dementia are beginning to be represented in the caregiving literature (McDonnell & Ryan, 2014).

A Gallup survey found 72% of caregivers cared for a parent, mother-in-law, or father-in-law, and 67% of caregivers provided care for someone aged 75 years or older (Mendes, 2011). Moreover the percentage of caregivers caring for individuals over 85 years of age has increased across all surveys of informal caregivers conducted by National Alliance for Caregiving & AARP (2004). Many caregivers of older people are themselves growing older (National Alliance for Caregiving & AARP, 2012).

On average, family caregivers of individuals with dementia provide care for 5 years; however, this can range upwards to 10 or 20 years. In early dementia, family caregivers may spend an average of 85 hours per month providing care. As dementia progresses and with the advanced stage, caregivers may spend over 250 hours per month providing care (Freedman & Spillman, 2014).

Caregiving is universal; it occurs across all race, ethnic, and cultural groups. Attitudes toward caregiving are largely based in part on cultural and family systems and can have a direct impact on the caregiving experience. For example, Asian American caregivers in the United States provide more caregiving hours than white, African American, and Hispanic caregivers. Hispanic and African American caregivers tend to underutilize resources. A comparison among African American, white American, and Hispanic caregivers found that 75% of Hispanic patients and 60% of African American patients lived with the family of the primary caregivers. African American and Hispanic caregivers are more likely than white caregivers to reduce their work hours to care for sick relatives and rely more on informal caregiving from friends and relatives and have larger social support networks than the white families. This increased sense of obligation to provide care for older family members is associated with more caregiving hours, greater resignation about caregiving, higher levels of caregiver strain, and a larger reduction in household income than that reported by white caregivers (Cox & Monk, 1996). The decision to reduce work hours rather than place a relative in a nursing home is associated with increased psychological, social, and financial burden (Covinsky et al., 2001).

> Most care for people with dementia is provided by informal, unpaid, family caregivers who include spouses, adult children, and friends.

WHAT DO CAREGIVERS DO?

The vast array of specialized knowledge and skills required by families to care for persons living with dementia is mind-boggling and

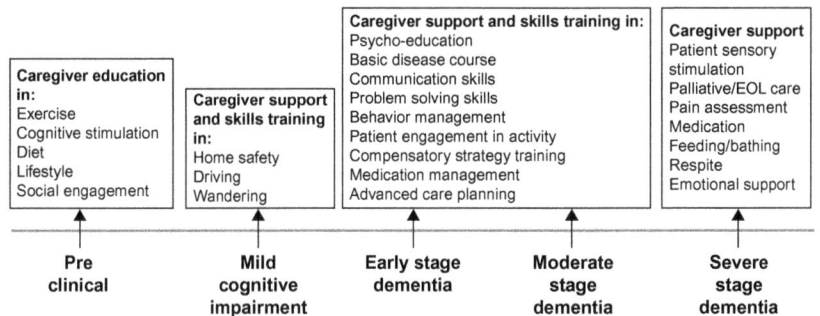

FIGURE 5-1 Caregiver needs across the dementia trajectory.

families rarely receive any preparation or training. Typically the roles assumed by families are incrementally assumed starting with episodic support and ending with fully time supervision and hands-on care. The care they provide may be sporadic or occur every day, and be of short- or long-term duration (Schulz & Eden, 2016).

Fig. 5-1 shows how caregiving typically follows a relatively linear trajectory with care tasks increasing incrementally with disease progression and as persons with dementia experience cognitive and functional declines and behavioral symptoms. That is tasks required of caregivers are cumulative and each dementia stage brings new challenges, in the early stages of dementia; as caregivers begin to observe memory and behavior changes in their family member, they must learn the dance of maintaining the person's dignity and autonomy while increasingly providing needed support.

The trajectory first begins with emerging awareness of the caregiver that there is a problem (Fortinsky & Downs, 2014). With this awareness that one is becoming a caregiver comes an array of overwhelming questions about what one should expect in order to meet the needs of the person with dementia. Typically, there are social role changes as the caregiver shifts from usual participation in life activities to a focus on caregiving. The caregiving tasks in the early stages of dementia may include assistance with housework, preparing meals, and transportation (Black et al., 2013). Tasks may also include paying bills and providing guidance or help with making major decisions such as financial or long-term planning (Wolff, Spillman, Freedman, & Kasper, 2016). Caregiving tasks also involve medical skills such as monitoring the individual's clinical symptoms and medications, as well as communicating with health professionals, and providing emotional support. This early stage is also punctuated with families providing episodic care such as accompanying the person with dementia to doctor visits or fulfilling transitional care needs such as coordinating among doctors and care settings (hospital to home).

The level of support increases as the disease progresses, starting with support for instrumental activities of daily living (household, financial, and social activities) and expanding to include personal care and eventually almost constant supervision. The extent of need and the types of care needed, and their progression over time, depend on many factors such as the clinical profile (types and severity of cognitive impairments and psychological symptoms, which may vary by type of dementia), the presence of comorbid physical and psychological problems, the custom and habits of the person with dementia, the person's personality and significant relationships.

As dementia progresses, caregivers become increasingly involved in activities of daily living such as dressing, bathing, and eating. In the moderate disease stage, caregivers must now learn how to navigate complex health care and social services systems and assume the role of surrogate decision maker for the person with dementia (Spillman, Wolfe, Freedman, & Kasper, 2014), all while maintaining constant supervision over safety and well-being (Gitlin & Wolff, 2011). In addition, caregivers become responsible for managing complex behavioral symptoms that are common in dementia such as agitation, irritability, apathy, and wandering, which in turn may be distressful and potentially harmful to the person with dementia and the caregiver.

In the advanced stages, caregivers take on the total physical care of the, person for whom they care, including bathing and feeding, incontinence care, and planning for the end of life. In this stage, caregivers usually need the assistance of professional care if the person continues living in the community. Since the disease progresses slowly, family members have often been providing care for many years and are under high levels of stress. The effects of high stress levels are intensified by the chronic fatigue associated with providing long hours of care without periods of relief. Dementia does not progress in isolation of aging and as such, most persons with dementia have or will experience other medical problems particularly in the advanced stages that can add to the time and complexity of caregiving. This may include medication management (65%) and skin/wound care (35%). These tasks are being carried out in the home, not in the medical settings, and caregivers are being called upon to carry out an array of nursing or medical tasks that previously would have been provided only by licensed or certified professionals in hospitals and nursing homes (Reinhard & Feinberg, 2015; Reinhard, Levine, & Samis, 2014).

As end-of-life approaches, decision may involve hospitalizations, placement into a long-term care facility or enrollment in a hospice program (Givens, Lopez, Mazor, & Mitchell, 2012). One of the most disruptive transitions to occur during the course of dementia caregiving is the decision to place a family member in a nursing home (Gaugler, 2014).

Although admission to a nursing home can be considered the end of caregiving, several qualitative and quantitative studies have implied that dementia caregivers' emotional distress and negative mental health may worsen after the institutionalization of a family member (Davies & Nolan, 2006; Grant et al., 2002). Family members often continue to provide care after a relative's move to a nursing home (Gaugler, 2005). Negative interactions between family caregivers and the formal caregivers in the nursing home can have powerful and negative impacts on family members (Almberg, Grafstrom, Krichbaum, & Winblad, 2000). Upon the end of life, some caregivers experience complicated grief and benefit from professional counseling. All caregivers go through the process and hard work of bereavement and must reframe their roles and craft a new purpose and flow of their daily lives. This can take time and can be challenging.

It is important to note that family members do not provide caregiving in isolation from the other roles and responsibilities in their lives and caregiving is differentially experienced based on gender, race, location and other factors. For example, male caregivers tend to demonstrate a more task-oriented approach to care, whereas female caregivers use more emotion-oriented coping methods and favor a more independent approach to caregiving, accessing less formal services and supports than their male counterparts (Baker & Robertson, 2008). Male caregivers have been reported to struggle with the transition to the caregiving role due to the "feminine" nature of many caregiving tasks (Baker & Robertson, 2008). Male caregivers spend fewer hours performing personal care tasks than female caregivers (Brazil, Thabane, Foster, & Bédard, 2009) and often find tasks such as cooking and cleaning difficult. How these trends may shift in terms of changing gender roles and the closing gender gap in life expectancy remains unknown.

> Caring for a family member is a mutual and interrelated experience between caregiver and the person living with dementia within their social and cultural space.

WHAT ARE THE CONSEQUENCES OF CAREGIVING?

Despite many common experiences, the consequences of caregiving are highly variable. The diversity of families, the timing of entry into the caregiving role, and the duration of the role in relation to the overall life course of the caregiver, all shape the caregiving experience. For example, many persons with dementia receive care from more than one family caregiver, and some caregivers may help more than one older adult.

Under ideal circumstances, the caregiver may be able to balance the responsibilities of these competing roles—such as caring for a child or employment demands and their caregiving responsibilities. Over time, however, caregiving exacts an immense toll on families and involves physical, social, financial, and emotional costs (Peacock, Hammond-Collins, & Forbes, 2014.)

The financial toll that caregiving places on families is especially underrecognized and underappreciated. According to the Institute of Medicine Report [IOM] (2009), "Family members, friends, and other unpaid caregivers provide the backbone for much of the care that is received by older adults in the United States." The value of unpaid family caregivers in the United States in 2010 was estimated to be 71.5 million, twice that of 35.1 million in 2000 (Coughlin, 2010). Many caregivers must leave their jobs in order to maintain the person they care for at home, and this increased financial burden on the family is typically overlooked. It is estimated that it costs $74/day or $49,00 per year for family caregivers to provide care (Jutkowitz et al., 2017).

> Caregivers provide $249,000 of support in terms of time and out of pocket costs over the typical 5 year course of dementia caregiving (Jutkowitz et al., 2017).

Caregiving also takes a physical toll. Caregivers of people with dementia self-report poorer health outcomes, lower well-being scores, and poorer quality of life than non-caregivers. They also experience worse health outcomes, including obesity, higher metabolic risk, higher levels of stress hormones, compromised immune response, antibodies, greater medication use, and greater cognitive decline (Schulz & Martire, 2004).

Caregiving also exacts an emotional toll. It is not uncommon for caregivers to report symptoms of depression and anxiety that can lead to episodes of clinical depression and impaired quality of life in 40% of dementia caregivers (Zarit, Femia, Kim, & Whitlach, 2010). Family caregivers often neglect their own health, which can lead to a worsening in a preexisting illness or increased vulnerability to stress-related illnesses (Son et al., 2007; Vitaliano, Zhang, & Scanlan, 2003; Yueh-Feng Lu & Austrom, 2005). Data on anxiety disorders in dementia caregivers are scarce but suggest that one in three caregivers suffers from such a disorder. Pilot studies in Africa, Latin America, and South and South-East Asia revealed that the levels of depression and anxiety among caregivers of people with dementia in low-income countries were at least as high as those seen in high-income countries (Prince et al., 2007). In the same study, the presence of behavioral and psychological symptoms of dementia was strongly associated with caregiver strain.

Certain risk factors place some caregivers at increased risk for poor outcomes. This is particularly true for spousal caregivers who are at increased risk for frailty (Dassel & Carr, 2016). Caregivers who have a history of major medical or psychiatric illnesses, and those with preexisting financial strain are also at increased risk for increased burden and strain (Roth, Fredman, & Haley, 2015). Caregivers who provide care to individuals with severe behavioral symptoms are also at increased risk for poor health outcomes (Schoenmakers, Buntinx, & Delepeleire, 2010).

Gender and the quality of the relationship also affects the consequences of caregiving. Female caregivers tend to report a higher degree of caregiver burden and psychological distress (Bookwala & Schulz, 2000). However, male caregivers may be reluctant to disclose feelings of burden or distress due to traditional views of masculinity that idealize self-reliance. Male caregivers are less likely to request formal assistance (Black, Schwartz, Caruso, & Hannum, 2008). One possible explanation may be due to the constraints of holding traditional masculine values (Baker et al. 2010). Several studies to date have examined the effects of caregiving on aspects of relationship quality when a partner or spouse has dementia (Clare et al., 2012). Winter, Gitlin, and Dennis (2011) reported that the quality of the relationship prior to the onset of dementia was significantly associated with desire to institutionalize the person living with dementia for male caregivers, but not females.

Nonetheless, and despite the array of negative consequences, caregivers also demonstrate resilience, adaptability, and report positive outcomes. Numerous surveys suggest that caregiving instills confidence, a renewed sense of purpose, and an opportunity to "give back" (Evercare, 2007) with some minority groups, such as African American caregivers reporting more positive outcomes than others (Roth et al., 2016). Family members report that caregiving provided lessons on dealing with difficult situations, brought them closer to their loved one, and assured them that the person with dementia is well cared for. Researchers have also noted that caregivers who are able to account for positive effects of caregiving and who feel confidence in their role are at lower risk for burden and depression and better overall mental health. For example, van der Lee and colleagues (2014) found that a sense of competence or self-efficacy was associated with less caregiver burden.

WHAT DO CAREGIVERS NEED?

Despite the health care system's tremendous reliance on families, family caregivers are typically provided little, if any, information and training to carry out the complicated medical procedures, personal care, and care coordination tasks they are expected to provide. For example, a survey of 307 caregivers found that only 32% of caregivers reported being confident in managing dementia-related problems, only 19% knew how to access community services to help provide care, and only 28% indicated that the individual's provider helped them work through dementia care problems (Jennings et al., 2015). In another survey, although not just of dementia caregivers, half (51%) of family caregivers reported that they provide medical/nursing tasks without any prior preparation, 21% wanted more help or information about incontinence, and 60% of the caregivers reported learning how to manage at least some medications without any training (Reinhard, Levine, & Samis, 2012). Caregiving often involves interacting with numerous health care providers, back- and-forth transitions from hospital to home or rehabilitation facility, move to a senior residence or assisted living facility, placement in a nursing home, and ultimately end-of-life care (Belden, Russonello, & Stewart, 2001), all of which the caregiver receives little, if any preparation.

RESEARCH IMPLICATIONS

While this chapter broadened our lens from the person living with dementia to the family caregiver, the research has yet to capture the full reality for most families and particularly families from different races, ethnicities and cultures. The research has focused primarily on a self-identified "primary" caregiver, whereas most family care situations involve a system of shared and shifting responsibilities and the diversity of families has also not been well captured in the research literature. Furthermore, we need to broaden our focus from examining single caregivers performing select tasks to include the full range of family members who may become involved in care and the often complex division of labor among families involved in a much fuller spectrum of care activities. Moving from a person-centered to a family-centered model of care as well as recognizing the heterogeneity of families is needed in order to shift the narrow medical focus views of families as only "key informants" to "key members" of the health care team.

Family-centered programs and models do exist although the role of the family caregiver in these programs varies. Some programs actively involve the family caregiver, while in other programs, their role is more passive and care planning primarily occurs through a nurse, case manager, or social worker (Bass et al., 2013). Yet, when family caregivers participate as an engaged member of the health care team, nursing home admissions for older adults with dementia can decline. When family caregivers participate in the hospital discharge process, rehospitalization rates and lengths of stay decline (Rodakowski et al., 2017; Gitlin & Wolff, 2011).

THE FUTURE OF CAREGIVING

With an increasingly mobile society, more people are going to be faced with the dilemma of providing care to a relative with dementia from a distance (Watari et al., 2006). Distance caregiving can create barriers to providing effective and timely care; caregivers must seek out and arrange services for their relative (Collins, Holt, Moore, & Bledsoe, 2003), and while providing physical care is exhausting, long-distance care can cause more psychological stress (Koerin & Harrigan, 2003). Understanding when help is required is more difficult when distance caregivers may not see the person in need of care on a regular basis and may not be aware of deteriorations in their parents' physical and mental health (Joseph & Hallman, 1998). Most long-distance caregivers reported at least one negative impact on employment, and over half reported that they had given up family time, vacations, hobbies, or other leisure activities (Koerin & Harrigan, 2003). These studies show how more attention is needed to support family caregivers living at a distance.

Alongside these shifts in proximity of caregivers is the increasing multiethnicity and multiculturalism in most societies. This calls for the need to learn how to understand, respect, and address cultural difference how to best support caregivers. Given the increasing diversity of our older adult population and their caregivers, attention to cultural factors influencing the caregiving experience is essential (Napoles, Chadiha, Eversley, & Moreno-John, 2010; Weiner, 2008).

The time has come for society to acknowledge the significant contributions of family caregivers. They are the mainstay of support for individuals living with dementia and yet are provided little training and assistance. More than simple recognition, caregivers need meaningful support to help them care for individuals with dementia and to maintain their own health, financial security, and well-being. In the next chapter, we present evidence-based strategies for preparing dementia-ready caregivers.

KEY POINTS

- Family caregiving is universal occurring across all socioeconomic levels and race/ethnic/cultural groups.
- Most persons with dementia are cared for by one or more family members, defining families in the broadest sense as individuals with a personal.
- Women who are married and employed and between the ages of 45 and 64 years are most likely to be family caregivers.
- There is a growing number of male caregivers and families caregiving from a long distance.

- Caregivers' tasks increase overtime and include episodic and long-term care and support include physical care (bathing, feeding, and dressing) housekeeping, medication management, behavioral symptom management, and providing emotional support—tasks for which they are provided little if any training or support.

What Actions Can be Taken Now

- Offer support to family caregivers and recognize that they are the primary source of support for persons living with dementia
- As a family caregiver, insist on being recognized in medical encounters as a key informant
- Appreciate and respect the cultural factors that influence family caregiving of persons living with dementia
- Upon diagnosis, consult with vetted websites such as ADEAR, National Institute on Aging, Alzheimer's Association for more disease information

---

References

Almberg, B., Grafstrom, M., Krichbaum, K., & Winblad, B. (2000). The interplay of institution and family caregiving: Relations between patient hassles, nursing home hassles and caregivers' burnout. *International Journal of Geriatric Psychiatry, 15*(10), 931–939. Available from https://doi.org/10.1002/1099-1166(200010)15:10 < 3c3c931::AID-GPS219 > 3e3e3.0.CO;2-L.

Alzheimer's Association. (2012). *2012 Alzheimer's disease facts & figures*. Retrieved from https://www.alz.org/downloads/facts_figures_2012.pdf.

Alzheimer's Association. (2016). *2016 Alzheimer's disease facts & figures*. Retrieved from https://www.alz.org/documents_custom/2016-facts-and-figures.pdf.

Baker, K. L., & Robertson, N. (2008). Coping with caring for someone with dementia: Reviewing the literature about men. *Aging & Mental Health, 12*(4), 413–422. Available from https://doi.org/10.1080/13607860802224250.

Baker, K. L., Robertson, N., & Connelly, D. (2010). Men caring for wives or partners with dementia: Masculinity, strain and gain. *Aging & Mental Health, 14*(3), 319–327. Available from https://doi.org/10.1080/13607860903228788.

Bass, D. M., Judge, K. S., Lynn Snow, A., Wilson, N. L., Morgan, R., Looman, W. J., & Kunik, M. E. (2013). Caregiver outcomes of partners in dementia care: Effect of a care coordination program for veterans with dementia and their family members and friends. *Journal of the American Geriatrics Society, 61*(8), 1377–1386. Available from https://doi.org/10.1111/jgs.12362.

Belden., Russonello., & Stewart. (2001). *In the middle: A report on multicultural boomer coping with family and aging issues*. Washington, DC: AARP. Retrieved from https://assets.aarp.org/rgcenter/il/in_the_middle.pdf.

Black, B. S., Johnston, D., Rabins, P. V., Morrison, A., Lyketsos, C., & Samus, Q. M. (2013). Unmet needs of community-residing persons with dementia and their informal caregivers: Findings from the maximizing independence at home study. *Journal of the American Geriatrics Society, 61*(12), 2087–2095. Available from https://doi.org/10.1111/jgs.12549.

Black, H. K., Schwartz, A. J., Caruso, C. J., & Hannum, S. M. (2008). How personal control mediates suffering: Elderly husbands' narratives of caregiving. *The Journal of Men's Studies*, *16*(2), 177–192. Available from https://doi.org/10.3149/jms.1602.177.

Bookwala, J., & Schulz, R. (2000). A comparison of primary stressors, secondary stressors, and depressive symptoms between elderly caregiving husbands and wives: The caregiver health effects study. *Psychology and Aging*, *15*(4), 607–616. Available from https://doi.org/10.1037/0882-7974.15.4.607.

Brazil, K., Thabane, L., Foster, G., & Bédard, M. (2009). Gender differences among Canadian spousal caregivers at the end of life. *Health & Social Care in the Community*, *17*(2), 159–166. Available from https://doi.org/10.1111/j.1365-2524.2008.00813.x.

Brody, E. M. (1981). "Women in the middle" and family help to older people. *The Gerontologist*, *21*(5), 471–480. Available from https://doi.org/10.1093/geront/21.5.471.

Brown, J. W., Chen, S., Mitchell, C., & Province, A. (2007). Help-seeking by older husbands caring for wives with dementia. *Journal of Advanced Nursing*, *59*(4), 352–360. Available from https://doi.org/10.1111/j.1365-2648.2007.04290.x.

Chow, T. W., Pio, F. J., & Rockwood, K. (2011). An international needs assessment of caregivers for frontotemporal dementia. *Canadian Journal of Neurological Sciences/Journal Canadien Des Sciences Neurologiques*, *38*(5), 753–757. Available from https://doi.org/10.1017/S0317167100054147.

Clare, L., Nelis, S. M., Whitaker, C. J., Martyr, A., Markova, I. S., Roth, I., & Morris, R. G. (2012). Marital relationship quality in early-stage dementia. *Alzheimer Disease & Associated Disorders*, *26*(2), 148–158. Available from https://doi.org/10.1097/WAD.0b013e318221ba23.

Collins, W. L., Holt, T. A., Moore, S. E., & Bledsoe, L. K. (2003). Long-distance caregiving: A case study of an African-American family. *American Journal of Alzheimer's Disease & Other Dementiasr*, *18*(5), 309–316. Available from https://doi.org/10.1177/153331750301800503.

Coughlin, J. (2010). Estimating the impact of caregiving and employment on well-being. *Outcomes & Insights in Health Management*, *2*(1), 1–7.

Covinsky, K. E., Eng, C., Lui, L.-Y., Sands, L. P., Sehgal, A. R., Walter, L. C., & Yaffe, K. (2001). Reduced employment in caregivers of frail elders: Impact of ethnicity, patient clinical characteristics, and caregiver characteristics. *The Journals of Gerontology Series A: Biological Sciences and Medical Sciences*, *56*(11), M707–M713. Available from https://doi.org/10.1093/gerona/56.11.M707.

Cox, C., & Monk, A. (1996). Strain among caregivers: Comparing the experiences of African American and Hispanic caregivers of Alzheimer's relatives. *The International Journal of Aging and Human Development*, *43*(2), 93–105. Available from https://doi.org/10.2190/DYQ1-TPRP-VHTC-38VU.

Dassel, K. B., & Carr, D. C. (2016). Does dementia caregiving accelerate frailty? Findings from the health and retirement study. *The Gerontologist*, *56*(3), 444–450. Available from https://doi.org/10.1093/geront/gnu078.

Davies, S., & Nolan, M. (2006). "Making it better": Self-perceived roles of family caregivers of older people living in care homes: A qualitative study. *International Journal of Nursing Studies*, *43*(3), 281–291. Available from https://doi.org/10.1016/j.ijnurstu.2005.04.009.

Evercare. (2007). *Family caregivers—What they spend, what they sacrifice*. National Alliance for Caregiving. Retrieved from http://www.caregiving.org/data/Evercare_NAC_CaregiverCostStudyFINAL20111907.pdf.

Fortinsky, R. H., & Downs, M. (2014). Optimizing person-centered transitions in the dementia journey: A comparison of national dementia strategies. *Health Affairs*, *33*(4), 566–573. Available from https://doi.org/10.1377/hlthaff.2013.1304.

Freedman, V. A., & Spillman, B. C. (2014). Disability and care needs among older Americans. *Milbank Quarterly*, *92*(3), 509–541. Available from https://doi.org/10.1111/1468-0009.12076.

Gallego-Alberto, L., Losada, A., Márquez-González, M., Romero-Moreno, R., & Vara, C. (2017). Commitment to personal values and guilt feelings in dementia caregivers. *International Psychogeriatrics, 29*(1), 57–65. Available from https://doi.org/10.1017/S1041610216001393.

Gaugler, J. E. (2005). Family involvement in residential long-term care: A synthesis and critical review. *Aging & Mental Health, 9*(2), 105–118. Available from https://doi.org/10.1080/13607860412331310245.

Gaugler, J. E. (2014). The turning point. *Journal of Applied Gerontology, 33*(5), 519–521. Available from https://doi.org/10.1177/0733464814537026.

Gitlin, L. N., & Wolff, J. (2011). Family involvement in care transitions of older adults: What do we know and where do we go from here? *Annual Review of Gerontology and Geriatrics, 31*(1), 31–64. Available from https://doi.org/10.1891/0198-8794.31.31.

Givens, J. L., Lopez, R. P., Mazor, K. M., & Mitchell, S. L. (2012). Sources of stress for family members of nursing home residents with advanced dementia. *Alzheimer Disease & Associated Disorders, 26*(3), 254–259. Available from https://doi.org/10.1097/WAD.0b013e31823899e4.

Grant, I., Adler, K. A., Patterson, T. L., Dimsdale, J. E., Ziegler, M. G., & Irwin, M. R. (2002). Health consequences of Alzheimer's caregiving transitions: Effects of placement and bereavement. *Psychosomatic Medicine, 64*(3), 477–486. Available from https://doi.org/10.1097/00006842-200205000-00012.

Institute of Medicine Report [IOM]. (2009). *Building the health care force.* Washington, DC: National Academies Press.

Jennings, L. A., Reuben, D. B., Evertson, L. C., Serrano, K. S., Ercoli, L., Grill, J., & Wenger, N. S. (2015). Unmet needs of caregivers of individuals referred to a dementia care program. *Journal of the American Geriatrics Society, 63*(2), 282–289. Available from https://doi.org/10.1111/jgs.13251.

Joling, K. J., Windle, G., Dröes, R.-M., Meiland, F., van Hout, H. P. J., MacNeil Vroomen, J., & Woods, B. (2016). Factors of resilience in informal caregivers of people with dementia from integrative international data analysis. *Dementia and Geriatric Cognitive Disorders, 42*(3–4), 198–214. Available from https://doi.org/10.1159/000449131.

Joseph, A. E., & Hallman, B. C. (1998). Over the hill and far away: Distance as a barrier to the provision of assistance to elderly relatives. *Social Science & Medicine, 46*(6), 631–639. Available from https://doi.org/10.1016/S0277-9536(97)00181-0.

Jutkowitz, E., Kuntz, K. M., Dowd, B., Gaugler, J. E., MacLehose, R. F., & Kane, R. L. (2017). Effects of cognition, function, and behavioral and psychological symptoms on out-of-pocket medical and nursing home expenditures and time spent caregiving for persons with dementia. *Alzheimer's & Dementia, 13*(7), 801–809. Available from https://doi.org/10.1016/j.jalz.2016.12.011.

Koerin, B. B., & Harrigan, M. P. (2003). P.S. I love you: Long-distance caregiving. *Journal of Gerontological Social Work, 40*(1–2), 63–81. Available from https://doi.org/10.1300/J083v40n01_05.

Lawton, M. P. (1983). The varieties of wellbeing. *Experimental Aging Research, 9*(2), 65–72. Available from https://doi.org/10.1080/03610738308258427.

McDonnell, E., & Ryan, A. A. (2014). The experience of sons caring for a parent with dementia. *Dementia, 13*(6), 788–802. Available from https://doi.org/10.1177/1471301213485374.

Mendes, E. (2011). *Most caregivers look after elderly parent: Invest a lot of time. Gallup.com.* Retrieved from http://news.gallup.com/poll/148682/caregivers-look-elderly-parent-invest-lot-time.aspx.

Metlife Mature Market Institute. (2011). *The MetLife study of caregiving costs to working caregivers: Double jeopardy for baby boomers caring for their parents.* Retrieved from http://www.caregiving.org/wp-content/uploads/2011/06/mmi-caregiving-costs-working-caregivers.pdf.

Napoles, A. M., Chadiha, L., Eversley, R., & Moreno-John, G. (2010). Reviews: Developing culturally sensitive dementia caregiver interventions: Are we there yet? *American Journal of Alzheimer's Disease & Other Dementias, 25*(5), 389−406. Available from https://doi.org/10.1177/1533317510370957.
National Alliance for Caregiving & AARP. (2004). *Caregiving in the U.S. 2004.*
National Alliance for Caregiving & AARP. (2012). *Caregiving in the U.S. 2012.*
National Alliance for Caregiving & AARP. (2015). *Caregiving in the U.S. 2015.*
O'Shaughnessy, C. (2014). National spending for long-term services and supports (LTSS), 2012.
Peacock, S. C., Hammond-Collins, K., & Forbes, D. A. (2014). The journey with dementia from the perspective of bereaved family caregivers: A qualitative descriptive study. *BMC Nursing, 13*(1), 42. Available from https://doi.org/10.1186/s12912-014-0042-x.
Prince, M., Patel, V., Saxena, S., Maj, M., Maselko, J., Phillips, M. R., & Rahman, A. (2007). No health without mental health. *The Lancet, 370*(9590), 859−877.
Reinhard, S. C., & Feinberg, L. F. (2015). The escalating complexity of family caregiving: Meeting the challenge. *Family Caregiving in the New Normal,* 291−303.
Reinhard, S. C., Levine, C., & Samis, S. (2012). *Home alone: Family caregivers providing complex chronic care.* Washington, DC: AARP Public Policy Institute.
Reinhard, S. C., Levine, C., & Samis, S. (2014). *Family caregivers providing complex chronic care to their spouses.* Washington, DC: AARP Public Policy Institute.
Rodakowski, J., Rocco, P. B., Ortiz, M., Folb, B., Schulz, R., Morton, S. C., & James, A. E. (2017). Caregiver integration during discharge planning for older adults to reduce resource use: A meta-analysis. *Journal of the American Geriatrics Society, 65*(8), 1748−1755. Available from https://doi.org/10.1111/jgs.14873.
Roth, D. L., Fredman, L., & Haley, W. E. (2015). Informal caregiving and its impact on health: A reappraisal from population-based studies. *The Gerontologist, 55*(2), 309−319. Available from https://doi.org/10.1093/geront/gnu177.
Roth, D. L., Sheehan, O. C., Huang, J., Rhodes, J. D., Judd, S. E., Kilgore, M., & Haley, W. E. (2016). Medicare claims indicators of healthcare utilization differences after hospitalization for ischemic stroke: Race, gender, and caregiving effects. *International Journal of Stroke, 11*(8), 928−934. Available from https://doi.org/10.1177/1747493016660095.
Schoenmakers, B., Buntinx, F., & Delepeleire, J. (2010). Factors determining the impact of care-giving on caregivers of elderly patients with dementia. A systematic literature review. *Maturitas, 66*(2), 191−200. Available from https://doi.org/10.1016/j.maturitas.2010.02.009.
Schulz, R., & Eden, J. (Eds.), (2016). *Families caring for an aging America.* Washington, DC: National Academies Press. Available from https://doi.org/10.17226/23606.
Schulz, R., & Martire, L. M. (2004). Family caregiving of persons with dementia: Prevalence, health effects, and support strategies. *The American Journal of Geriatric Psychiatry, 12*(3), 240−249.
Son, J., Erno, A., Shea, D. G., Femia, E. E., Zarit, S. H., & Parris Stephens, M. A. (2007). The caregiver stress process and health outcomes. *Journal of Aging and Health, 19*(6), 871−887. Available from https://doi.org/10.1177/0898264307308568.
Spillman, B., Wolfe, J., Freedman, V., & Kasper, J. (2014). *Informal caregiving for older American: An analysis of the 2011 National Study of Caregiving.* US Department of Health and Human Services. Retrieved from https://aspe.hhs.gov/system/files/pdf/77146/NHATS-IC.pdf.
van der Lee, J., Bakker, T. J. E. M., Duivenvoorden, H. J., & Dröes, R.-M. (2014). Multivariate models of subjective caregiver burden in dementia: A systematic review. *Ageing Research Reviews, 15,* 76−93. Available from https://doi.org/10.1016/j.arr.2014.03.003.

Vitaliano, P. P., Zhang, J., & Scanlan, J. M. (2003). Is caregiving hazardous to one's physical health? A meta-analysis. *Psychological Bulletin*, *129*(6), 946−972. Available from https://doi.org/10.1037/0033-2909.129.6.946.

Watari, K., Wetherell, J. L., Gatz, M., Delaney, J., Ladd, C., & Cherry, D. (2006). Long distance caregivers. *Clinical Gerontologist*, *29*(4), 61−77. Available from https://doi.org/10.1300/J018v29n04_05.

Weiner, M. F. (2008). Perspective on race and ethnicity in Alzheimer's disease research. *Alzheimer's & Dementia*, *4*(4), 233−238. Available from https://doi.org/10.1016/j.jalz.2007.10.016.

Winter, L., Gitlin, L. N., & Dennis, M. (2011). Desire to institutionalize a relative with dementia: Quality of premorbid relationship and caregiver gender. *Family Relations*, *60*(2), 221−230. Available from https://doi.org/10.1111/j.1741-3729.2010.00644.x.

Wolff, J. L., Spillman, B. C., Freedman, V. A., & Kasper, J. D. (2016). A national profile of family and unpaid caregivers who assist older adults with health care activities. *JAMA Internal Medicine*, *176*(3), 372. Available from https://doi.org/10.1001/jamainternmed.2015.7664.

Yueh-Feng Lu, Y., & Austrom, M. G. (2005). Distress responses and self-care behaviors in dementia family caregivers with high and low depressed mood. *Journal of the American Psychiatric Nurses Association*, *11*(4), 231−240. Available from https://doi.org/10.1177/1078390305281422.

Zarit, S. H., Femia, E. E., Kim, K., & Whitlatch, C. J. (2010). The structure of risk factors and outcomes for family caregivers: Implications for assessment and treatment. *Aging & Mental Health*, *14*(2), 220−231. Available from https://doi.org/10.1080/13607860903167861.

CHAPTER 6

How We Can Support Families

The problem is [patients and family caregivers] are expected to operate this kind of stuff, which obviously, in years past, has been relegated to nurses and skilled professionals. Now, we're expected to do these things. No one wants to take the time to train us, and work side by side with us, until we have it down pat. **Family caregiver as reported in Institute for Healthcare Improvement / National Patient Safety Foundation, Cambridge and Boston, MA, 2017.**

If these interventions were drugs, it is hard to believe that they would not be on the fast track to approval. The magnitude of benefit and quality of evidence supporting these interventions considerably exceed those of currently approved pharmacologic therapies [for dementia]. **Kenneth E. Covinsky, MD, MPH, Editorial, Annals of Internal Medicine, 2006.**

Most people living with dementia stay at home, either in their own long-term residence or that of a family member. Some individuals, although the numbers are not known, may float between households, living in one family member's home for part of the year, and that of another for another part of the year. Regardless of living environment, families provide most of the long-term care for people living with dementia from time of diagnosis to end-of-life, estimated to be over 80% of the care needed throughout the disease process. The role of family caregivers in providing care is universal, occurring across all countries, socioeconomic levels, race, ethnic, and cultural groups and has become an expectation of health care systems and society (Gitlin & Hodgson, 2015; World Health Organization, 2012; World Health Organization, 2014). In the United States, an estimated 15 million families provide care to persons living with dementia (Alzheimer's Association, 2017).

As discussed in the previous chapter, compared to families caring for individuals without cognitive impairment, families of persons living with dementia spend more time caregiving, have more care responsibilities, report a wider range of needs and stressors including emotional and physical and have much higher out-of-pocket costs (Jutkowitz et al., 2017a; Jutkowitz et al., 2017b; Moon & Dilworth-Anderson, 2015; Pinquart & Sörensen, 2003). Thus, dementia is a family affair. To assure quality of life for persons living with dementia, we must broaden our lens from a strictly medical approach focusing on the person to one that includes the family as well—it is a condition of the family. Understanding the consequences of dementia caregiving (see Chapter 5: Family Member as Care Partner) and the implications for providing families what they need, when they need it, and how they prefer to receive assistance, education, support (this chapter), is paramount. This chapter builds on the previous and discusses ways to think about providing care and services to families and the range of approaches, strategies, programs available from over 40 years of research. Our fundamental message in this chapter is that although more research is absolutely necessary for developing and/or adapting approaches that address the wide ranging needs of families, there are actions that can be taken now that would go a long way to improving dementia care and helping family caregivers.

ASSUMPTIONS FOR PROVIDING CARE AND SERVICES TO FAMILIES

We start our discussion by identifying a set of assumptions based on the research for guiding the design of care and services that can address the far ranging and changing needs of families (Feinberg, 2017; Gitlin & Hodgson, 2015). As shown in Box 6-1, the first important assumption is that the needs of families are not monolithic. They vary widely based on any number of conditions and their unique constellation including but not limited to factors associated with: the person living with dementia, their disease stage, health condition, and care needs and preferences; the living environment including the physical features of home and community as well as proximity and access to help, services, respite, and geographic location of family members; where in a caregiver's life course caregiving begins; employment status and time available for caregiving; marital status, and social network; financial resources; and own physical and emotional health and well-being, cultural considerations including family organization, decision-making, coping mechanisms, value, and beliefs including understandings of dementia. All of these factors inform what families are able to absorb and contend with, making dementia care and delivering supportive services a complex matter.

A related point is that each disease stage brings with it new challenges such that caregivers often state that they need specific knowledge and skills when they perceive they need it and not before (or after).

> **Box 6-1**
> **Ten Basic Assumptions**
>
> - Needs of families change over time
> - Needs of families differ based on a range of factors including those associated with person living with dementia, resources, living environments, at what point in the life course caregiving begins, access to care and services
> - Comprehensive assessment of a caregiver/family to evaluate their needs, preferences, values, employment status, and availability is basis for developing care plans
> - One size does not fit all
> - Tailoring to needs, circumstances, preferences, and readiness is critical
> - Repeated exposures to information and skills is important to help families learn and integrate new approaches into daily care routines
> - Learning through doing (having opportunities for guided practice) is preferred
> - Multicomponent approaches are more potent and impact multiple outcomes
> - Caregiver-centered and caregiver-directed approaches work best when providing specific knowledge and skills to address self-identified care challenges
> - There are many outcomes of importance to families over and above reducing their own distress or feelings of burden and these should be identified through systematic assessment and addressed

Thus, the timing of when to introduce specific information and strategies to be effective is critical; if too much information is provided too early, it cannot be absorbed and may not be found to be useful.

It logically follows then that one size does not fit all. That is, there will not be one single magic bullet, "pill," strategy, or program that can address all needs of all families at all stages of the disease; rather multiple strategies will need to be advanced, although a coordinated, comprehensive "package" of such strategies should be the goal. Yet another important assumption is that families need repeated exposures to information about dementia. The complexity of the disease process and often nuanced cognitive, behavioral, and functional changes can be confusing. Furthermore, some research suggests that families are able to absorb knowledge and skills more effectively by learning through doing; prescriptive or didactic approaches may be helpful for some caregivers, but most including formal caregivers, learn best through observing and then practicing specific strategies as it concerns managing complex behavioral manifestations and functional changes (Belle et al., 2006). Exposure to support over time is critical to impact certain outcomes such as being able to keep person living with dementia at home and avoid nursing home placement. However, brief support can also eliminate situational stressors as well as provide immediate knowledge and skills to address targeted problem areas identified by families. Of importance and as stated above, effective care and services must start with an assessment, and then address those needs caregivers themselves identify as critical to them at that moment in time. Strategies, approaches, and programs must match caregiver needs (Zarit, 2017). A caregiver-centered and caregiver-directed approach is most effective when trying to help families address the most pressing challenges they are managing at a given point in time. Unfortunately, there continues to be a mismatch between what caregivers may need and what programs offer. For example, although financial and physical strain are both strong predictors of risk for nursing home placement (Spillman & Long, 2009), very few tested interventions for family caregivers address these issues (Cornman-Levy, Gitlin, Corcoran, & Schinfeld, 2001). The final assumption is that there are many important outcomes that we need to achieve with our approaches, programs, services, strategies—and the importance of any one of these outcomes may vary according to the caregiver's particular needs, preferences, and personal care goals. It follows from a family-centered and directed approach that it should also be determined what caregivers themselves seek to achieve from a particular approach, service, program, e.g., what their own goals are for making life better for them and the person living with dementia. Box 6-2 lists some of the key outcomes that are of importance to families, although there is limited research that identifies outcomes families themselves seek. As we advance our understanding of the nuances of family caregiving among culturally diverse communities, other outcomes of importance will be identified.

PATHWAYS FOR SUPPORTING FAMILY CAREGIVERS

There are various pathways by which we may positively impact the outcomes for family caregivers listed in Box 6-2. Fig. 6-1 below outlines the direct and indirect pathways leading towards positive outcomes for families. It suggests that a strategy/program/service/ intervention may directly target and impact the family member(s) or alternatively, may target and impact the person living with dementia which in turn may then

> **Box 6-2**
> **Key Outcomes Valued by Caregivers**
>
> - Respite, time for self
> - Improved self-care and health
> - Reduced frustrations, upset, depression, and distress
> - Enhanced knowledge and skills
> - Aging in place at home
> - Better communication and less discord among family members
> - Improved communications and coordination with health professionals
> - Knowing how to advocate and interact with health professionals
> - Confidence managing day-to-day
> - Reduced social isolation
> - Improved well-being
> - Better balance between caregiving and other responsibilities including work
> - Flexible work opportunities/employer support
> - Knowing where to go for help and resources
> - Strong social network for instrumental and emotional support
> - Improved quality of life of person living with dementia

indirectly benefit the caregiver or both pathways may be the preferred approach, that is impacting both caregivers and persons with dementia with gains in one positively leading to improvements in the other.

There is scant evidence to indicate which pathway is most impactful and for which types of outcomes and families as well as for which disease stage or etiology. Some evidence and perhaps common sense suggests that if the primary desired outcome is a reduction in depressive symptoms in a family caregiver, then a program directed at the caregiver may be most effective such as offering counseling, instruction in coping strategies, or implementation of other evidence-based depression approaches. However, if the source of depression is from being overwhelmed by caregiving responsibilities, it may be that reducing physical and emotional care burdens impacts mood.

In turn, if the desired outcome for a caregiver is to obtain more time for him/herself, then targeting the person living with dementia by for example the use of adult day services may be the pathway that is most effective in providing respite. Impacting both the caregiver and person with dementia (dyadic focus) in turn may be most effective if desired outcomes are dual fold. For example, a goal may be to both reduce and manage challenging behaviors of the person living with dementia and the upset of the caregiver. The pathway being considered to evince

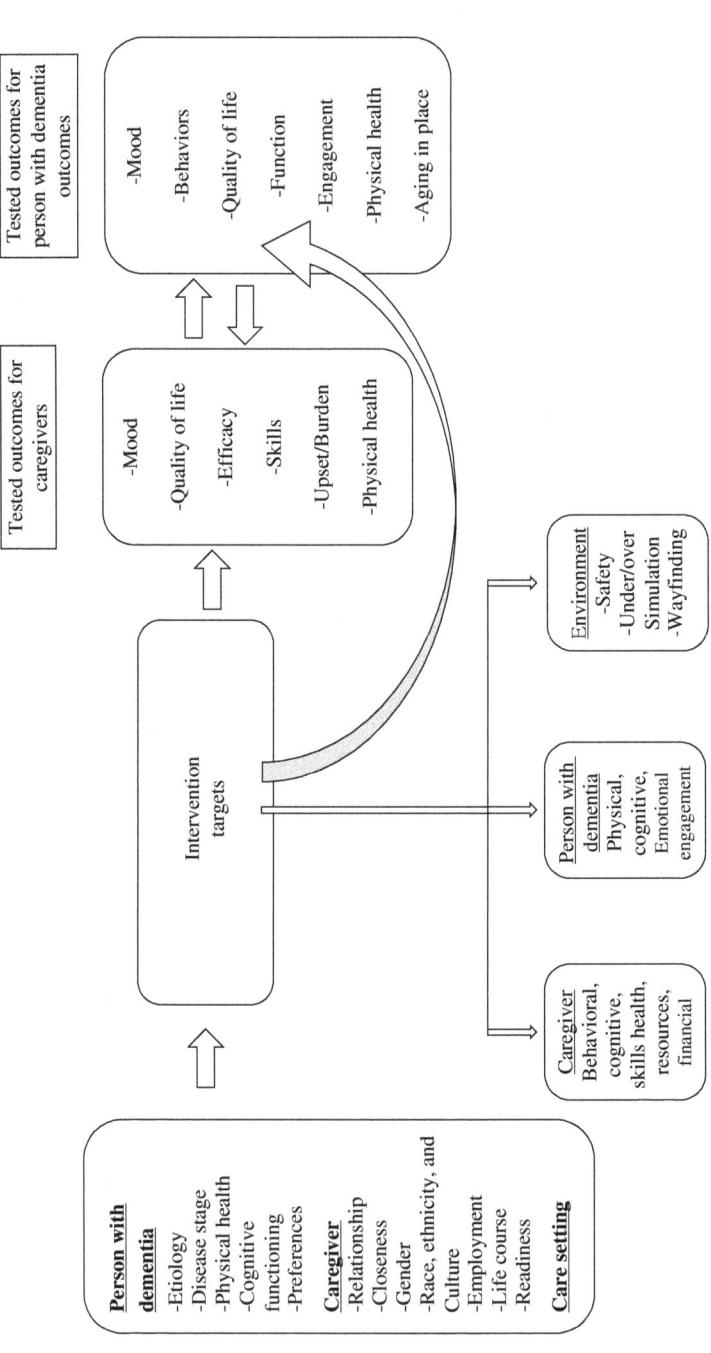

FIGURE 6-1 Direct and indirect pathways for supporting family caregivers and persons living with dementia. Adapted from Gitlin L.N., & Hodgson N. (2015). Caregivers as therapeutic agents in dementia care: The evidence-base for interventions supporting their role. In J.E. Gaugler, & R.L. Kane (Eds.), Family caregiving in the new normal (pp. 305–356). San Diego: Academic Press.

a particular outcome should be explicitly articulated in order to assure efficiency in intervention delivery and to maximize impact(s).

LOOKING BACKWARDS TO MOVE FORWARD

To date, in the United States, there is not a systematic uniform approach to identifying caregivers and providing families with education and support in care settings in which they interact including primary care, social services, clinics, or community-based programs directed towards older adults (e.g., senior centers and adult day services). Nevertheless, there has been over 40 years of research developing and evaluating caregiver interventions. It is helpful to reflect upon the history of caregiver intervention research as looking backwards can inform what we know works and how best to move forward. A look backwards reveals that there are in fact many proven approaches that could be helpful to families, yet they have not been widely implemented or accessible to families. An immediate goal should be to scale these interventions for widespread implementation, determine the payment model, and integrate them into different medical and service settings (Gitlin, Marx, Stanley, & Hodgson, 2015). We return to this point later on in this chapter.

Caregiver intervention research over these past 40 plus years can be categorized as representing four overlapping phases, each building on the other chronologically, and demonstrating increasing methodological sophistication and better outcomes (Callahan, Kales, Gitlin, & Lyketsos, 2013). The first wave of caregiver interventions (roughly between 1960s and early 1990s) mostly focused on providing families with education, coping strategies, and respite to reduce caregiver distress and avoid or delay nursing home placement. Findings from these initial studies, taken as a whole, yielded mixed results with small to no benefits reported (Knight, Lutzky, & Macofsky-Urban, 1993). Many lessons were learned from this initial foray including that individualized approaches tended to yield better outcomes than groups, interventions were poorly characterized precluding replication, fidelity was not assessed making it difficult to discern if implementation was consistent and as intended, samples were homogeneous (mostly spouses), and outcome measures were typically distal from the intent or content of interventions and too global (Callahan et al., 2013; Pruchno & Gitlin, 2012).

A discernable second wave of intervention studies (from early 1990s to late 2000s) followed with these studies employing more rigorous trial designs and yielding better outcomes. Yet limitations of this corpus included homogenous samples, inadequate characterization of delivery characteristics and oversight of implementation from a fidelity perspective and a continued focus on stress and burden, nursing home placement, and caregiving at the moderate stage of dementia. The next wave of randomized controlled studies (late 1990s to early 2000s) was even more robust and began to involve diverse study samples (mostly white, African American, and Latino caregivers). A key outcome of interest at this stage was reducing nursing home placement with the New York University Caregiver Intervention (Mittelman, Ferris, Shulman, Steinberg, & Levin, 1996), being one of the first trials to show significant reductions in placement and hence cost savings.

Meta-analyses began to emerge showing that intervention benefits could be achieved although effect sizes were small (Pinquart & Sörensen, 2006). Emerging in this historic period was the National Institute of Health supported Resources for Enhancing Alzheimer's Caregiver Health (REACH I) initiative. This initiative was developed to try to determine definitively which approach could benefit caregivers most. REACH I involved six different interventions ranging from psycho-educational group and individual counseling, skills training in behavioral management and problem-solving, technology-based education, environmental modification, and supportive programs (Gitlin et al., 2003). Each site included its own outcome measures specific to its intervention focus and also shared a core battery of measures in order to compare outcomes of interventions across sites using common metrics. There were important design improvements from previous studies such that the REACH initiative (I and II) sets a new methodological bar for caregiver intervention studies. This included for example attending to and documenting fidelity, standardizing treatment manuals and training, and documentation of implementation processes. The interventions demonstrated different outcomes among diverse families (white, African American, and Latino) including improvements in skills, mastery, efficacy, and well-being. Taken as a whole and using a meta-analytic approach, the interventions showed significant reductions in caregiver upset with behavioral symptoms but not caregiver depression or delay in nursing home placement (Gitlin et al., 2003). REACH I was followed by REACH II which involved testing a multicomponent intervention which included the essential active components of the previous six site-specific interventions. Improvements included a tailoring approach based on a systematic assessment of a caregiver's risk profile and needs (Czaja et al., 2009). Findings showed positive benefits in a quality of life construct for Latino, white, and spousal African American caregivers, reduced prevalence of depression but no statistically significant differences in nursing home placement rates at 6 months (Belle et al., 2003; Belle et al., 2006). Still, the intervention focused on moderate stage dementia and used an overarching stress process model with main outcomes focusing on deficit reductions.

Finally, a fourth, more current discernable phase of intervention development is now underway (roughly 2006 to present). In this current phase, novel approaches are being developed to address caregiver needs across the disease continuum from early stage to end of life. These approaches include but are not limited to evaluating care management models (Callahan et al., 2011), community-based care management models (Bass et al., 2013; Samus et al., 2014), technologies for delivering programs (Czaja, Loewenstein, Schulz, Nair, & Perdomo, 2013), adapting existing evidence-based programs for different populations, cultural and linguistic groups (Gaugler, Reese, & Mittelman, 2013), developing interventions to address a wider range of outcomes than that previously considered (see Box 6-2), advancing interventions using a usability perspective or one in which end users and stakeholders are integral to the process of developing the intervention (Gitlin & Czaja, 2015; Onken, Carroll, Shoham, Cuthbert, & Riddle, 2014), and developing interventions for specific clinical sites (Wolff et al., 2017).

BEGIN WITH ASSESSMENT

As the needs of families differ depending upon a wide range of circumstances, factors, and time, assessment is the first step for providing any type and level of support to caregivers (Feinberg, 2003).

A comprehensive definition of assessment is as follows:

"...a systematic process of gathering information about a caregiving situation to identify the specific problems, needs, strengths, and resources of the family caregiver, as well as the ability of the caregiver to contribute to the needs of the care recipient. Effectively assessing and addressing caregiver needs can maintain the health and well-being of caregivers, sustain their ability to provide care, prevent or postpone nursing home placement, and produce better outcomes for the care recipient" (Feinberg & Houser, 2012).

Key to this definition is the term "systematic" in which information is captured uniformly, purposefully, and thoroughly to understand caregiver needs and ways to address them. As per our discussion in Chapter 5, Family Member as Care Partner, various studies assessing unmet needs of caregivers suggest that most caregivers report one or more unmet needs for themselves and that of the person living with dementia (Black et al., 2013), with needs changing and escalating with disease progression (Hodgson, Gitlin, Winter, & Hauck, 2013). Most report on the needs of caregivers in the United States and elsewhere (Dimakopoulou, Sakka, Efthymiou, Karpathiou, & Karydaki, 2015) suggest that families need education about the disease and seek skills for managing functional decline and behavioral symptoms as well as assuring home safety. Additionally, studies highlight the need of a substantial number of caregivers for mental health attention and addressing their own health problems.

While various needs assessments are used in research studies, few have been evaluated specifically for their psychometric properties or validated for use with different family caregivers. Nevertheless, there are assessments available for use and a few exemplars are shown in Table 6-1.

As suggested in Table 6-1, most existing assessment tools are general, addressing a wide range of areas of need and not dementia-specific. The few dementia-specific assessment tools tend to address select areas of need and target mostly families caring for individuals with moderate dementia. Although not shown in Table 6-1, assessment tools are currently being advanced as part of care coordination models. Although not readily accessible to agencies or clinical arenas, they are quite promising with a few being developed for electronic data capture (Samus et al., 2014). Furthermore, assessments used in research studies to capture needs are also helpful and can potentially be adopted for integration in clinical settings (Bass et al., 2013; Black et al., 2013; Bangerter, Griffin, Zarit, & Havyer, 2017). There is much room for research development in this area to advance tools that are brief, well validated, and that can be used in various clinical and social service contexts and are applicable to diverse family caregivers and contexts of care. Feinberg's insights in 2003 remain relevant today:

> "Because support for family caregivers is an emerging area of debate in long-term care, there is no consensus on a consistent approach to assessing family care or on what should be included in a comprehensive caregiver assessment tool. The complexities of caregiving and the varied tasks performed, however, make the case for implementing caregiver assessment as part of long-term care policy and practice." (Feinberg, 2003, p. 21).

When and where should assessment occur? Assessment should occur at any time when there is an expectation that a family member is needed to participate in the support or care of a person living with dementia. This may be at the time that a diagnosis is shared with the family and thereafter with continuous medical monitoring or with any change in the status of the caregiver or the person living with dementia. It can occur in all care and clinical settings, including the physician's office, upon hospital and rehabilitation admission and discharge, and in nursing homes and assisted living facilities in addition to social service settings (adult day, senior centers, Medicaid Waiver programs, Managed Care, and so forth).

TABLE 6-1 Exemplar Caregiver Assessments

Assessment name	Domains assessed	Item description
American Medical Association (AMA). Caregiver Self-Assessment [online]. Available at http://web.mit.edu/workplacecenter/hndbk/docs/questionnaire.pdf. Accessed August 23, 2017.	Not dementia specific Caregiver stress and depression	18-items. Caregivers are asked to respond either "Yes" or "No" to a series of statements For Item 17, family caregivers are asked to rate their level of stress on a 1–10 basis. For Item 18, they are asked to rate their perception of their current health in comparison to their health 1 year ago.
California Caregiver Resource Centers. Uniform Assessment Tool [online]. Available at https://www.caregiver.org/sites/caregiver.org/files/pdfs/tk_california_assessment_tool.pdf. Accessed August 23, 2017.	Includes items specific to dementia caregiving 1. Demographic information of caregivers and care receivers (such as marital status and income); 2. Caregiver characteristics (such as work status, health, level of burden, depression score, relationship to care receiver, hours per week of caregiving, and hours of unpaid help received weekly from others); and 3. Care receiver characteristics (such as behavioral and functional problems).	11 items and also incorporates other scales such as the Revised Memory and Problem Behavior Checklist (Teri et al., 1992).

(Continued)

TABLE 6-1 (Continued)

Assessment name	Domains assessed	Item description
The C.A.R.E. Tool (C.A.R.E. = Caregiver's Aspirations, Realities, and Expectations) Keefe, Guberman, Fancey, Barylak, & Nahmiash (2008)	Not dementia-specific. Areas of assessment include physical care, housework, supervision/support, crisis planning, and future planning.	The CARE Tool contains 10 main sections. Each section of the CARE Tool enables caregivers to express their feelings related to caregiving and contextualize the caregiving experience in their own words. Specific definitions and guidelines accompany each section of the tool to guide practitioners' interpretation of the information received and to ensure that the tool accurately identifies caregivers' needs. In the summary section of the tool, practitioners are instructed to indicate levels of caregiver difficulty in 15 identified areas related to the caregiving situation, rated on a scale of 1 (little or no difficulty) to 4 (extreme difficulty).
Minnesota Long-Term Care Consultation Services Assessment Form Minnesota Department of Human Services. Available at https://www.bluecrossmn.com/carecoordination/public/6_25_ltcc_assessment_dhs.pdf. Accessed on August 23, 2017.	Addresses work status, care burden, services and support, and health domains.	13 domains are covered with multiple questions in each.
Perceived Change for the Better Index Aravena, Albala, & Gitlin (2017) Gitlin, Winter, Dennis, & Hauck (2006)	Validated brief index specific to dementia caregiving which identifies areas improving or worsening from which to target support.	13-items reflecting three domains: management of dementia; affective well-being and somatic concerns. Caregivers indicate for each item whether it is getting worse, staying the same, or improving.

REACH II Risk Appraisal Measure Czaja et al. (2009)	Specific to moderate dementia Depression, burden, self-care and health behaviors, social support, safety, and patient problem behaviors	16-items that indicate areas of risk for which the caregiver could benefit from intervention
Rosalynn Carter Institute for Caregiving. Family Caregiver Assessment. Available at http://www.rosalynncarter.org/UserFiles/File/RCI_FCA.pdf. Accessed on August 23, 2017.	Not specific to dementia Burden, unmet needs, support, caregiving challenges.	The Rosalynn Carter Institute Family Caregiver Assessment is an instrument specifically designed to assess the psychosocial needs of family caregivers. It should be used by professionals providing services or assistance to families in which there are persons with serious illnesses or disabilities. There are two sections: basic screening details about the caregiver and person being cared for; and type of supports available to caregiver as well as their level of burden and needs.
Washington State. CARE Tool. Available at https://www.caregiver.org/sites/caregiver.org/files/pdfs/tk_washington_assessment_tool.pdf. Accessed on August 23, 2017.	Obtains information about caregiver, support services, stress barriers, and relationship strain/burden.	18 items which is part of a Washington State comprehensive assessment tool.

Assessment can take the form of a simple question or a set of questions, a brief or long interview to evaluate areas of risk, well-being, knowledge and needs, and whether the caregiver is able to participate in the care that is being expected by the clinical care setting. The type of assessment will depend upon clinical context in which it is being conducted (at hospital discharge, intake for adult day), the purpose of the assessment (to assess caregiver well-being and support needs or to assess capabilities of carrying out a specific care task such as wound care or medication dispensing), who administers the assessment (nurse, psychologist, occupational therapist (OT), and physician assistant), time available for the assessment, and how the information obtained will be used (to help family derive an action plan, plan for the future, or address immediate unmet needs).

For example, asking a straightforward question about how a family caregiver is doing in a physician's office can be critical for deriving an understanding of the family context of a patient with dementia (Gitlin & Hodgson, 2016). A common objection of caregivers is that health and human service professionals (either their own physician, that of the person they care for or other providers) do not ask them how they are doing, what they do, and what help they may need to assure their continued well-being and that of the person living with dementia (Schulz & Eden, 2016). Asking a caregiver how he/she is doing, and then providing reassurance, support, education, and referral can have a positive impact. Also, asking about care responsibilities, sources of support and assistance, and how he/she is managing and their own health and stress are important follow-up questions. A simple intervention based on these questions might be to help the caregiver find ways to obtain respite, take care of their own health, and to make recommendations to connect with local resources (e.g., the Alzheimer's Association, adult day services, the National Family Caregiver Support Program offered by the local Area Agency on Aging). This should be the fundamental, minimum that any clinical, health care, or social service setting could engage in as well as other organizations in contact with families including community-based villages, faith-based organizations, senior centers, and so forth.

From a family-centered dementia care perspective, asking how the caregiver of a person living with dementia is faring and about his or her immediate needs is the only ethical and moral stance that a clinician or health and human service professional can assume (Barnard & Yaffe, 2014; Cohen, 2000; Gitlin & Hodgson, 2016). These simple questions are important not only to determine the well-being of the caregiver but also to evaluate whether the person living with dementia is at risk and needs additional supports. As the caregiver's poor health can pose a risk to the person living with dementia, asking can be considered a moral obligation of any clinician to assure the safety and well-being of the person living with dementia who is their patient or client.

As will be discussed below, many different caregiver support programs have been developed, evaluated, and found to effectively support family caregivers. Most of these tested programs begin by taking stock of who the caregiver is, their needs, and the care context, and then tailoring the intervention/strategies/treatment plan by targeting solutions to the identified care challenges. While this approach is a mainstay of multicomponent tailored interventions, the needs assessments used, with the exception of the REACH Risk Appraisal Measure (Czaja et al., 2009), have not been validated or published for use by others independently of the intervention/program itself; nevertheless, as they cause.

EVIDENCE-BASED APPROACHES: WHAT WORKS?

So given this evolving history of caregiver intervention research, what works and what lessons have we learned? Systematic reviews and meta-analyses have been conducted to summarize the many intervention studies published over the past 10 years. A review of reviews shows a total of 7 meta-analyses and 17 systematic reviews ($n = 24$) of randomized controlled trials (RCTs) published between 1966 and 2013. Since then other systematic reviews as well have been generated. Taken as a whole, sample sizes across studies included in these reviews ranged from 4 to 8095, an average of 50 caregivers per study. Although reviews often included the same trials, we estimate that there were 200 unique caregiver programs tested (Gitlin & Hodgson, 2015).

Although there is not an agreed-upon classification of or way to group tested interventions into meaningful categories, we identify six broad types outlined in Box 6-3.

Box 6-3
Types of Caregiver Interventions

- Professional support (counseling, depression therapies)
- Care management
- Psychoeducation
- Skills training (Behavioral management)
- Psychotherapy
- Self-care/relaxation training
- Multicomponent (combination of above)

The primary outcomes of this corpus of studies mostly focused on caregiver's knowledge, burden, self-efficacy, psychological morbidity (anxiety/depression), and with regard to the person with dementia, behavioral symptoms, functional dependence, and time to nursing home placement.

Programs can be further categorized as being "general" or "targeted" (Gitlin, Kales, Lyketsos, 2012). A general caregiver program typically provides education, and coping strategies and other needed skills; Savvy is an example of this approach (Griffiths, Whitney, Kovaleva, & Hepburn, 2016; Hepburn, Tornatore, Center, & Ostwald, 2001; Hepburn, Lewis, Sherman, & Tornatore, 2003). A targeted program typically focuses on a particular problem area such as caregiver depression, caregiver lack of sleep) or a particular care challenge (managing behavioral symptoms). Project ACT with its focus on providing caregivers specific knowledge and skills for managing caregiver-identified behavioral symptoms of the person living with dementia is an example of a targeted approach (Gitlin, Winter, Dennis, Hodgson, & Hauck, 2010a). Some programs use a combination of a generalized and targeted approach such as the REACH II (Belle et al., 2006) or COPE programs (Gitlin, Winter, Dennis, Hodgson, & Hauck, 2010b).

Table 6-2 summarizes the effectiveness of interventions that have been evaluated in systematic reviews and meta-analyses and per the key outcomes reported in these studies (Gitlin & Hodgson, 2015). As shown, the average pooled effect size (d) of interventions was relatively modest although benefits are certainly demonstrated. Taken together, multicomponent interventions or approaches that address multiple

TABLE 6-2 Average Pooled Effect Sizes Across Reviews (d)

Outcome	Pooled effect sizes
Reducing caregiver burden	Range of 0.01–0.52, with multicomponent interventions showing the largest effect for this outcome.
Improving caregiver knowledge	Range of 0.05–0.51 with interventions providing caregiver education showing the largest effect
Reducing caregiver anxiety	Range of 0.16–0.50 with relaxation training showing the largest benefit.
Reducing caregiver depression	Range of 0.31–0.68 with psychoeducation approaches demonstrating the largest benefit.
Delaying time to nursing home placement	Average effect (odds ratio; OR) was in the range of 0.43–0.99 (mean OR = 0.66) with multicomponent interventions and those involving individual and family counseling having the largest benefit.

concerns and areas (e.g., education, skills, or stress reduction) appear to have the largest effects.

Of importance is that studies do not report that the interventions being tested result in any adverse effects. A study evaluating a cognitive–behavioral intervention found negative outcomes such that both intervention and control groups declined similarly over time (Chang, 1999); negative outcomes for burden were also reported in Schoenmakers, Buntinx, and DeLepeleire's (2010) study on respite care. Yet, a significant limitation of this body of research is that most interventions/programs target family caregivers of persons living with moderate to severe dementia with few focusing on early stage and end-of-life or including families from diverse race/ethnic backgrounds. This is problematic in that research clearly shows that families begin to experience anxiety and depression early on and could benefit from education and how to prepare for the future; also families continue to need support even if the person with dementia resides in assisted living or nursing homes. Attention to the development and evaluation of approaches across the disease trajectory is an important research direction. However, Fig. 6-2 displays the potential care and services that family caregivers may benefit from at each disease stage based on evidence as to the unmet needs typically encountered by family caregivers.

EXEMPLARS

It is not possible to list or summarize the over 200 and growing proven caregiver interventions. In Table 6-3, we list a few select and promising interventions that were previously tested in clinical randomized trials, shown to be effective on various measured outcomes, and which are now being translated and evaluated for their implementation in different clinic, health system, or web-based contexts. Note, however, this is not an exhaustive table and many efforts are currently underway to move proven programs into real-world contexts (Feinberg, 2017). This remains a moving target so to speak without yet a centralized location for families, clinicians, and agencies to learn about proven approaches.

The interventions listed in Table 6-3 mostly focus on families providing hands-on care for persons at the moderate disease stage. Shared components typically include education about dementia and behavioral symptoms, positive coping and stress reduction techniques, problem solving and brainstorming, referrals to local resources, validation, and support.

Here we describe three exemplar programs that are currently being evaluated to illustrate the differential delivery characteristics of

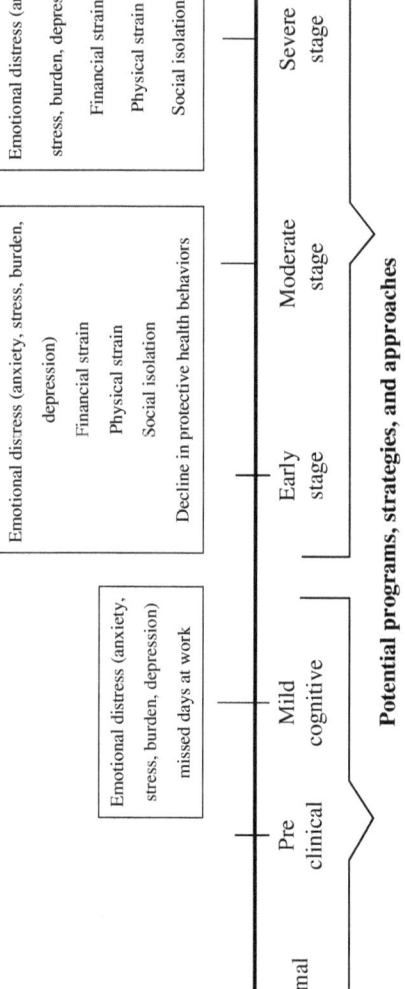
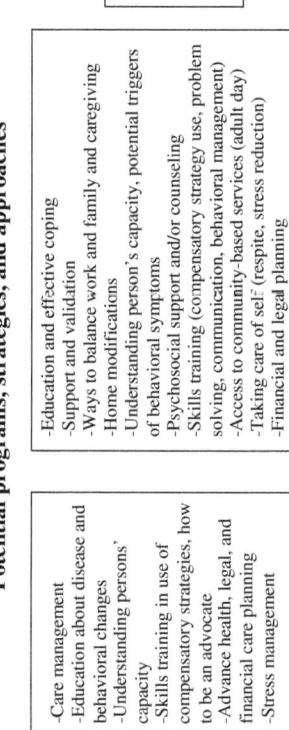

FIGURE 6-2 Clinical trajectory of dementia, potential consequences of caregiving, and strategies for supporting families.

TABLE 6-3 Select Caregiver Interventions Tested in RCTs and Being Translated for Widespread Dissemination

Program	Targeted population	Interventionists	Number of sessions/duration	Description	Key outcomes
COPE (Gitlin et al., 2010a)	Persons living with dementia and family caregivers	Occupational therapist (10 sessions) and Advance Practice Nurse (1 face-to-face, 1 telephone session)	Up to 12 sessions over 4 months	The COPE program sought to support capabilities of persons with dementia by reducing environmental stressors and enhancing caregiver skills. Training in problem solving, communication, engaging persons in activities, and simplifying tasks and environments was tailored to address caregiver identified concerns and patient capabilities. OTs also conducted cognitive and functional testing to identify strengths and deficits in attention, initiation and perseveration, construction, conceptualization, and memory of person with dementia, the readiness and stress of caregivers, and level of safety, clutter of environment.	Person with dementia: Functional dependence, quality of life, frequency of agitated behaviors, and engagement for patients Caregivers: well-being, confidence using activities, and ability to keep person at home.
MIND (Samus et al., 2014)	Persons living with dementia or cognitive disorder and a "study partner" willing to participate in all visits	Interdisciplinary care team comprising nonclinical community workers (coordinators) linked to an RN and a geriatric psychiatrist.	18 months of care coordination with a median of five in-person visits and 21 phone contacts	The manualized care coordination protocol consisted of four key components: identification of needs and individualized care planning to match the priorities and preferences of the patient and family; provision of dementia education and skill-building strategies; coordination, referral, and linkage to services; and care monitoring. Care components are individually tailored to current unmet needs and updated based on emergent needs of participants and caregivers.	Primary outcomes: time to transfer out of the home; unmet care needs. Secondary outcomes: quality of life of caregiver, person with dementia, behavioral symptoms, and depression of persons with dementia.

(Continued)

TABLE 6-3 (Continued)

Program	Targeted population	Interventionists	Number of sessions/duration	Description	Key outcomes
Mittelman NYU Caregiver Intervention (Mittelman et al., 1993)	Spouses caring for a person with dementia	Counselors with advanced degrees in Social Work or allied professions	Two individual/four family counseling sessions in first 4 months; Participation in weekly support group and ad hoc counseling	• Two individual counseling sessions tailored to each caregiver's specific situation • Four family counseling sessions with the primary caregiver and family members selected by that caregiver • Participation in a weekly support group • Ad hoc counseling	Studies of the NYU Spouse–Caregiver have looked at caregiver depression, appraisal of behavior problems, and time to nursing home placement.
Partners in Dementia Care (PDC) (Bass et al., 2014)	Caregivers of veterans with dementia living in the community	Two half-time care coordinators and two part-time care coordinator assistants delivered at each intervention site. The two care coordinators and assistants worked as a team, with one shared electronic care coordination information system.	Ongoing, initial assessment first 4 weeks of enrollment; action plan taking weeks or months; ongoing monitoring up to 20 contacts over 12 months, with reassessment every 6 months	Partners in Dementia Care is a coaching model driven by consumer choice, with care coordinators helping find solutions to concerns that are the priorities of veterans and caregivers. PDC followed a set of standardized protocol that required a minimum of one contact between care coordinators and consumers per month; more frequent contacts occurred as needed. The protocol also required care coordinators to discuss with veterans or caregivers a broad range of medical and nonmedical concerns, although the specific content of assistance was customized for consumers' preferences and needs.	Caregiver perception of unmet needs; strains in role captivity, physical health strain, and relationship strain; depression; and number of support resources.

Project ACT (Gitlin, Winter, Dennis, & Hauck, 2007)	Stressed family caregivers providing in-home care to persons with moderate stage dementia with behavioral symptoms	OT and Advanced Practice Nurse (NU)	14 sessions over 6 months	• Three initial assessment visits by OT/NU • Eight skills building sessions with OT • Three telephone maintenance of skills calls A nonpharmacological home-based intervention that modifies the environment and other potential behavioral triggers to reduce the frequency of occurrence of targeted behaviors and associated caregiver distress.	Primary patient outcome was frequency of the problem behavior targeted by caregivers as most distressful to them. Primary caregiver outcomes included caregiver upset with and confidence in managing the target problem behavior.
REACH II (Belle et al., 2006)	Caregivers and their care recipients With Alzheimer disease or related disorders	Intensively trained interventionists, with robust monitoring and review	12 in-home and telephone sessions over 6 months	• 9 in-home sessions for 1.5 hours • 3 half-hour telephone sessions • 5 structured telephone support group sessions The REACH II intervention was designed to maximize outcomes by systematically targeting several problem areas, tailoring the intervention to respond to the needs of each individual, and actively engaging the caregiver in the intervention process.	The primary outcome was a quality-of-life indicator comprising measures of 6-month caregiver depression, burden, self-care, and social support and care recipient problem behaviors. Secondary outcomes were the prevalence of caregiver clinical depression and institutional placement of care

(Continued)

TABLE 6-3 (Continued)

Program	Targeted population	Interventionists	Number of sessions/duration	Description	Key outcomes
REACH II Adapted (REACH VA) (Nichols, Martindale-Adams, Burns, Graney, & Zuber, 2011)	Stressed caregivers of patients with dementia	Clinical staff members from 24 VA Medical Center Home-Based Primary Care programs in 15 states	12 in-home and telephone sessions over 6 months	• Nine in-home sessions for 1 hour • Three half-hour telephone sessions • Five 1-hour structured telephone support group sessions There were three differences in implementation from REACH II to REACH VA. First, computer-assisted screen telephones were not used in REACH VA due to expense. Second, for REACH VA, because the interventionists were located at multiple facilities and would not always have access to dementia experts, all behavioral strategies were listed in a caregiver notebook. Third, the 21-item REACH VA risk appraisal, a component of overall risk assessment, was streamlined from the 51-item REACH II risk appraisal.	Caregiver outcomes included differences between baseline and 6-month follow-up for measures of caregiving risk. Clinical variables included burden, depression, health, health behaviors, and number of and bother with care recipient behaviors. Caregiving variables included safety, social support, caregiving difficulties, caregiving frustrations, daily time spent on duty, and daily time spent providing actual care. recipients at 6-month follow-up.
Savvy (Hepburn et al., 2003)	Family and professional caregivers	Trained workshop facilitator as guided by a trainer's manual	Six 2-hour sessions over 6 weeks	The program focuses on helping caregivers think about their situation objectively and providing them with the knowledge, skills, and attitudes they need	Caregiver relational deprivation, role captivity, competence,

STAR-C (Teri, McCurry, Logsdon, & Gibbons, 2005)	Family caregivers and care recipients with AD	Consultants were master-level health care professionals	Eight weekly sessions followed by four monthly phone calls	Consultants conducted training with caregivers to ensure that they could talk freely without frequent interruptions or fear of upsetting the persons for whom they were providing care. First three treatment sessions focused on teaching caregivers the rationale and use of the ABC problem-solving approach to behavior change. Subsequent sessions focused on improving caregiver communication, increasing pleasant events as a means to improve care recipients' mood, and developing strategies to enhance caregiver support. Monthly follow-up calls reinforced behavior management, communication, and caregiver support strategies for new problems.	to manage stress and carry out the caregiving role effectively. Caregiver depression; sleep quality; stress and burden; feelings of competence Person with dementia; behavioral disturbance; quality of life

mastery, loss of self, and distress.

programs and how they are being implemented in three different contexts: the home (COPE), an agency (Adult Day Service Plus), and via an online web-based application (WeCareAdvisor).

Home-based Program: The COPE program (Care of Persons with Dementia in their Environments) includes these elements and goes one step further. It involves up to 10 sessions conducted by an advance practice nurse (2 sessions) and an occupational therapist (8 sessions) over 4 months. Occupational therapists initially interview caregivers to identify participant routines, previous and current roles, habits and interests, and to identify challenging care concerns that families want to address. The occupational therapist also conducts cognitive and functional performance tests to identify capacities and deficits in cognitive functioning, including attention, initiation/perseveration, construction, conceptualization, memory, planning, and problem solving, as well as in physical functioning, including fall risks and mobility performance of persons living with dementia. The OTs then provide to and review with caregivers a written report that summarizes assessment results. This provides caregivers an important understanding of the preserved abilities of persons living with dementia versus only learning about what persons can no longer be performed. Based on this understanding, caregivers are provided specific strategies to address the areas that they self-identify and prioritize as most challenging. Strategies may include ways to modify home environments, simplify daily activities, and communicate effectively to support participant capabilities, use problem-solving to identify solutions for caregiver-identified concerns (e.g., behavioral challenges, difficulties managing patient self-care), and use stress reduction techniques to lower their own distress. For each targeted concern jointly identified by caregivers and OTs, a written plan as part of the clinical trial protocol, referred to as a "COPE prescription" is devised describing treatment goals, participant capacities, and specific strategies for the caregiver to implement.

In a separate home visit, the nurse provides caregivers with information to help them identify and monitor common health-related concerns (pain detection, hydration, constipation, and medication management). In addition, the nurse works with the caregiver to help them become effective medical advocates and introduces advance care planning and the importance of them taking care of themselves. The nurse also obtains blood/urine samples from persons with dementia, and assesses for signs of pain and dehydration. Laboratory evaluations include complete blood count, blood chemistry, and thyroid testing of serum samples, and culture and sensitivity of urine samples. Medications are also reviewed for polypharmacy and dosing appropriateness. The purpose of these clinical tests is to rule out underlying medical conditions, infections, or medication issues that may be negatively contributing to functioning and behavioral symptoms at home. The nurse informs caregivers by telephone of laboratory results within 48 hours and mails two copies of the results to caregivers (one for their records and the other copy to share with participants' physicians). For positive laboratory results, the nurse faxes results to the physician (upon caregiver agreement as part of the Consenting process) and discusses with them directly. All COPE dyads receive exposure to each treatment component (clinical interview and assessments, home safety check and recommendations, education, support, targeting three to five caregiver challenges, tailored strategies for caregiver identified problem areas, nurse assessment, and education). Specific issues discussed and COPE prescriptions devised are tailored to address each caregiver's self-identified concerns, participant capabilities, and home environmental factors. In addition to laboratory results, results from the assessments conducted by the OT and the COPE prescriptions are provided in written documents. Box 6-4

Box 6-4
Case Example of COPE Program—How It Works

Background: Mrs. B, an 85 year old African-American with moderate dementia, lives with her daughter. She exhibits challenging behavioral symptoms (resistance to care, pacing, repetitive vocalizations, shadowing and high anxiety) and is dependent in dressing and grooming. She sits in front of the TV most days and is disengaged. The daughter is worried about her mother's quality of life and she is afraid to leave the home to shop or go to her part-time job. Prescribed medications have not decreased her mother's behaviors and she had side effects. The daughter had high readiness to try new strategies and wanted to work on her mother's anxiety, resistance to bathing, and lack of activity in the COPE program. **COPE Program**: Based on assessments (sessions 1–2), the OT identified that Mrs. B is able to follow simple verbal cues, respond to visual cues, has good upper body strength and endurance and can participate in simply activities for up to 30 minutes. The OT observes that the daughter's communications are too complex, the home is cluttered, and the tub is slippery. The OT also discerns that Mrs. B was previously a homemaker, involved in her church and enjoyed cooking. The nurse found no underlying medical infections but expressed concern about polypharmacy and the possibility of pain when

continued

Box 6-4 (cont'd)
Mrs. B ambulated. The nurse (sessions 3–4) showed the daughter how to detect pain and reviewed questions to ask her mother's physician. The OT (sessions 5–12) next provided the daughter with education about dementia, how her mother's behaviors and functional changes are a consequence of disease (vs. intention), and techniques to reduce her own stress. Different activities were developed graded to her mother's interests and abilities and the daughter was taught how to help Mrs. B initiate and participate in them. The OT helped the daughter remove unnecessary objects from the bathroom and helped her to secure bathroom equipment (grab bar, tub bench and hand-held shower). The OT modeled verbal and tactile cueing and trained the daughter how to bring Mrs. B to the shower and sit her on the tub bench. **Outcomes**: By 4-months, the daughter reported more time to herself, less distress, and increased pleasure and engagement in activities by Mrs. B. Her anxiety was reduced and she was less resistant to bathing. The daughter used better communication and simplification strategies resulting in Mrs. B's greater independence in other activities of living. She also met with Mrs. B's doctor to review medications and evaluate her ambulation. The daughter was more hopeful about continuing to care for her mother and keeping her at home.

presents a case from the COPE trial illustrating its approach and outcomes.

The COPE program was initially tested in a randomized trial which showed that at 4 months COPE resulted in statistically significant reductions in functional disability, targeted challenging behaviors, and improved caregiver wellbeing. At 9 months caregivers in the COPE program compared to an education-only control group were more likely to report being able to keep their family member at home, improved quality of life for that person, and greater confidence in their abilities to manage day-to-day (Gitlin et al., 2010b; Hodgson et al., 2013). COPE is now being evaluated in community-based and Medicaid Waiver programs in Connecticut (Fortinsky et al., 2016).

Community-based Program: The Adult Day Service Plus (ADS Plus) program provides family caregivers of older adults with dementia enrolled in ADS with education, skills, referrals, support, and approaches for taking care of themselves. This 12-month program can be delivered by any staff member of an adult day service with experience working with families. In the first 3 months of the program, staff work with caregivers in person on site for up to eight sessions to identify their care challenges and provide specific, easy-to-use strategies at home. Similar to COPE, family caregivers learn problem solving and simplification strategies (how to simplify communications and the home environment) to support daily functioning of the ADS older adult client. After 3 months, staff check in with the caregiver every other week for the next 3 months to see how they are doing, if new care challenges have emerged, and to provide additional strategies when needed. Between 6 and 12 months, staff continue to check in with caregivers once a month to evaluate if new care challenges have emerged and how to address them, and provide ongoing support and validation. All sessions are either on site when a family member drops off or picks up the ADS client for whom they care. ADS Plus provides a safety net for caregivers who can schedule appointments as needed and as care challenges emerge. An initial pilot in three settings showed significant reductions in nursing home placement, more days using ADS and reduced caregiver distress. We showed that via regular, structured contact with family members by a designated ADS staff member, ADS Plus effectively addresses the diverse and ongoing needs of caregivers of ADS client with dementia and complex conditions (Gitlin et al., 2006; Reever, Mathieu, Dennis, & Gitlin, 2004).

In both the COPE and ADS Plus programs, key common lessons caregivers learn through discussion, demonstrations, hands-on practicing are shown in Table 6-4.

The findings from this pilot have led to the development and testing of a larger scale pragmatic trial, funded by the National Institute on Aging, which involves over 30 ADS organizations nationally throughout the United States. This new trial, led by Drs. Gitlin and Gaugler (University of Minnesota), will also serve as a model for how to augment aging services with a systematic caregiver-focused supportive program in order to optimize benefits of the program for both the older adult client and family caregiver.

Web-based Program: Caregivers' comfort with and interest in technology and technology-based tools suggest that interventions delivering customized and evidence-based recommendations in real-time may be effective using this modality. Using technology to deliver strategies and support on demand may be of particular relevance to families and formal caregivers who are managing behavioral symptoms in persons living with dementias in real time, as it can provide strategies on demand support (Werner et al., 2017). Recent reports indicate that nearly all caregivers (97%) are comfortable with computers, and 80% are comfortable with tablets and cell phones (AARP, 2016). Additionally, three-quarters of caregivers have used the Internet to access health information related to caregiving and 71% believe that they could benefit by using these tools to save time, reduce stress, help their relatives feel

TABLE 6-4 Common Lessons Caregivers Learn in Face-to-Face Supportive Programs

Caregiver's orientation	What caregiver learns
My husband is doing this to spite me (Behaviors are intentional).	Behaviors are not intentional but part of the disease process and may be triggered by an unmet need
I want my mother to learn how to remember better and do what she used to be able to do.	New learning particularly in the moderate disease stage is not possible. Gear activities to what the person can do and where they are at. Being engaged in an activity that is set up to meet capabilities can be very meaningful for the person living with dementia.
I don't want my husband washing dishes or folding the clothing as he does it all wrong	Relax the rules. There is no right or wrong way of doing an activity as long as the person is safe. Creating opportunities for the person living with dementia to have a meaningful role and participate in everyday tasks can restore a sense of control and purpose.
I want to enable my father to make choices and so I ask him what he wants to do.	Open-ended questions can be confusing. Provide two choices and simplify directions.
Caregiving is stressful and I am overwhelmed	Use simple deep breathing or other stress reduction techniques and develop routines that allow time for yourself.

safer, and increase their own feelings of self-efficacy (National Alliance for Caregiving, 2011). Used to inform families contending with other chronic conditions, online platforms in particular may be useful to connect families to each other, and provide vetted, accurate, and useful information.

WeCareAdvisor is an online platform developed from a usability perspective that involved seeking input from key stakeholders and end users including family caregivers, physicians and nurses who care for persons living with dementia (Kales et al., 2017; Kales, Gitlin, & Lyketsos, in, press; Werner et al., 2017). The tool consists of three components: "daily tips," basic information about dementia and behaviors ("Caregiver Survival Guide"), and an algorithm (DICE—Describe, Investigate, Create, and Evaluate) to help families identify contributors to behavioral symptoms from which to create a treatment plan. A personal tool navigator is also identified who reflects the basic characteristics of the caregiver based on the information he/she provides when setting up the tool (Gitlin, Cigliana, Cigliana, & Pappa, 2017).

Daily tips are delivered every day to a user's email. Users can also view all tips on the online platform if they choose. Tips were developed by the research team to reflect the best evidence for the common and daily challenges that caregivers experience. Messages concern tips for good dementia care or offer general support to caregivers. They are also designed to encourage the caregiver to interact with the WeCareAdvisor on their own on a regular basis to address behavioral symptoms as well as to support and motivate caregivers. Basic information about dementia and behavioral symptoms are provided in a section on the online platform referred to as the Caregiver Survival Guide. The research team developed the content of the Guide based on the best evidence, education materials previously developed and tested in randomized trials, and clinical experience. The guide also includes over 1000 strategies for addressing behavioral symptoms that were identified from the literature and best clinical practices. The heart of WeCareAdvisor is an algorithm for identifying behaviors and potential contributors from which a customized treatment plan is generated. The algorithm, referred to as DICE (Describe, Investigate, Create, Evaluate) and described in detail elsewhere (Kales, Gitlin, & Lyketsos, 2014; Kales, Gitlin, & Lyketsos, 2015), was developed by a consensus panel of dementia care experts (Kales et al., 2017). DICE involves the following steps. The first is to describe the behavior. This involves asking family caregivers to choose the most problematic behavioral category (e.g., agitation, aggression, depression, and irritability) they wish to work on and then to respond to a series of questions concerning how often the targeted behavior occurs, if the behavior reflects sudden onset, if the caregiver or the person with dementia is in danger as a result of the behavior, how stressed the caregiver is as a result of the behavior and the context in which the behavior occurs (e.g., only at night? When too many people are around?). The second step, referred to as investigate, seeks to identify potential modifiable contributors to the targeted behavioral symptom. This involves the caregiver answering a series of questions concerning the person with dementia's medication use, changes in medical status, safety, and pain, their living environment (e.g., is it overstimulating, is there sufficient light), as well as the caregiver's own level of stress and well-being. In the third step, create, a customized "prescription" based on the information the caregiver provided in the previous steps is generated that provides strategies in four areas: health and safety; for the person with dementia; for the caregiver; and for the environment. Caregivers are encouraged to print the prescriptions to share with their health providers and other family members and to try tips for a week. After 1 week of use, caregivers receive an email reminder to use the tool to complete the final step of DICE by evaluating the effectiveness of each tip in reducing or managing the targeted behavior. If the strategy was not effective, caregivers are asked a series of questions to help them problem solve possible reasons why (e.g., not enough time to try, just did not work). Caregivers are able to obtain additional strategies for the targeted behavior or choose a new behavior to work on any time they wish. Additionally, families can refer to the Caregiver Survival Guide to review all possible tips whenever they choose.

WeCareAdvisor is still under development. However, an initial test of its feasibility and acceptability with 57 family caregivers is very promising. After 1-month of tool use, caregivers in the treatment arm using the tool showed greater improvement in distress as compared to controls (-3.71 points, $t = -2.33$, $P = 0.02$), adjusting for site and baseline distress. After 1 month of tool use, the waitlist group also showed significant improvement in distress (-3.72 points, $t = -2.66$, $P = 0.01$), stress (-0.41 points, $t = -2.19$, $P = 0.04$), and confidence (4.38 points, $t = 4.56$, $P < 0.0001$). The level of acceptability was very high with most caregivers indicating the tool was not too time consuming to use, was helpful, and they would recommend its use to others (Kales et al., being submitted).

LESSONS LEARNED

From this large body of research, important lessons can be gleaned for moving forward evidence-based and evidence-informed care and services for family caregivers. First, noteworthy is that there are different pathways ways in which we can positively impact family caregivers. As noted above and in Fig. 6-1, approaches, services, programs, and interventions may target the family caregiver, the person living with dementia, the physical environment, or a combination thereof. For example, an intervention targeting the caregiver may seek to address caregiver cognitions (coping, cognitive framing), behaviors (communications), or skills (ways of setting up tasks, coordinating care); an intervention targeting the person living with dementia may seek to address poor sleep, underlying medical conditions, physical health, depression, anxiety, poor quality of life, cognitive or social engagement; and an intervention targeting the physical living environment may seek to reduce clutter, provide adequate stimulation, and enhance way finding. An intervention may also involve any combination of these targets. The domain targeted will depend upon the need of the caregiver and desired outcome. However, it is unclear as to which domain or combination to target to optimize benefit in a given area.

Second, the evidence suggests that programs, services, interventions may be delivered using various modalities (listed in Box 6-5), with some approaches initially tested as face-to-face, now being adapted for delivery via other modalities such as through telephone or web-based platforms (Griffths, Kovaleva, Higgins, Langston, & Hepburn, 2018). There is growing evidence that each of these forms of delivery may

Box 6-5
Modalities by Which to Deliver Care and Support to Caregivers

- In person (at home, community agency, clinic, or service setting)
- Telephone
- Online web-based platform
- Computer asynchronous or synchronous
- Video conferencing
- Mailings
- In groups
- Combinations of above

TABLE 6-5 What Works and What Does Not When Providing Education to Caregivers

What works	What does not work
Using a conversational approach	Lecturing
Applying the information to the specific situation of the caregiver	Being prescriptive and didactic
Providing information as needed	Providing a lot of information at one time
Repeated exposure to the information	Providing information only one time
Taking the lead from the caregiver as to how much information and type of information that want and can absorb at that time	Providing written brochures and materials if caregiver is not ready to receive, has low literacy, or is not interested in learning the information
Checking in with caregiver to make sure they understand the information and determining how they are applying it	Assuming caregiver understands about dementia and behavioral symptoms even if they have read materials

have a positive impact; however, it is not clear which approach is preferred by whom and whether certain delivery approaches benefit some caregivers but not others. Yet another lesson learned is that services/supports will need to be offered using a variety of modalities to enable caregivers to access what they want, when they want it, and how they wish to receive it. Optimizing choice and control are important.

Previous intervention studies also serve as a guide post as to what works and what does not when delivering services (whatever type) to family caregivers. For example, Table 6-5 outlines key principles to follow when providing education to family caregivers.

Yet another lesson from previous research concerns the core treatment principles that should guide service delivery to families. These

TABLE 6-6 Core Treatment Principles of Face-to-Face Programs for Caregivers

Core principle	Explanation
Family-centered and family directed	<ul><li>Meet caregivers where they are</li><li>Work on areas of most immediate concern to families</li></ul>
Customize strategies	<ul><li>Tailor strategies to abilities and interests of persons living with dementia</li><li>Tailor education and strategies to caregiver readiness and identified care challenges</li><li>Consider environmental factors that support or deter daily function of caregiver and person living with dementia</li></ul>
Culturally relevant	<ul><li>Strategies fit previous/current roles, habits and beliefs</li><li>Problem solving based</li><li>Identifying strategies and activities that are acceptable and/or meaningful to the person living with dementia and/or family caregiver</li></ul>
Build rapport and trust and demonstrate respect	<ul><li>A strong therapeutic alliance characterized by rapport and trust is important in order for caregivers to feel comfortable sharing some of the most challenging and possibly intimate issues that they may confront (e.g., toileting, sexual problems, feelings of intense guilt, depression, and suicidal ideation)</li></ul>
Engage caregiver and offer choices and assure their control in decision-making	<ul><li>Caregivers are in the forefront of providing everyday care and have important knowledge about what may work and what may not in caregiving. Involving caregivers as care partners, offering choices and assuring that they remain in control of decision-making can reinforce rapport, trust and respect</li></ul>
Understand level of readiness of caregiver to change their own behaviors and/or environments	<ul><li>Caregivers may have varying degrees of readiness to learn about dementia and strategies that require them to change their own behaviors, communications and approaches. Assessing caregiver readiness and tailoring one's approach to the caregiver is more effective than using a one size fits all strategy</li></ul>
Involve trained staff skilled in understanding caregiving experience and dementia care	<ul><li>Given complexities of dementia caregiving and family dynamics, providing knowledge and specific strategies and skills requires a trained workforce.</li></ul>

(Continued)

TABLE 6-6 (Continued)

Core principle	Explanation
Active engagement of persons with dementia and caregivers	• Engage caregivers versus lecturing; use the principle of learning through doing • Take lead from caregiver and what they are ready and able to work on, think about and engage in • Modify delivery of intervention protocol if needed (e.g., phone vs home visit, or spend more time in one area than another depending upon family needs

core principles listed below in Table 6-6 are those that underlie the COPE program and are similar to those guiding delivery of other effective interventions, and particularly when working with family caregivers of persons with moderate dementia where more hands-on care is needed (Nichols et al., 2011; Nichols, Martindale-Adams, Burns, Zuber, & Graney, 2016; Zarit & Femia, 2008).

DO ALL CAREGIVERS NEED SUPPORT?

All families need access to basic support in the form of education about the disease, planning for the future and knowledge of resources from time of diagnosis on (Schulz & Eden, 2016). All families also need to be assessed for their capacity to provide care or administer any type of medical intervention. However, not all families may need intense hands-on supportive services and skills. A recent evaluation of Memory Care Home Solutions, a community-based service for families of persons with dementia living at home in St. Louis, Missouri and surrounding area, found that families appropriately self-identified the type and level of services they needed. An evaluation of 717 caregivers enrolled in the service over a 2-year period indicated that families were managing on average 11.64 (SD = 4.64) behavioral symptoms and high functional dependence (6 IADLs; 2 ADLs). Caregivers were offered a choice of either a Basic or Enhanced program. The Basic program involved about a 3-hour consultative service with a social worker or OT in the home to address immediate care challenges. At the conclusion of the Basic, caregivers were offered the option of receiving an additional five home visits by an OT to work on challenge care issues in more depth. Caregivers choosing a more intensive Enhanced service ($N = 314$, 44.9%) tended to be older ($P = 0.025$) and spouses ($P = 0.002$), reported greater distress with behaviors ($P = 0.051$), and managed higher dependence

(ADLs, $P = 0.018$; IADLs, $P = 0.002$) than caregivers opting for Basic service ($N = 403$, 56.2%). As caregivers in Basic and Enhanced had similar benefits, having caregivers self-identify the level of support they perceive they need appears to be an effective organization approach. Moreover, even when families were offered opportunities to obtain additional service contacts over 12 months, they exercised this option judiciously. Only a little more than a quarter of families in the Basic service self-initiated additional calls for assistance, and 40.4% of those in the Enhanced service sought additional assistance. Yet, these unscheduled calls for both groups were under 30 minutes, demonstrating that brief, intermittent support appears to be what caregivers sought, even for those with more care challenges. From a policy perspective, this is good news and refutes the "woodwork" phenomenon or fear that if services are offered, everyone will take advantage of them regardless of their level of need and possibly extend beyond the resources of funders and service providers. This evaluation suggests that not all families will seek continuous supportive services and that when on-going support is offered, families self-modulate use of this option (Gitlin, Cigliana, Cigliana & Papa, 2017). Also, this evaluation showed that even brief supportive services resulted in fewer adverse health-related events (emergency room visits, hospitalizations, falls, and emergency medical calls) of persons living with dementia.

ETHICAL CONSIDERATIONS

A discussion of ways to support family caregivers as we have provided thus far in this chapter may implicitly lead one to conclude that it is the full responsibility of families to absorb costs and care in dementia. However, that is not our intent nor do we endorse that it is only the responsibility of families to support people living with dementia. While it is imperative that we advance better services and supports for families, a critical question for all of us is one of policy, and involves societal and organizational level factors of our social ecological model. Here the essential questions are these: Whose responsibility is it? What is the right balance between familial and societal responsibilities? It may not be possible for families to absorb all the care and associated costs associated with living with dementia progress, and thus, how do we assure quality of life throughout the disease process for individuals living with dementia and family members?

Balancing familial and societal responsibilities is an imperative and a significant ethical and policy issue that will be answered based on a nation's view of whether health and long-term care is considered a human right and thus a societal concern or whether it is considered a privilege and hence an individual's sole responsibility.

Attention to family caregivers should be mandatory as their health and well-being are critical to providing care to persons living with dementia. Regardless of ethical framework employed or societal/cultural value placed on health, health and human service professionals and society at-large are morally and ethically obligated to reach out to family caregivers despite barriers in health care systems that may make it challenging to do so. As the health and well-being of family caregivers (see Chapter 5: Family Member as Care Partner) are integrally bound to the health and well-being of persons living with dementia, reaching out to and supporting caregivers not only helps everyone.

KEY POINTS

This chapter has made the following key points:

1. Although more research is needed, there are approaches, programs, services, interventions that can help families now.
2. In working with a family caregiver, begin with assessment of their needs, care preferences, and caregiving goals.
3. Agencies can use different strategies for bringing the evidence to families; either implementing in its entirety a proven program and assuring fidelity; adapting the program for a particular setting and evaluating outcomes; integrating key stand-alone protocols.
4. Not all family caregivers need intensive services; however, all family caregivers need education, access to resources as needed, and skills to manage the complexities of dementia care.
5. We have an ethical and moral responsibility to reach out to families to assess and address their unmet needs.
6. We must obtain the right balance between family and societal responsibility as the costs and emotional and physical toll currently is imbalanced, placing families at great peril.

What Can Be Done Now

- Identify the preferred ways families wish to be referred (e.g., some may not identify as a caregiver) to provide appropriate support
- Ask caregivers how they are doing, what care tasks they do and what they need
- Use a formal assessment to identify unmet needs

- Offer caregivers referrals to local resources including educational websites or to address legal issues, financial and/or power of attorney concerns
- If a health system or social service agency, identify and implement an evidence-based program
- If unable to offer a full evidence-based program, provide caregivers with proven strategies (problem solving, stress reduction, education, referrals and linkages, communication, and other simplification techniques)

References

AARP. (2016). *Caregivers & technology: What they want and need*. Retrieved from http://www.aarp.org/content/dam/aarp/home-and-family/personal-technology/2016/04/Caregivers-and-Technology-AARP.pdf.

Alzheimer's Association. (2017). *2017 Alzheimer's disease facts & figures*. Retrieved from https://www.alz.org/documents_custom/2017-facts-and-figures.pdf.

Aravena, J. M., Albala, C., & Gitlin, L. N. (2017). Measuring change in perceived well-being of family caregivers: Validation of the Spanish version of the Perceived Change Index (PCI-S) in Chilean dementia caregivers. *International Journal of Geriatric Psychiatry*. Available from https://doi.org/10.1002/gps.4734.

Bangerter, L. R., Griffin, J. M., Zarit, S. H., & Havyer, R. (2017). Measuring the needs of family caregivers of people with dementia: An assessment of current methodological strategies and key recommendations. *Journal of Applied Gerontology*. Available from https://doi.org/10.1177/0733464817705959, 73346481770595.

Barnard, D., & Yaffe, M. J. (2014). What is the physician's responsibility to a patient's family caregiver? *The Virtual Mentor: VM, 16*(5), 330–338. Available from https://doi.org/10.1001/virtualmentor.2014.16.05.ecas1-1405.

Bass, D. M., Judge, K. S., Lynn Snow, A., Wilson, N. L., Morgan, R., Looman, W. J., & Kunik, M. E. (2013). Caregiver outcomes of Partners in Dementia Care: Effect of a care coordination program for veterans with dementia and their family members and friends. *Journal of the American Geriatrics Society, 61*(8), 1377–1386. Available from https://doi.org/10.1111/jgs.12362.

Bass, D. M., Judge, K. S., Snow, A. L., Wilson, N. L., Morgan, R. O., Maslow, K., & Kunik, M. E. (2014). A controlled trial of Partners in Dementia Care: Veteran outcomes after six and twelve months. *Alzheimer's Research & Therapy, 6*(1), 9. Available from https://doi.org/10.1186/alzrt242.

Belle, S. H., Czaja, S. J., Schulz, R., Zhang, S., Burgio, L. D., Gitlin, L. N., & Ory, M. G. (2003). Using a new taxonomy to combine the uncombinable: Integrating results across diverse interventions. *Psychology and Aging, 18*(3), 396–405. Available from https://doi.org/10.1037/0882-7974.18.3.396.

Belle, S. H., Burgio, L., Burns, R., Coon, D., Czaja, S. J., Gallagher-Thompson, D., & Zhang, S. (2006). Enhancing the quality of life of dementia caregivers from different ethnic or racial groups: A randomized, controlled trial. *Annals of Internal Medicine, 145*(10), 727–738.

Black, B. S., Johnston, D., Rabins, P. V., Morrison, A., Lyketsos, C., & Samus, Q. M. (2013). Unmet needs of community-residing persons with dementia and their informal caregivers: Findings from the Maximizing Independence at Home Study. *Journal of the*

American Geriatrics Society, 61(12), 2087–2095. Available from https://doi.org/10.1111/jgs.12549.

Callahan, C. M., Boustani, M. A., Weiner, M., Beck, R. A., Livin, L. R., Kellams, J. J., & Hendrie, H. C. (2011). Implementing dementia care models in primary care settings: The Aging Brain Care Medical Home. *Aging & Mental Health, 15*(1), 5–12. Available from https://doi.org/10.1080/13607861003801052.

Callahan, C. M., Kales, H. C., Gitlin, L. N., & Lyketsos, C. G. (2013). *The historical development and state of the art approach to design and delivery of dementia care services. Designing and delivering dementia services* (pp. 17–30). Oxford, UK: John Wiley & Sons, Ltd. Available from https://doi.org/10.1002/9781118378663.ch2.

Chang, B. L. (1999). Cognitive-behavioral intervention for homebound caregivers of persons with dementia. *Nursing Research, 48*(3), 173–182. Available from https://doi.org/10.1097/00006199-199905000-00007.

Cohen, C. A. (2000). Caregivers for people with dementia. What is the family physician's role? *Canadian Family Physician Medecin de Famille Canadien, 46*, 376–380.

Cornman-Levy, D., Gitlin, L. N., Corcoran, M. A., & Schinfeld, S. (2001). Caregiver aches and pains: The role of physical therapy in helping families provide daily care. *Alzheimer's Care Quarterly, 2*(1), 47–55.

Czaja, S. J., Gitlin, L. N., Schulz, R., Zhang, S., Burgio, L. D., Stevens, A. B., & Gallagher-Thompson, D. (2009). Development of the risk appraisal measure: A brief screen to identify risk areas and guide interventions for dementia caregivers. *Journal of the American Geriatrics Society, 57*(6), 1064–1072. Available from https://doi.org/10.1111/j.1532-5415.2009.02260.x.

Czaja, S. J., Loewenstein, D., Schulz, R., Nair, S. N., & Perdomo, D. (2013). A videophone psychosocial intervention for dementia caregivers. *The American Journal of Geriatric Psychiatry, 21*(11), 1071–1081. Available from https://doi.org/10.1016/j.jagp.2013.02.019.

Dimakopoulou, E., Sakka, P., Efthymiou, A., Karpathiou, N., & Karydaki, M. (2015). Evaluating the needs of dementia patients' caregivers in Greece: A questionnaire survey. *International Journal of Caring Sciences, 8*(2).

Feinberg, L. (2017). From research to standard practice: Advancing proven programs to support family caregivers of persons living with dementia. *Insight On The Issues*(127)).

Feinberg, L., & Houser, A. N. (2012). *Assessing family caregiver needs: Policy and practice considerations*. Washington, DC: AARP Public Policy Institute.

Feinberg, L. F. (2003). The state of the art of caregiver assessment. *Generations, 27*(4), 24–32.

Fortinsky, R. H., Gitlin, L. N., Pizzi, L. T., Piersol, C. V., Grady, J., Robison, J. T., & Molony, S. (2016). Translation of the Care of Persons with Dementia in their Environments (COPE) intervention in a publicly-funded home care context: Rationale and research design. *Contemporary Clinical Trials, 49*, 155–165. Available from https://doi.org/10.1016/j.cct.2016.07.006.

Gaugler, J. E., Reese, M., & Mittelman, M. S. (2013). Effects of the NYU caregiver intervention-adult child on residential care placement. *The Gerontologist, 53*(6), 985–997. Available from https://doi.org/10.1093/geront/gns193.

Gitlin, L., & Czaja, S. (2015). *Behavioral intervention research*. New York: Springer Publishing Company.

Gitlin, L. N., Belle, S. H., Burgio, L. D., Czaja, S. J., Mahoney, D., Gallagher-Thompson, D., & Ory, M. G. (2003). Effect of multicomponent interventions on caregiver burden and depression: The REACH multisite initiative at 6-month follow-up. *Psychology and Aging, 18*(3), 361–374. Available from https://doi.org/10.1037/0882-7974.18.3.361.

Gitlin, L. N., Cigliana, J., Cigliana, K., & Pappa, K. (2017). Supporting family caregivers of persons with dementia in the community: Description of the "Memory Care Home Solutions" program and its impacts. *Innovation in Aging, 1*(1). Available from https://doi.org/10.1093/geroni/igx013.

Gitlin, L. N., & Hodgson, N. (2015). Caregivers as therapeutic agents in dementia care: The evidence-base for interventions supporting their role. In J. E. Gaugler, & R. L. Kane (Eds.), *Family caregiving in the new normal* (pp. 305–356). San Diego: Academic Press.

Gitlin, L. N., & Hodgson, N. A. (2016). Who should assess the needs of and care for a dementia patient's caregiver? *AMA Journal of Ethics, 18*(12), 1171–1181. Available from https://doi.org/10.1001/journalofethics.2016.18.12.ecas1-1612.

Gitlin, L. N., Kales, H. C., & Lyketsos, C. G. (2012). Nonpharmacologic management of behavioral symptoms in dementia. *JAMA, 308*(19), 2020. Available from https://doi.org/10.1001/jama.2012.36918.

Gitlin, L. N., Kales, H. C., Marx, K., Stanislawski, B., & Lyketsos, C. (2017). A randomized trial of a web-based platform to help families manage dementia-related behavioral symptoms: The WeCareAdvisor™. *Contemporary Clinical Trials, 62,* 27–36. Available from https://doi.org/10.1016/j.cct.2017.08.001.

Gitlin, L. N., Marx, K., Stanley, I. H., & Hodgson, N. (2015). Translating evidence-based dementia caregiving interventions into practice: State-of-the-science and next steps. *The Gerontologist, 55*(2), 210–226. Available from https://doi.org/10.1093/geront/gnu123.

Gitlin, L. N., Reever, K., Dennis, M. P., Mathieu, E., & Hauck, W. W. (2006). Enhancing quality of life of families who use adult day services: Short- and long-term effects of the Adult Day Services Plus Program. *The Gerontologist, 46*(5), 630–639. Available from https://doi.org/10.1093/geront/46.5.630.

Gitlin, L. N., Winter, L., Dennis, M. P., & Hauck, W. W. (2006). Assessing perceived change in the well-being of family caregivers: Psychometric properties of the Perceived Change Index and response patterns. *American Journal of Alzheimer's Disease & Other Dementias, 21*(5), 304–311. Available from https://doi.org/10.1177/1533317506292283.

Gitlin, L. N., Winter, L., Dennis, M. P., & Hauck, W. W. (2007). A non-pharmacological intervention to manage behavioral and psychological symptoms of dementia and reduce caregiver distress: Design and methods of project ACT. *Clinical Interventions in Aging, 2*(4), 695–703. Available from https://doi.org/10.2147/CIA.S1337.

Gitlin, L. N., Winter, L., Dennis, M. P., Hodgson, N., & Hauck, W. W. (2010a). A biobehavioral home-based intervention and the well-being of patients with dementia and their caregivers. *JAMA, 304*(9), 983. Available from https://doi.org/10.1001/jama.2010.1253.

Gitlin, L. N., Winter, L., Dennis, M. P., Hodgson, N., & Hauck, W. W. (2010b). Targeting and managing behavioral symptoms in individuals with dementia: A randomized trial of a nonpharmacological intervention. *Journal of the American Geriatrics Society, 58*(8), 1465–1474. Available from https://doi.org/10.1111/j.1532-5415.2010.02971.x.

Griffiths, P. C., Whitney, M. K., Kovaleva, M., & Hepburn, K. (2016). Development and implementation of Tele-Savvy for dementia caregivers: A Department of Veterans Affairs clinical demonstration project. *The Gerontologist, 56*(1), 145–154. Available from https://doi.org/10.1093/geront/gnv123.

Griffths, P. C., Kovaleva, M., Higgins, M., Langston, A. H., & Hepburn, K. (2018). Tele-Savvy: An online program for dementia caregivers. *American Journal of Alzheimer's Disease & Other Dementias.* Available from https://doi.org/10.1177/1533317518755331.

Hepburn, K. W., Lewis, M., Sherman, C. W., & Tornatore, J. (2003). The Savvy Caregiver Program: Developing and testing a transportable dementia family caregiver training program. *The Gerontologist, 43*(6), 908–915. Available from https://doi.org/10.1093/geront/43.6.908.

Hepburn, K. W., Tornatore, J., Center, B., & Ostwald, S. W. (2001). Dementia family caregiver training: Affecting beliefs about caregiving and caregiver outcomes. *Journal of the American Geriatrics Society*, *49*(4), 450–457. Available from https://doi.org/10.1046/j.1532-5415.2001.49090.x.

Hodgson, N., Gitlin, L. N., Winter, L., & Hauck, W. W. (2013). Caregiver's perceptions of the relationship of pain to behavioral and psychiatric symptoms in older community residing adults with dementia. *The Clinical Journal of Pain*, 1. Available from https://doi.org/10.1097/AJP.0000000000000018.

Jutkowitz, E., Kane, R. L., Dowd, B., Gaugler, J. E., MacLehose, R. F., & Kuntz, K. M. (2017a). Effects of cognition, function, and behavioral and psychological symptoms on Medicare expenditures and health care utilization for persons with dementia. *The Journals of Gerontology: Series A*, *72*(6), 818–824. Available from https://doi.org/10.1093/gerona/glx035.

Jutkowitz, E., Kane, R. L., Gaugler, J. E., MacLehose, R. F., Dowd, B., & Kuntz, K. M. (2017b). Societal and family lifetime cost of dementia: Implications for policy. *Journal of the American Geriatrics Society*, *65*(10), 2169–2175. Available from https://doi.org/10.1111/jgs.15043.

Kales, H. C., Gitlin, L. N., & Lyketsos, C. G. (2014). Management of neuropsychiatric symptoms of dementia in clinical settings: Recommendations from a multidisciplinary expert panel. *Journal of the American Geriatrics Society*, *62*(4), 762–769. Available from https://doi.org/10.1111/jgs.12730.

Kales, H. C., Gitlin, L. N., & Lyketsos, C. G. (2015). Assessment and management of behavioral and psychological symptoms of dementia. *BMJ*, *350*. Available from https://doi.org/10.1136/bmj.h369, h369–h369.

Kales, H.C., Gitlin, L.N., & Lyketsos, C.G. (in press). Outcomes of a pilot test of the WeCareAdvisor: A web-based tool to help family caregivers manage behavioral symptoms.

Kales, H. C., Gitlin, L. N., Stanislawski, B., Marx, K., Turnwald, M., Watkins, D. C., & Lyketsos, C. G. (2017). WeCareAdvisor™: *The development of a caregiver-focused, web-based program to assess and manage behavioral and psychological symptoms of dementia*. *Alzheimer Disease & Associated Disorders*, *31*(3), 263–270. Available from https://doi.org/10.1097/WAD.0000000000000177.

Keefe, J., Guberman, N., Fancey, P., Barylak, L., & Nahmiash, D. (2008). Caregivers' aspirations, realities, and expectations: The CARE tool. *Journal of Applied Gerontology*, *27*(3), 286–308. Available from https://doi.org/10.1177/0733464807312236.

Knight, B. G., Lutzky, S. M., & Macofsky-Urban, F. (1993). A meta-analytic review of interventions for caregiver distress: Recommendations for future research. *The Gerontologist*, *33*(2), 240–248. Available from https://doi.org/10.1093/geront/33.2.240.

Mittelman, M. S., Ferris, S. H., Steinberg, G., Shulman, E., Mackell, J. A., Ambinder, A., & Cohen, J. (1993). An intervention that delays institutionalization of Alzheimer's disease patients: Treatment of spouse-caregivers. *The Gerontologist*, *33*(6), 730–740. Available from https://doi.org/10.1093/geront/33.6.730.

Mittelman, M. S., Ferris, S. H., Shulman, E., Steinberg, G., & Levin, B. (1996). A family intervention to delay nursing home placement of patients with Alzheimer disease. A randomized controlled trial. *JAMA*, *276*(21), 1725–1731. Available from https://doi.org/10.1001/jama.1996.03540210033030.

Moon, H., & Dilworth-Anderson, P. (2015). Baby boomer caregiver and dementia caregiving: Findings from the National Study of Caregiving. *Age and Ageing*, *44*(2), 300–306. Available from https://doi.org/10.1093/ageing/afu119.

National Alliance for Caregiving. (2011). *e-Connected family caregiver: Bringing caregiving into the 21st Century*. Bethesda: UnitedHealthcare. Retrieved from http://www.caregiving.org/data/FINAL_eConnected_Family_Caregiver_Study_Jan%202011.pdf.

Nichols, L. O., Martindale-Adams, J., Burns, R., Graney, M. J., & Zuber, J. (2011). Translation of a dementia caregiver support program in a health care system—REACH VA. *Archives of Internal Medicine, 171*(4). Available from https://doi.org/10.1001/archinternmed.2010.548.

Nichols, L. O., Martindale-Adams, J., Burns, R., Zuber, J., & Graney, M. J. (2016). REACH VA: Moving from translation to system implementation. *The Gerontologist, 56*(1), 135–144. Available from https://doi.org/10.1093/geront/gnu112.

Onken, L. S., Carroll, K. M., Shoham, V., Cuthbert, B. N., & Riddle, M. (2014). Reenvisioning clinical science. *Clinical Psychological Science, 2*(1), 22–34. Available from https://doi.org/10.1177/2167702613497932.

Pinquart, M., & Sörensen, S. (2003). Differences between caregivers and noncaregivers in psychological health and physical health: A meta-analysis. *Psychology and Aging, 18*(2), 250–267. Available from https://doi.org/10.1037/0882-7974.18.2.250.

Pinquart, M., & Sörensen, S. (2006). Helping caregivers of persons with dementia: Which interventions work and how large are their effects? *International Psychogeriatrics, 18*(4), 577. Available from https://doi.org/10.1017/S1041610206003462.

Pruchno, R., & Gitlin, L. N. (2012). Family caregiving in late life: Shifting paradigms. In R. Blieszner, & V. H. Bedford (Eds.), *Handbook of families and aging* (pp. 515–541). Westport, CT: Praeger Publishers. Available from https://doi.org/10.5860/choice.50-4731.

Reever, K. E., Mathieu, E., Dennis, M. P., & Gitlin, L. N. (2004). Adult day services plus: Augmenting adult day centers with systematic care management for family caregivers. *Alzheimer's Care Today, 4*(4), 332–339.

Samus, Q. M., Johnston, D., Black, B. S., Hess, E., Lyman, C., Vavilikolanu, A., & Lyketsos, C. G. (2014). A multidimensional home-based care coordination intervention for elders with memory disorders: The Maximizing Independence at Home (MIND) pilot randomized trial. *The American Journal of Geriatric Psychiatry, 22*(4), 398–414. Available from https://doi.org/10.1016/j.jagp.2013.12.175.

Schoenmakers, B., Buntinx, F., & DeLepeleire, J. (2010). Supporting the dementia family caregiver: The effect of home care intervention on general well-being. *Aging & Mental Health, 14*(1), 44–56. Available from https://doi.org/10.1080/13607860902845533.

Schulz, R., & Eden, J. (Eds.), (2016). *Families caring for an aging America*. Washington, DC: National Academies Press. Available from https://doi.org/10.17226/23606.

Spillman, B. C., & Long, S. K. (2009). Does high caregiver stress predict nursing home entry? *INQUIRY: The Journal of Health Care Organization, Provision, and Financing, 46*(2), 140–161. Available from https://doi.org/10.5034/inquiryjrnl_46.02.140.

Teri, L., McCurry, S. M., Logsdon, R., & Gibbons, L. E. (2005). Training community consultants to help family members improve dementia care: A randomized controlled trial. *The Gerontologist, 45*(6), 802–811. Available from https://doi.org/10.1093/geront/45.6.802.

Teri, L., Truax, P., Logsdon, R., et al. (1992). Assessment of behavioral problems in dementia: The revised memory and behavior problems checklist (RMBPC). *Psychology and Aging, 7*, 622–631.

Werner, N. E., Stanislawski, B., Marx, K. A., Watkins, D. C., Kobayashi, M., Kales, H., & Gitlin, L. N. (2017). Getting what they need when they need it. *Applied Clinical Informatics, 8*(1), 191–205. Available from https://doi.org/10.4338/ACI-2016-07-RA-0122.

World Health Organization. (2012). *Dementia: A public health priority*. Geneva, Switzerland: WHO Press. Retrieved from http://apps.who.int/iris/bitstream/10665/75263/1/9789241564458_eng.pdf?ua=1.

World Health Organization. (2014). *Dementia: A public health priority*. Geneva, Switzerland: WHO Press. Retrieved from https://extranet.who.int/agefriendlyworld/wp-content/uploads/2014/06/WHO-Dementia-English.pdf.

Wolff, J. L., Guan, Y., Boyd, C. M., Vick, J., Amjad, H., Roth, D. L., & Roter, D. L. (2017). Examining the context and helpfulness of family companion contributions to older adults' primary care visits. *Patient Education and Counseling, 100*(3), 487–494. Available from https://doi.org/10.1016/j.pec.2016.10.022.

Zarit, S. H. (2017). Past is prologue: How to advance caregiver interventions. *Aging & Mental Health*, 1–6. Available from https://doi.org/10.1080/13607863.2017.1328482.

Zarit, S., & Femia, E. (2008). Behavioral and psychosocial interventions for family caregivers. *AJN, American Journal of Nursing, 108*(Supplement), 47–53. Available from https://doi.org/10.1097/01.NAJ.0000336415.60495.34.

CHAPTER 7

Formal Caregivers: The Role of the Interprofessional Team

> When you take your loved one to be tested, they should inform you of the resources available ... they should tell you what to expect, where to go and what to do ... nobody tells you what to expect in different stages ... they tell you what to expect when you have a baby, but nobody tells you what to do when you reach that stage of life ... they just don't tell you **Anonymous from Loukissa, Farran, & Graham, 1999.**
>
> The dementia challenge will only be met if the work is underpinned by a workforce equipped to provide good quality dementia care **Alzheimer's Society, UK.**

Persons living with dementia and their family caregivers need support and coordinated care provided by a trained and competent healthcare team (Silverstein & Maslow, 2006). Regrettably, we are faced with national workforce shortages that have become the biggest future challenges for aging societies throughout the world. In this chapter, we move from the role of the family caregiver to that of professional or formal caregivers. We refer to formal caregivers as those paid healthcare team members who provide assessment, education, support, hands-on care, and supervision to persons living with dementia and their family caregivers, and are part of an interprofessional team.

Case Snapshot—Mrs. M

Mrs. M and her daughter are preparing for a visit to the memory care clinic. Mrs. M had a one-year history of "being very forgetful", "easily frustrated" and had "trouble finding words for things, even familiar objects". Before the visit, they were sent a letter telling them to expect a one-hour meeting and describing the interdisciplinary team members they would encounter. "I'm nervous for this visit. Although I am glad to get this letter, I'm not sure what they'll be able to accomplish in one-hour", her daughter stated, hesitantly.

Once they arrive for their appointment Mrs. M is greeted by a nurse practitioner who completes a physical assessment and review of symptoms while her daughter is interviewed by the nurse to collect a history regarding the onset and progression of her mother's cognitive, mood, behavior and functional symptoms. Mrs. M is then escorted to a meeting with a geriatric psychiatrist for neuropsychological testing. At the same time, her daughter meets with the social worker who conducts a psychosocial interview and needs assessment. Following these assessments Mrs. M and her daughter meet with the team to review their findings and develop a tailored care plan based on their identified needs. The entire visit is completed in 70 minutes and Mrs. M and her daughter state that they feel they have a clear plan for moving forward.

The case of Mrs. K and her daughter is not fabricated, but unfortunately it is not typical. Most persons with dementia do not experience the model of care presented above. More commonly, individuals living with dementia see multiple individual healthcare providers separately. The majority of older adults with memory problems first present to their primary care provider where they might receive an evaluation after several weekly visits involving an office-based team of nurses or social workers, if such a team is available. Alternatively, the primary care provider might refer the older adult to a neurologist, geriatrician, or psychiatrist. However, these providers often have limitations on the amount of time they can spend on each office visit. Each of these providers may duplicate an assessment or repeat a test that was previously ordered, and never convene as a team to discuss a plan of care with them or their family. This lack of coordination has resulted in medical errors, poor transitions in care, and poor satisfaction (IOM, 2008).

It is vitally important that the workforce of formal caregivers be enhanced in both ability and size to meet the critical needs of the increasing number of persons living with dementia and their family caregivers (Box 7-1). To ensure quality dementia care, formal caregivers must be educated and trained in key competencies of dementia care that are the focus of this chapter (Chenoweth, Jeon, Merlyn, & Brodaty, 2010).

The current education and training of most formal caregivers is insufficient to prepare these practitioners to provide quality care to

> **Box 7-1**
> **Why We Need a Well-Prepared Dementia Care Workforce**
>
> - Growing heterogeneity of older population with dementia
> - Increasing prevalence of older adults with more complex needs related to chronic diseases
> - Complexity of skills and knowledge required to provide comprehensive care
> - Specialization within health professions and fragmentation of disciplinary knowledge
> - Need for continuity of care and standard communication across treatment settings

individuals with dementia (Gitlin & Hodgson, 2016). Regrettably, the number of educational programs in dementia care has declined precipitously in recent years. One-third of staff in long-term care and one half of all nursing staff in hospitals have not received any dementia care training (Hughes, Bagley, Reilly, Burns, & Challis, 2008). The leading categories of training needs reported by formal caregivers who work in dementia care settings are in managing behaviors nonpharmacologically (92.3%), enhancing patient safety (89.7%), coping with care challenges (84.2%), and involving patients in activities (81.6%). Although many formal caregivers believed their care contributed a great deal to well-being, approximately 75% reported frustrations and being overwhelmed by dementia care (Marx et al., 2014). Moreover, the majority of formal caregivers receive low pay, have low status, and no clear career path. These factors have led to high rates of job dissatisfaction, high turnover rates and a lack of healthcare providers choosing to work in dementia care (Hallberg et al., 2016).

Most formal caregivers are trained and socialized in single practitioner delivery models, yet in reality, formal caregivers are all part of interprofessional care teams composed of different healthcare disciplines working together towards common goals to meet the needs of persons with dementia and their family caregivers (Keough & Huebner, 2000). The work of each team member is based on their scope of practice and information shared in order to support one another's work and coordinate processes. (Lamb, Zimring, Chuzi, & Dutcher, 2010). We use the term "interprofessional practice" to refer to this preferred model of dementia care to address the need for prepared and supported workforce in dementia care.

In this chapter, we discuss the interprofessional team in the context of formal caregiving and address three fundamental questions:

- What is an interprofessional approach to formal caregiving for persons with dementia and their families?
- Why is an interprofessional approach to dementia care important?
- What skills do formal caregivers need to practice as part of an interprofessional care team?

A well-prepared dementia care workforce is urgently needed to provide care to the growing population of older adults with dementia.

WHAT IS AN INTERPROFESSIONAL APPROACH TO FORMAL CAREGIVING?

For individuals living with dementia and in particularly, for those also living with complex, multiple conditions with medical, psychological, and social needs, teams are more effective in assessing needs and creating an effective plan than having any one professional work alone (Brown, Vassar, Connor, & Vickrey, 2013). Teams need to be structured to maximize the skills and abilities of every formal caregiver (in addition to of course the individual and family member) and include clear goals with measurable outcomes. Interprofessional care involves the use of a team approach consisting of many different types of formal caregivers who collaborate to identify and meet the needs of individuals and their families from their unique perspective. Successful interprofessional teams are often described as having "fluid boundaries" to address a multitude of symptoms, problems, and needs (Galvin, Valois, & Zweig, 2014). As shown in Fig. 7-1, the person with dementia and family caregiver are included as core members of the interprofessional team.

Interprofessional Teams are typically composed of physicians, nurses, physician assistants, social workers, chaplains, other health professionals such as occupational therapists, physical therapists, speech therapists, rehabilitation specialists, social workers, and support staff. Table 7-1 describes the roles and responsibilities of the core members of an interprofessional dementia care team.

At a practical level, interprofessional teams are involved in the assessment and planning of care, making independent and joint decisions about approaches to care, and providing direct services individually or jointly with other team members to meet the needs of the person with dementia and their family (AACN, 2011). The team members can meet informally, formally, and virtually, and use various structures and tools to meet, communicate, coordinate, and monitor care.

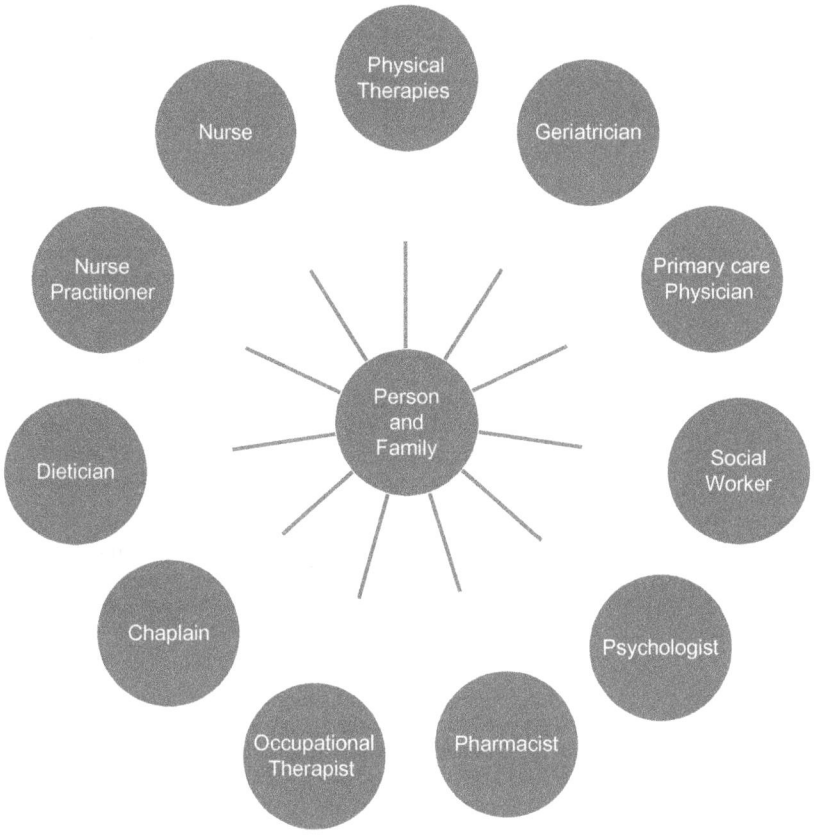

FIGURE 7-1 The interprofessional care team.

TABLE 7-1 Interdisciplinary Team Members Role in Care of Person With Dementia[a]

Team member	Role in care
Nurse	Provide personal care and assist in activities of daily living. Manage illness-related symptoms. Perform prescribed treatments and give treatments and medications with knowledge of actions, interactions, and polypharmacy issues. Provide milieu for therapeutic communication and coping strategies. Advocate for patients. Teach families, caregivers, and patients. Develop care plan in collaboration with interprofessional team members and access various resources available for patients.

(Continued)

TABLE 7-1 (Continued)

Team member	Role in care
Nurse practitioner	Provide uncomplicated ongoing health care and collaborate with physicians and other disciplines to develop plan of care. Provide educational sessions to staff about caring for person with dementia. Provide counseling sessions or facilitate support groups for family members
Primary care physician	Recognition of change in cognitive function; routine diagnostic evaluation, counseling of patient and family, imitate, and or monitor medical therapy. Refer to specialized medical health professions and community resources and provide longitudinal support for patient and family.
Geriatrician	Provider expert evaluation, diagnosis, and management of unusual or complex dementia presentations; special expertise in managing behavioral symptoms and comorbid illness; expert in community resources home care and residential care settings. Ongoing support for patient/family.
Geriatric psychiatrist	Expert in evaluation and diagnosis of full spectrum of cognitive disorders and behavioral manifestations of dementia and related psychiatric disorders. Recommends and monitors medication therapy, counsels patient/family and coordinates with other providers overall plan of care.
Physician assistant	Under the supervision of a physician; recognition of change in cognitive function; routine diagnostic evaluation, education, and counseling of patient and family; initiate, and/or monitor medical therapy. Refer to specialized medical health professions and community resources and provide longitudinal support for patient and family.
Social worker	Conduct comprehensive, strength-based assessment of individual and caregiver to develop care plan. Link to community resources to address unmet needs. Coordinate community care with hospital and nursing facility discharge planners. Provide case management. Educate and counsel throughout disease process. Advocacy activities per need. Establish and facilitate client and caregiver support groups.
Nursing assistant	Assists the team assessing the daily physical and emotional needs of persons with dementia. Assists persons with dementia in meeting daily care needs.
Psychologist	Perform neuropsychological assessments for mild cognitive impairment or dementia. Provide psychotherapy and group therapy. Provide end-of-life counseling.
Pharmacist	Optimize pharmacotherapeutic regiment to reduce or eliminate dementia-causing drugs. Recommend therapeutic options and monitor for adverse effects. Provide medication-related information to patient and caregiver. Provide assistance for improving medical adherence.

(Continued)

TABLE 7-1 (Continued)

Team member	Role in care
Occupational therapist	Evaluate preserved capabilities and functional performance and determine the type of assistance, compensatory strategy, and environmental modification needed to successfully and safely complete activities. Provide caregiver training in problem solving, task simplification, communication, and stress-reduction techniques to ease caregiver's burden.
Physical therapist	Provide interventions such as education and training to both the person with dementia and the caregivers to maximize ADLs, function and mobility, promote a safe environment, and to reduce risk of injuries and falls. Work effectively with the interdisciplinary team to support the highest attainable quality of life for the person with dementia and the caregivers.
Chaplain	Assesses spiritual, cultural, and emotional needs. Provides prayer and supports practice of spiritual traditions.
Speech therapist	Assesses speech and swallowing capacity, recommends dietary modifications based on assessment, and provides therapy to assist with communication challenges.
Recreation therapist	Assesses and provides for the daily activity and recreations needs of individuals.
Dietitian	Encourage independent eating, educate on the importance of fluid intake, and provide foods that are ethnically and culturally appropriate. Gives advice and counseling on nutrition and diet.
Family member of choice (caregiver)	Provide nuances of behavior and physical states of person with dementia. Help team define realistic goals. Shares effective strategies for interacting with patient. Caregivers can sense how receptive patient will be with treatment plan.
Individual with dementia	Provides insights on his/her daily routines, needs, abilities, interests, and preferences

[a]Other members of the team may include dentist, respiratory therapist, optometrist, podiatrist, and orthotist/prosthetist.

WHY IS INTERPROFESSIONAL CARE IMPORTANT?

An interprofessional team approach has been shown to improve chronic disease management and to prevent medical error (Bodenheimer, Wagner, & Grumbach, 2002; Chodosh et al., 2012). In persons living with dementia, interprofessional care has significantly improved reports concerning the quality of care and in behavioral and psychological symptoms

> **Box 7-2**
> **Benefits of an Interprofessional Team Approach to Dementia Care**
>
> - Effective use of health care resources
> - Effective assessments of needs
> - Less duplication of effort, more efficiency
> - Reduced clinical error
> - Increased formal caregiver, individual and family caregiver satisfaction
> - Better problem solving, morale, and coordination among team members
> - Improved care

of dementia in individuals in primary care (Callahan et al., 2006; Lee et al., 2014) (Box 6-2). Callahan and colleagues conducted a randomized trial of an interprofessional collaborative model of care compared with usual care. The foundation of this study was the use of an interprofessional team lead by an advanced practice nurse. Patients in the interprofessional program had fewer behavioral problems and fewer depression symptoms than those in the usual care group (Callahan et al., 2006).

Lee et al. tested a memory care clinic within a primary care practice that included a "family health" team composed of the physician, registered nurses, a social worker, and a pharmacist with a geriatrician available for consultation. They reported a high level of satisfaction with care by individuals living with dementia and families and a reduction in medication errors (Lee et al., 2014).

More recently, Tan et al. demonstrated that a team approach to interprofessional dementia care increased dementia screening and management in physicians, nurses, social workers, and pharmacists (Tan et al., 2017) A systematic review of interprofessional dementia educational interventions concluded that interprofessional programs are essential for promoting high quality, person-centered care (Brody & Galvin, 2013). The core benefits of interprofessional teams are listed in Box 7-2.

> Empirical evidence supports the effectiveness of an interprofessional team approach to improving dementia care and enhancing the satisfaction of individuals with dementia, their family, and formal caregivers.

WHAT SKILLS DO FORMAL CAREGIVERS NEED TO PRACTICE AS PART OF AN INTERPROFESSIONAL CARE TEAM?

The effectiveness of interprofessional teams is dependent on a number of factors, including the team members' knowledge of one another's roles; the scope of practice; mutual trust and respect among the team members; commitment in building relationships; and willingness to cooperate and collaborate (Oandasan et al., 2004; Zwarenstein, Goldman, & Reeves, 2009) (Table 7-2). One significant barrier to interprofessional dementia care practice is the lack of universal and agreed-upon competencies (Costley, 2016).

Competencies refer to a set of skills that demonstrate the capability of healthcare providers to effectively deliver care and are derived from a select set of relevant attributes defined by a combination of "knowledge, skills, and attitudes." No one attribute is sufficient to describe an individual or profession as competent. Rather, a combination of knowledge, skills, and attitudes is necessary for an individual or profession to be regarded as "competent" (Traynor, Inoue, & Crookes, 2011).

Much of the work in defining dementia-based competencies has been to define core, profession-specific, dementia competencies in the disciplines of medicine (Bodenheimer et al., 2002), nursing (AACN, 2010), social work (Damron-Rodriguez, Lawrance, Barnett, & Simmons, 2006), and pharmacy (Burke et al., 2008). These profession-specific core competencies and their sources are presented in Table 7-3.

While there is growing literature addressing discipline-specific competencies, there is variability and a general lack of agreement for establishing a core competency framework for dementia care across all formal

TABLE 7-2 Dementia-specific Interprofessional Competencies

- Demonstrates a working knowledge of dementia care services and treatment for persons with dementia and their family caregivers.
- Describes the role and responsibility of one's discipline as it pertains to the care of persons with dementia to other professionals and family caregivers.
- Recognizes the limits of one's discipline in terms of competencies, roles, and responsibilities.
- Demonstrates respect for the unique contributions of other disciplines in the care of persons with dementia and their family.
- Demonstrates an understanding of the continuum of care and services needed for persons with dementia and their families across the disease trajectory.
- Collaborates with other members of the interprofessional team.

Adapted from Oandasan, I, D'Amour, D., Zwarenstein, M. ... Tregunno, D. (2004). Interdisciplinary education for collaborative, patient-centered practice: Research findings report. Ottawa: Health Canada.

TABLE 7-3 Discipline-specific Core Competencies in Dementia Care

	Nurse	Physician	Social worker	Pharmacist
Source	Recommended baccalaureate competencies and curricular guidelines for geriatric nursing care (AACN, 2010)	Minimum geriatric competencies for internal or family medicine residents (Williams et al., 2010)	Hartford Practicum Partnership Program Geriatric Social Work Competency Scale (Damron-Rodriguez et al., 2006)	Pharmacy practice competencies across three core domains (Burke et al., 2008)
Distinct core competencies	Use valid reliable tools to assess the functional, physical, cognitive, psychological, social, and spiritual status. Assess living environment, with attention to functional, physical, cognitive, psychological, and social changes. Assess family knowledge of skills necessary to deliver care. Recognize and manage geriatric syndromes. Recognize benefits of interprofessional team.	Use a validated screening tool for delirium, dementia, depression, substance abuse. Recognize delirium as a medical emergency. Evaluate and formulate differential diagnosis and examination for individuals with changes in affect, cognition, and behavior.	Assess cognitive functioning and mental health status. Administer and interpret standardized assessment and diagnostic tools. Link to resources and services. Educate on wellness and disease management.	Provide administration techniques to enhance adherence. Monitor for therapeutic benefit/risk. Evaluate actual or potential effect of drug–drug, drug–disease, and drug–food interactions.

caregivers and settings of care (Alzheimer's Australia, 2007; National Guideline Clearinghouse, 2007). Despite the lack of consensus, there are sufficient similarities across the discipline specific competencies that can be generalized across all dementia care practitioners. These are summarized in Box 7-3. While more work in this area is still needed, several countries, including Japan and Scotland, have begun to integrate dementia competencies in generalist frameworks as minimum standards for formal caregivers (Hallberg et al., 2013; Japanese Nursing Association, 2004).

> **Box 7-3**
> **Common Dementia Competencies Across All Practitioners**
>
> - Demonstrate a working knowledge of dementia
> - Recognize, prevent, and manage distressing behaviors
> - Adapt communication to cognitive/emotional and interpersonal needs of the person with dementia
> - Assist with daily living
> - Promote an optimal environment
> - Provide ethical and person-centered care;
> - Implement nonpharmacologic strategies to promote quality of life
> - Respond to the needs of family caregivers
> - Promote health and well-being

CONCLUSION

Preparing a skilled and effective dementia workforce is an international concern; yet there remains limited understanding of how this can be achieved. Given the current and future shortage of licensed health providers with specialty training in dementia care, innovative new models of health service delivery are necessary. One strategy may be in exploring the role of community health workers for persons living at home with dementia. The benefits of community health worker model include associations with health care systems, shared ethnicity, language, and socioeconomic status with community residing persons with dementia (Litzelman et al., 2017).

While nationally agreed-upon frameworks for dementia educational content exist, there are no agreed-upon requirements for continuing professional development education or training. As a consequence low levels of dementia knowledge remain commonplace among formal caregivers. A greater understanding and consideration of what effective dementia education and training for this workforce entails is necessary. Innovative strategies to enhance workforce training, through the use of technology and online education, is one promising approach (Cartwright, Franklin, Forman, & Freegard, 2015; Gitlin & Hodgson, 2016). Regardless of the training strategy, compensation for those formal caregivers who provide direct care must be increased to improve the quality of care they provide and to attract a sufficient workforce.

The current workforce of formal caregivers of persons with dementia has been trained to practice in a silo, single professional healthcare delivery model. However, individuals living with dementia have complex medical, psychological, and social needs that require interprofessional teams who share responsibility for the individual and their family caregivers. Without an immediate and significant commitment to developing an interprofessional health care workforce to address this challenge, the care received by Mrs. M. and her daughter will be scarce and most individuals with dementia and their families will receive inadequate care.

KEY POINTS

- The proportion of health care workers receiving dementia care training is low.
- Interdisciplinary teams are groups of health care practitioners of different disciplines who work together collaboratively with close communication and coordination to optimize care for persons with dementia and their family caregivers.
- Each member of an interdisciplinary team brings a unique set of skills, knowledge, and experiences to support and augment the team and deliver quality dementia care.

What Actions Can be Taken Now

- Professional associations and educational programs should institute training in dementia specific competencies for all health care providers working with individuals living with dementia and their family caregivers
- Promote collaborative, interprofessional care models as the standard of formal caregiving
- Develop measures capturing the use of interprofessional teams and their outcomes on health and wellbeing of individuals living with dementia and families as well as satisfaction of team members

References

Alzheimer's Australia. (2007). *Quality Dementia Care: Practice in Residential Aged Care Facilities for all Staff*. Retrieved from https://www.dementia.org.au/sites/default/files/20090200_Nat_QDC_QDC1PracResAgedCareFacAll.pdf.

American Association of Colleges of Nursing (AACN) (2011). *Core competencies for interprofessional collaborative practice: Report of an expert panel*. Washington, DC, [online]. Available at http://www.aacn.nche.edu/education-resources/ipecreport.pdf Accessed September 03, 2017.

American Association of Colleges of Nursing., & John, A. (2010). *Recommended baccalaureate competencies and curricular guidelines for geriatric nursing care*. Washington DC: American Association of Colleges of Nursing.

REFERENCES

Bodenheimer, T., Wagner, E. H., & Grumbach, K. (2002). Improving primary care for patients with chronic illness. *JAMA, 288*(15), 1909. Available from https://doi.org/10.1001/jama.288.15.1909.

Brody, A. A., & Galvin, J. E. (2013). A review of interprofessional dissemination and education interventions for recognizing and managing dementia. *Gerontology & Geriatrics Education, 34*(3), 225−256. Available from https://doi.org/10.1080/02701960.2013.801342.

Brown, A. F., Vassar, S. D., Connor, K. I., & Vickrey, B. G. (2013). Collaborative care management reduces disparities in dementia care quality for caregivers with less education. *Journal of the American Geriatrics Society, 61*(2), 243−251. Available from https://doi.org/10.1111/jgs.12079.

Burke, J. M., Miller, W. A., Spencer, A. P., Crank, C. W., Adkins, L., Bertch, K. E., ... Valley, A. W. (2008). Clinical pharmacist competencies. *Pharmacotherapy, 28*(6), 806−815. Available from https://doi.org/10.1592/phco.28.6.806.

Callahan, C. M., Boustani, M. A., Unverzagt, F. W., Austrom, M. G., Damush, T. M., Perkins, A. J., ... Hendrie, H. C. (2006). Effectiveness of collaborative care for older adults with alzheimer disease in primary care. *JAMA, 295*(18), 2148. Available from https://doi.org/10.1001/jama.295.18.2148.

Cartwright, J., Franklin, D., Forman, D., & Freegard, H. (2015). Promoting collaborative dementia care via online interprofessional education. *Australasian Journal on Ageing, 34*(2), 88−94. Available from https://doi.org/10.1111/ajag.12106.

Chenoweth, L., Jeon, Y.-H., Merlyn, T., & Brodaty, H. (2010). A systematic review of what factors attract and retain nurses in aged and dementia care. *Journal of Clinical Nursing, 19*(1−2), 156−167. Available from https://doi.org/10.1111/j.1365-2702.2009.02955.x.

Chodosh, J., Pearson, M. L., Connor, K. I., Vassar, S. D., Kaisey, M., Lee, M. L., & Vickrey, B. G. (2012). A dementia care management intervention: Which components improve quality? *The American Journal of Managed Care, 18*(2), 85−94.

Costley, A. W. (2016). Exploring skills-based competencies through geriatric care management modules. *Gerontology & Geriatrics Education, 37*(4), 329−341. Available from https://doi.org/10.1080/02701960.2014.990151.

Damron-Rodriguez, J., Lawrance, F. P., Barnett, D., & Simmons, J. (2006). Developing geriatric social work competencies for field education. *Journal of Gerontological Social Work, 48*(1−2), 139−160. Available from https://doi.org/10.1300/J083v48n01_10.

Galvin, J. E., Valois, L., & Zweig, Y. (2014). Collaborative transdisciplinary team approach for dementia care. *Neurodegenerative Disease Management, 4*(6), 455−469. Available from https://doi.org/10.2217/nmt.14.47.

Gitlin, L. N., & Hodgson, N. A. (2016). Online training—Can it prepare an eldercare workforce? *Generations (Special Issue on Workforce Development), 40*(1), 71−81.

Hallberg, I. R., Leino-Kilpi, H., Meyer, G., Raamat, K., Martin, M. S., Sutcliffe, C., ... Karlsson, S. (2013). Dementia care in eight European countries: Developing a mapping system to explore systems. *Journal of Nursing Scholarship, 45*(4), 412−424. Available from https://doi.org/10.1111/jnu.12046.

Hallberg, I. R., Cabrera, E., Jolley, D., Raamat, K., Renom-Guiteras, A., Verbeek, H., ... Karlsson, S. (2016). Professional care providers in dementia care in eight European countries; their training and involvement in early dementia stage and in home care. *Dementia, 15*(5), 931−957.

Hughes, J., Bagley, H., Reilly, S., Burns, A., & Challis, D. (2008). Care staff working with people with dementia: Training, knowledge and confidence. *Dementia, 7*(2), 227−238. Available from https://doi.org/10.1177/1471301208091159.

Institute of Medicine. (2008). *Retooling for an aging America: Building the health care workforce.* Washington DC: National Academies Press. Retrieved from http://www.nationalacademies.org/hmd/~/media/Files/Report%20Files/2008/Retooling-for-an-Aging-Ame rica-Building-the-Health-Care-Workforce/ReportBriefRetoolingforanAgingAmericaBuild ingthehealthCareWorkforce.pdf.

Japanese Nursing Association. (2004). *Curriculum guideline outlining standards of education for certified expert nurses working with older adults in dementia care*. Tokyo: Japanese Nursing Association.

Keough, J., & Huebner, R. A. (2000). Treating dementia: The complementing team approach of occupational therapy and psychology. *The Journal of Psychology, 134*(4), 375–391. Available from https://doi.org/10.1080/00223980009598223.

Lamb, G., Zimring, C., Chuzi, J., & Dutcher, D. (2010). Designing better healthcare environments: Interprofessional competencies in healthcare design. *Journal of Interprofessional Care, 24*(4), 422–435. Available from https://doi.org/10.3109/13561820903520344.

Lee, L., Hillier, L. M., Heckman, G., Gagnon, M., Borrie, M. J., Stolee, P., & Harvey, D. (2014). Primary care–based memory clinics: Expanding capacity for dementia care. *Canadian Journal on Aging / La Revue Canadienne Du Vieillissement, 33*(3), 307–319. Available from https://doi.org/10.1017/S0714980814000233.

Litzelman, D. K., Inui, T. S., Schmitt-Wendholt, K. M., Perkins, A., Griffin, W. J., Cottingham, A. H., & Ivy, S. S. (2017). Clarifying values and preferences for care near the end of life: The role of a new lay workforce. *Journal of Community Health., 42*(5), 926–934. Available from https://doi.org/10.1007/s10900-017-0336-5.

Marx, K. A., Stanley, I. H., Van Haitsma, K., Moody, J., Alonzi, D., Hansen, B. R., & Gitlin, L. N. (2014). Knowing versus doing: Education and training needs of staff in a chronic care hospital unit for individuals with dementia. *Journal of Gerontological Nursing, 40* (12), 26–34. Available from https://doi.org/10.3928/00989134-20140905-01.

National Guideline Clearinghouse. (2007). *Brief summary: Caregiving strategies for older adults with delirium, dementia and depression*. Washington DC: NGC.

Oandasan, I., D'Amour, D., Zwarenstein, M., Barker, K., Purden, M., Beaulieu, M., & Tregunno, D. (2004). *Interdisciplinary education for collaborative, patient-centred practice: Research and findings report*. Ottawa: Health Canada.

Silverstein, N., & Maslow, K. (2006). *Improving hospital care for persons with dementia*. New York: Springer Pub. Co.

Tan, Z. S., Damron-Rodriguez, J., Cadogan, M., Gans, D., Price, R. M., Merkin, S. S., ... Chodosh, J. (2017). Team-based interprofessional competency training for dementia screening and management. *Journal of the American Geriatrics Society, 65*(1), 207–211. Available from https://doi.org/10.1111/jgs.14540.

Traynor, V., Inoue, K., & Crookes, P. (2011). Literature review: Understanding nursing competence in dementia care. *Journal of Clinical Nursing, 20*(13–14), 1948–1960. Available from https://doi.org/10.1111/j.1365-2702.2010.03511.x.

Williams, B. C., Warshaw, G., Fabiny, A. R., Nancy Lundebjerg, M. P. A., Medina-Walpole, A., Sauvigne, K., ... Leipzig, R. M. (2010). Medicine in the 21st century: recommended essential geriatrics competencies for internal medicine and family medicine residents. *Journal of Graduate Medical Education, 2*(3), 373–383.

Zwarenstein, M., Goldman, J., & Reeves, S. (2009). Interprofessional collaboration: Effects of practice-based interventions on professional practice and healthcare outcomes. *The Cochrane Database of Systematic Reviews*(3), , CD000072. Available from https://doi.org/ 10.1002/14651858.CD000072.pub2.

Further Reading

Alzheimer's Association Campaign for Quality Residential Care. (2009). *Dementia care practice recommendations for assisted living residences and nursing homes*. Chicago: Alzheimer's Association. Retrieved from https://www.alz.org/national/documents/brochure_DCPRphases1n2.pdf.

PART III

ABOUT LIVING ENVIRONMENTS

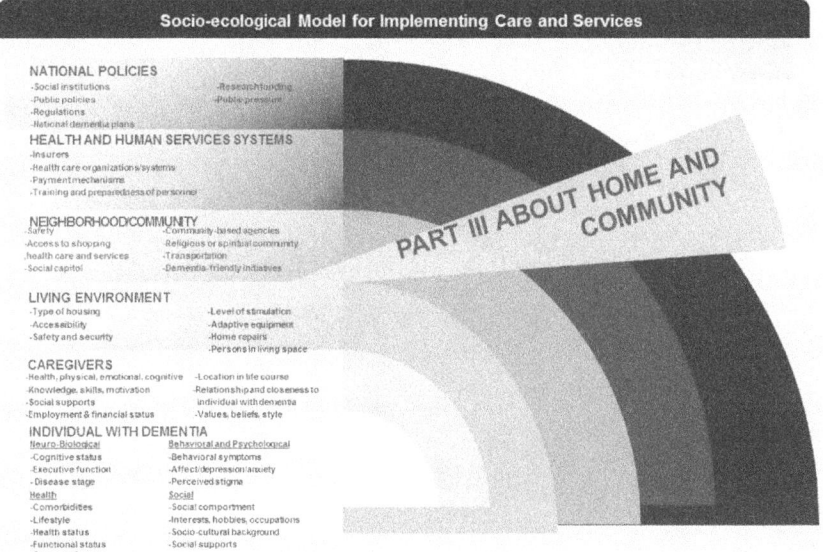

In Part III, we examine living environments, specifically, the home and community and their respective impacts on optimizing (or not) quality of life. We start with the home environment in Chapter 8, The Physical Home Environment: A Neglected Therapeutic Context, where most persons living with dementia reside and up to the end of life. Here the focus is on a safe, secure environment and one that supports daily function. The physical home environment is a neglected therapeutic modality in which simple and low-cost modifications can be implemented including home repairs to support the person living with dementia and caregivers. We specifically discuss safety concerns and home modifications that can make everyday life a bit easier. Of import is striking the right balance between autonomy and safety and security and making simple modifications over time as capabilities change.

Moving on to the larger context in which people reside, that of the immediate neighborhood and community (see Chapter 9: Living in the Community), we examine the constructs of dementia friendly and dementia capable and their respective principles. The community-based movement occurs at a local level but is a global phenomenon, and we can learn from the principles and actions of other global efforts.

CHAPTER

8

The Physical Home Environment: A Neglected Therapeutic Context

> *Creating a safe and comfortable home environment, plays an important role in ensuring better quality of life for people with dementia.* **Alzheimer's Australia.**
>
> *Challenges related to patient safety in the home are wide ranging and include fragmentation of care; household hazards; ill-prepared family caregivers; limited training and regulation of home care workers; inadequate communication among patients, caregivers, and providers; and misaligned payment incentives.* **Institute for Healthcare Improvement, 2017.**

Over the past 40 years there have been significant theoretical and empirical advances in the field of environmental gerontology, leading to a greater understanding of the importance of the physical and social environment for supporting persons living with dementia (Gitlin, 2017; Wahl, & Gitlin, in press). Although the home is the place where most persons living with dementia and their caregivers seek to remain for the duration of the disease, its role in comprehensive dementia care and how the home can support daily life has been mostly neglected (van Hoof, Kort, van Waarde, & Blom, 2010).

Most research efforts specific to living environments have sought to create and evaluate dementia appropriate living spaces in residential care settings either by trying to shift the culture of nursing homes from a medical to a socially-oriented model of care, or creating new living communities specifically designed to support health and well-being of persons living with dementia (Calkins, 2011; Davos, Byers, Nay, & Koch, 2009). Initial research on home environments primarily focused on residential satisfaction (Lawton & Simon, 1968), relocation decision-making, housing adaptations (Gitlin, 1998; Struyk & Katsura, 1988), and housing policies (Golant, 2003) with minimal consideration given to how the physical and social characteristics of homes either supported or not people living with dementia nor how its features and meanings effect the family members' experience of living with dementia (Gitlin, 2003; Gitlin, 2007).

Given the importance of "home" to individuals themselves and their family members, the focus of this chapter is specifically on this location. In Chapter 9, Living in the Community, we examine residential environments and in Chapter 10, Services and Settings of Care, we will consider the community as a living environment. In this chapter, we reflect upon the home as the immediate location in which a person living with dementia resides in a community. The home may be a long-term residence in an apartment, single dwelling, duplex or row, and/or the home of a family member/friend. How people who are living with dementia and their family members experience the home environment is relatively unknown. New research on unmet needs has identified home safety and specifically, caregiver concerns for safety which has helped to shed light on living conditions and how the home environment can serve as a therapeutic modality (Black et al., 2013).

We begin this chapter by considering key societal trends driving a renewed interest in the home and its consideration as the epicenter for dementia care. We then examine how home environments may positively and/or negatively impact people living with dementia, their caregivers, and health providers. We specifically examine home safety considerations, common home environmental modifications, and existing checklists and assessments that can guide an evaluation of a home for its support and safety of people living with dementia. Three fundamental questions we address are, What are some of the key safety concerns for persons living with dementia at home and their families and health providers? How can home environments positively support people living with dementia? What are some tools by which to evaluate the home for its safety and supportive characteristics from which to derive recommendations for care and services?

CRITICAL DRIVERS OF HOME AS AN EPICENTER FOR DEMENTIA CARE

Numerous critical societal trends have converged to make the home a possible epicenter for dementia care. These trends include changes in demography, the economics of health care, rise of portable, sophisticated technologies, and hospital and medical care models relying on the home as well as that staying put at home remains the persistent and almost universal desire of individuals and families. The push to stay at home is also buttressed by the lack of viable alternative housing stock, adequate alternative living options, and familial financial constraints, all of which may prohibit relocation to special care facilities or high technology-outfitted experimental communities, such as smart homes. The development and evaluation of different home-like arrangements is a critical research and housing industry need.

Of these trends, the primary driver for the home as epicenter of care remains demography, that is, the aging of the population, a phenomenon shared worldwide. In the United States, in just 12 years, by 2030, more than 20% (about 72.7 million) will be 65 years or older (National Academies of Sciences, Engineering, & Medicine, 2016). This represents a dramatic increase from 9.8% in 1970 and 13% in 2010. As age is the single strongest risk factor for cognitive impairment, these numbers are alarming. Of equal importance is that the fastest growing segment of the aging population is 80 years and older. It is this group that is most likely to experience cognitive changes and require some level of care or daily assistance.

The economics of moving or staying put also tip the balance to staying at home. Staying at home represents a big cost savings for the government that typically pays through Medicare and Medicaid for nursing home placements. Furthermore, with the movement from fee-for-service to prospective payment models capping coverage based on diagnosis and penalizing rehospitalizations, hospitals have become incentivized to develop outpatient practices and discharge people from hospital to home earlier (Carpenter, 2017). This in turn has pummeled rapid development forward of home health care (National Research Council, 2011). Furthermore, rapid advancements of a wide range of technologies have provided the vehicle for better home monitoring, telemedicine, and implementation of quite complex care in the home, previously only provided in hospital settings. Programs such as Hospital at Home, which is designed to provide hospital-level care to acutely ill older adults in their homes, represents an integration of these driving forces (Leff et al., 2005). This program, among others has found that recovery can be quicker at home, resulting in better sleep, less pain, and more rapid return of function. Finally, as a person's residence typically provides a great source of historical and biographical meaning, maintenance of cognitive and functional abilities, and a feeling of comfort and security, it is not surprising that surveys consistently report the almost universal desire to stay home under any circumstances (AARP, 2016; Wiles, Leibing, Guberman, Reeve, & Allen, 2012). Although aging-in-place surveys have not been specific to people living with dementia, there is evidence that most people do stay at home for the duration of the disease (Callahan, 2017).

As people with dementia also age with other health conditions, disease progression and comorbidities can conspire to make it extremely challenging to leave the home for doctor appointments or otherwise. This is yet another critical reason why it is important to consider how the home can serve as the epicenter for developing and implementing coordinated and systematic dementia care in this setting. Dr. Lyketsos, a world expert in dementia care, shares his thoughts about why the home must become the center for comprehensive dementia care, at the end of this chapter.

IMPACT OF HOME ENVIRONMENTS ON DAILY LIFE

The home is a complex environment composed of various realms including the physical, personal, social, cultural, and supra-personal (e.g., geographic proximity to transportation, shopping; Lawton, 1982; Lawton, 1999). Each of these environmental realms are imbued with objective implications, multiple and diverse personal meanings, history, and culture, and affect every day functioning for both persons living with dementia and their family members. As the home environment reflects objective conditions and is also subjectively experienced, both must be understood, evaluated, and considered in terms of their respective and interactive impact on daily life. Objective conditions for example include but are not limited to the number and size of rooms in a home, placement of bathrooms (first floor or otherwise), ease of wayfinding, number and condition of stairs, number of persons and their ages living in the household, location of the home in a community, and proximity to needed services including shopping.

We know from research on living environments of older adults in general that the home affords important subjective experiences including providing a sense of safety, security, maintenance of well-being (National Research Council, 2011), and for persons living with dementia, a sense of familiarity with and knowledge of objects and their placement, which in turns affords agency, control, and comfort.

To date, however, neither objective nor subjective aspects of home environments have been fully examined or are well understood for persons living with dementia either alone or with others. We know from research on aging in general that with age and associated age-related changes or progression of various diseases, the home typically takes on increasing importance. Older adults with significant chronic illnesses and/or functional challenges tend to turn inwards and their physical space for engagement typically becomes constricted to the home. The home becomes the principal context for socialization, leisure participation, and more recently, the delivery of health care (Gitlin, 2007; Samus et al. 2018). Most will spend the vast majority if not all of the day at home.

The home serves multiple purposes and these purposes may change with disease progression. As such, it is a complex setting imbued with history, culture, norms, beliefs and values, biographical identities, and explicit and veiled meanings. With the presence of other members of a family, such as children, the complexities increase as the home environment must absorb or accommodate varied and nuanced needs of all of its inhabitants, each of whom may have different goals, preferences, capacities, and daily needs. The case of Mrs. J is illustrative of some of the points above and highlights the central role that the home plays for persons living with dementia and their caregivers.

Case Snapshot—Mrs. J

Mrs. J is a widow with moderate dementia. She moved to her daughter's small apartment to live with her a few years ago after her husband's death and once it became challenging for her to take care of herself and home. As this was initially an unfamiliar living environment, she didn't know where common household objects were kept (e.g., cups kitchen or bathroom), which frustrated her and increased her anxiety. Her daughter works part time but mostly stays at home to attend to her mother. Mrs. J has a number of comorbidities and in particular has significant difficulties ambulating. She mostly sits in a lounge chair all day with nothing to do. Her daughter is concerned about her mother's quality of life. Also, she noticed that she has been using a commode placed by her chair with increasing frequency, about every 15 minutes and worries she might have a bladder infection. Yet taking her to the doctor is an arduous task so she is waiting to see what will happen. In the meantime, she has reduced her mother's fluid intake thinking that it might help to minimize the frequency of her toileting. With nothing to do and sitting all day, Mrs. J also has difficulty sleeping at night. With relatively little movement and boredom, she has been eating more. Her consequent weight gain has made it even more difficult for her to get up from the lounge chair and ambulate. The daughter tries to keep the apartment looking "normal" and with the exception of the commode, keeps any other medical objects related to care (e.g., walker, medicines, blood pressure cuff) out of sight in a closet. As her mother does not ambulate much, she has not been concerned about kitchen safety; yet when she is at work, her mother does try to make hot tea by using the oven or microwave. Occasionally, she has burned herself or left the oven on. The daughter has increasing concerns about her mother's safety and wellbeing, particularly when she leaves her mother home alone to go to work or attend to errands. She however has no other relatives, children or supports to rely on or who are available to her to help out.

In this case, we see that Mrs. J found it initially upsetting and disorienting to move from her own home to that of her daughter's; however, over time, her initial anxiety did subside. Nevertheless, she now lives in a small confined space although it is a loving and somewhat secure environment. Her daughter has established a "control" center for her mother such that needed objects are set up on a tray by her chair for easy reach that includes the TV remote, pitcher and glass of water, and a commode next to her chair. While the apartment may have been appropriate for Mrs. J initially, it is becoming increasingly hazardous, particularly when she spends time alone. Her ability to ambulate safely and to use the oven is becoming questionable. Preserving the home in its original set up is important to the daughter to maintain a sense of "normalcy"; yet this may not be the best set up for Mrs. J. For example, if Mrs. J is responsive to written notes, she may benefit from having signage throughout the apartment; one could be located on her bedroom door to signify it is her room, another sign could be placed on the microwave to remind her how to turn it on and off. The daughter should consider disabling the oven when she leaves the home. Of course the question remains whether Mrs. J is safe alone now at home. Consultation with an occupational therapist who can assess Mrs. J's cognitive functioning and home safety could provide important information for treatment planning. Finally, it is disconcerting that Mrs. J uses the commode with such frequency as well as that the daughter's response is to limit fluids. It is unclear whether Mrs. J has an underlying urinary infection or whether other factors may be contributing to this situation. For example, Mrs. J sits in her chair all day with nothing to do and having the commode in her full view. It is possible that this may be triggering her sense of a need to use the commode—it becomes an activity. Her daughter also needs to understand that limiting fluids can be dangerous, leading to dehydration, and that having fluids is not the underlying cause of the excessive commode use.

Furthermore, having her walker kept in plain sight next to the easy-chair in which she sits (versus in the closet) could be helpful for encouraging safe ambulation.

HOME SAFETY CONSIDERATIONS

Although the home affords a sense of security and safety, it can also pose significant obstacles, leading to unsafe conditions, suboptimal functioning, and poor quality of life (Black et al., 2013; Gitlin & Piersol, 2014). Obtaining the just-right-fit between persons, their competencies and living environments should be a top priority and significant treatment goal. This requires the systematic evaluation of homes, which occurs with changes in cognitive and functional status (discussed more below).

Safety is a highly valued commodity for families. Common safety concerns among family members include fear of an injurious fall of themselves or the person living with dementia, and getting the person up from the floor safely, that the person may exit the home and wander and become lost, of inappropriate use of the oven or other kitchen equipment, ingestion of house cleaning materials or other fluids, or of using tools that may be dangerous including kitchen knives, guns, or sharp objects. Nevertheless, families are rarely prepared for dementia or adequately versed in creating safe environments and modifying the home as the person's competencies change over time. Health professionals also rarely inquire about the objective conditions of home environments or refer families to a home care agency or occupational therapist to conduct a home safety evaluation.

People with dementia typically live at home with a significant number of home hazards; and the number and type of hazards can increase with disease progression. A survey of 313 individuals with cognitive impairments found that 90% had one or more home safety issues (Black et al., 2013; Hodgson, Black, Johnston, Lyketsos, & Samus, 2014). Another survey of 88 people living at home with dementia found an average of 8 home hazards with some individuals observed to have upwards of 27 safety concerns. Most hazards, in this survey, were found in the kitchens, followed by bathrooms and then bedrooms. About half of the family caregivers (52%) in the sample also indicated one or more unmet environmental need: of these, 30% ($n = 26$) indicated that the person they cared for needed adaptive equipment such as grab bars or tub benches; and 34% ($n = 30$) reported that the person with dementia had difficulty navigating the home with stair-climbing being the most frequently cited problem area (Gitlin, Hodgson, Piersol, Hess, & Hauck, 2014). Yet another survey of 22 families using an observational tool involving a walk-through of the home found an average of 12 hazards per household with bathrooms and bedrooms having the greatest number. The level of observed clutter was rated as moderate to high in key rooms (living room, kitchen, bedroom; Gitlin et al., 2002). Clutter refers to the presence of unnecessary objects in an area of a home which serve either as obstacles to navigation or understanding cues from the environment as to what tasks should be performed. For example, as to the latter, consider a kitchen table which has various objects on it including mail, bills needing payment, a newspaper, medications, and a place setting for a meal. These objects which are for disparate purposes may cause confusion as to what should be done in that space and be distracting to a person with dementia when they are eating. Unsafe conditions in homes are wide ranging as summarized in Box 8-1. Families express

---

Box 8-1
Home Safety Concerns

- Ambulating and wayfinding safely
- Injury from ingestion of dangerous substances (cleaning fluids)
- Unsecured throw rugs
- Access to stove
- Limited or no secured railings on staircases
- Unstable or unsupportive chairs without armrests
- Injury to self or others from sharp objects
- Fire or burns from in appropriate use of appliances (oven, toaster, microwave)
- Inability to appropriately respond to crisis
- Access to medications
- Susceptibility to financial scams
- Inappropriately letting people in the home
- Risk of and injury from falls due to throw rugs, broken tile, torn carpets, raised door thresholds, slippery floors, obstructed pathways
- Poor hydration and/or nutrition
- Risk of physical and/or emotional abuse
- Contamination when attending to wound care, toileting, medication dispensing
- Ingestion of rotten food
- Storing items (e.g., newspapers) in the oven
- Exiting home and getting lost
- Clutter heightening risk falls and confusion
- Steep stairs
- Slipper tubs—lack of grab bars
- No night lights
- Unattended home repair needs
- Too hot or too cold
- Smoking (especially at night in bed)
- Driving

concerns that the person being cared for may be at risk for falling, one of the most frequent reasons for hospitalization, exiting the home and wandering away, or using the oven inappropriately (Black et al., 2013; (Gitlin, & Corcoran, 2000). Yet, there are other home hazards that families may not be aware of such as having steep steps, no rails or rails that are loose and which do not cover all steps, or if a person has access to cleaning fluids that may inadvertently be digested or confused for some other purpose. Most people are poor reporters of the safety conditions of their homes primarily due to the lack of knowledge and insight as to what constitutes a hazard vis à vis the person for whom they care. Families are typically ill informed about what the person living with dementia is able to understand and is able to do, or adequately versed in how to modify the home environment to make it safe and supportive as the disease progresses.

As shown in Box 8-1, despite the potential number of safety concerns, of most importance is that they all can be addressed and safety should be a primary treatment goal in dementia care. Perhaps, one of the most difficult areas however to manage has to do with driving. While driving is not a hazard within the home, it remains a pressing safety concern that families and health providers have challenges effectively monitoring and controlling. Taking away keys to a car can be traumatic for all persons and discussion with a health provider as to when and how this should occur should commence with knowledge of the diagnosis. Often, the issue of driving is not addressed until there is an accident or an egregious mistake is made; yet waiting for an event can place all persons at risk warranting that a more preventive approach be assumed. It is of course difficult to decide when someone must stop driving as it is important to balance safety with autonomy as with all other decisions when modifying the home. Driving however must be evaluated, managed, and finally stopped with disease progression. A booklet from The Hartford provides excellent guidance in these matters and checklists to help evaluate when it is time for the person to stop driving (http://hartfordauto.thehartford.com/UI/Downloads/Crossroads.pdf).

Yet another very challenging issue concerns smoking. It may not be possible for a life-long smoker to quit; however, assuring a safe place for smoking is paramount. One concern is that the person living with dementia may smoke in bed and fall asleep with a lit cigarette or inappropriately dispose of a lit cigarette or match in the house. Controlling when, where, and how the person living with dementia smokes may be the only way to effectively manage these risks.

Hazards can be found in all rooms of homes although bathrooms and kitchens tend to have the most number of significant safety concerns (Gitlin et al., 2014). In addition to home hazards and other safety considerations (driving, traveling independently), home repairs may become increasingly difficult to keep up with although necessary to assure safe functioning at home (Fausset, Kelly, Rogers, & Fisk, 2011; Kelly, Fausset, Rogers, & Fisk, 2014; Szanton, Roth, Nkimbeng, Savage, & Klimmek, 2014).

In summary, attending to home safety is an important aspect of assuring the well-being of persons with dementia. With disease progression, safety risks increase and pose daily challenges. Furthermore, different features of the home and community (discussed in Chapter 9: Living in the Community) may become unsafe as capabilities decline or change. Enhancing home safety and preventing self-injury may involve putting into place simple environmental solutions. However, assuring safety should be balanced with ways to assure a person's autonomy, sense of control, agency, and personal choice. This can be challenging and pose ethical challenges for families and providers. While there is no one size fits all or easy solution, the goal should be to optimize safety by offering safe activities and environmental setups that also preserve dignity, comfort, and some level of control.

Noteworthy is that home safety is intimately tied to the capabilities of a person living with dementia. Conditions that are hazardous for one person may not be for another. Additionally, conditions that are safe at one point in time may pose as a hazard with disease progression. For example, placing medications on the kitchen table may be helpful to a person in the mild disease stage but presents as a hazard at a moderate–severe stage if the person is unable to recognize one medication from another or differentiate them from food or candy. Thus, home conditions pose dangers vis à vis what a person can navigate, understand, or interpret in the environment. Home safety must be contextualized and is associated with the capabilities of its inhabitants; conditions that are safe at one point in time may be hazardous at another point due to changes in the ability of the person to navigate and understand visual cues. Also, of importance but a neglected concern is that if home repairs are not kept up, deteriorated conditions can pose as serious hazards to a family.

THE HEALTH PROVIDER PERSPECTIVE

Providing assistance, support, or health care or other services at home may be invaluable for families. However, the home does present a unique set of challenges to service provision and for health and human service professionals. Key challenges are presented in Box 8-2 and include a wide range of considerations that can make it very challenging and unsafe for providers or the provision of health services (Gitlin & Piersol, 2014). Nevertheless, the concept of home as epicenter

> **Box 8-2**
> **Challenges Working in the Home for Health and Human Service Professionals**
>
> - Unsafe block or neighborhood
> - Lack of transportation and/or safe parking
> - Pets and other potential allergens
> - Other people in the home making care provision challenging
> - Lack of space for medical paraphernalia
> - Potential for contamination
> - Lack of internet access for documentation or setting up telemedicine technologies
> - Lack of or intermittent electricity
> - Lack of safe electrical plugs
> - Electrical plugs not in areas useful for medical equipment
> - Lack of running water
> - Intermittent or no telephone service
> - Inability to get into the home, particularly if person is bedbound and no one is home or available
> - Infestation including vermin, bed bugs and other insects
> - Extreme clutter and/or dirtiness

(versus primary care or memory clinic) for dementia care has much merit, especially as there is an increasing number of home-based intervention studies demonstrating positive impacts on quality of life, behavioral symptoms, and daily function (Gitlin, Choi, and Hodgson 2016); however, this is not currently the reality (Samus et al., 2018).

ENVIRONMENTAL ASSESSMENTS

Key to enhancing the safety of a home is conducting an assessment of its conditions including hazards as well as the adaptations put into place to support the daily functioning of persons living with dementia. Evaluating home environments should be an important component of comprehensive dementia care. Assessment of the home needs to be conducted at each juncture of the disease trajectory.

A home assessment involves a health professional, typically an occupational therapist, who performs a thorough walk through of a home using a standardized home assessment tool. In the United States, a home evaluation conducted by an occupational therapist, with a script from a physician, can be reimbursed through Medicare or paid out-of-pocket. While families can use simple checklists as a first line of defense in evaluating their home, occupational therapists are particularly trained to examine home conditions in terms of a person's capabilities as well as to make specific recommendations for assistive devices and home modifications that would be safe to make for all members of the household.

A number of environmental assessments have been developed that can be useful although a few are specifically devoted to households of people living with dementia. Table 8-1 lists a few helpful checklists that can be used by families or health professionals. These tools are evaluative in that home conditions are observed for their level of safety independently of a person and their particular abilities. Only through a skilled assessment approach from an occupational therapist can the link between capabilities and environmental conditions be adequately made.

TABLE 8-1 Select Home Environmental Assessments

Tool or resource	Where to obtain	Description
AARP Home Fit Guide	https://assets.aarp.org/www.aarp.org_/articles/families/HousingOptions/200590_HomeFit_rev011108.pdf	Information for keeping the home environment in optimal condition for comfort, safety, and livability for older adults wishing to stay in their homes. Includes sections on home livability, safety, maintenance, energy conservation, and resources for getting help.
American Academy of Orthopaedic Surgeons Home Safety Checklist	http://orthoinfo.aaos.org/topic.cfm?topic = A00123	Checklist of home safety tips by housing feature (e.g., stairs, bedroom, bathroom, etc.).
Center for Healthy Aging & National Council on Aging	https://www.ncoa.org/wp-content/uploads/cha_tools_checklists.pdf	List of helpful home safety checklists for use by consumers and health professionals and as part of fall prevention programs.
Check For Safety: A home fall prevention checklist for older adults	https://www.cdc.gov/HomeandRecreationalSafety/pubs/English/booklet_Eng_desktop-a.pdf	Consumer-oriented checklists to enhance home safety and prevent falls organized by each room of the home.

(*Continued*)

TABLE 8-1 (Continued)

Tool or resource	Where to obtain	Description
Home Environmental Assessment Protocol (for Dementia)	Tool available from author, Gitlin et al. (2002)	Room-by-room observation of potential hazards specific to individuals with dementia, and the presence/absence of adaptations to support daily functioning. Useful for both clinical and research purposes and can be used by health professionals or individuals trained in use of tool.
Home Falls and Accidents Screening Tool (HOME FAST)	Mackenzie, Byles, & Higginbotham (2002)	Designed to identify older people living at home in the community who are at risk of falls due to environmental issues in their home. The HOME FAST consists of 25 items covering a range of environmental and functional home safety concerns. Administered by an Occupational Therapist, OT assistant, or social worker.
Home Safety SmartCheck	http://www.homesafetysmartcheck.com/siteimages/2010/11/RoombyRoomOlderAdultNov11.pdf	A room-by-room safety checklist for older adults.
Home-Screen	Johnson, Cusick, & Chang (2001)	The Home-Screen was specifically designed as a nurse-administered instrument to identify environmental hazards and unsafe behavior and alert nurses to the need for specialized environmental assessment and behavior change. Items included seven environmental features: room clutter, good lighting for day and night, floor coverings, shoes worn in the home, toileting, and showering facilities.

(Continued)

TABLE 8-1 (Continued)

Tool or resource	Where to obtain	Description
Housing Enabler	http://www.enabler.nu/download.html	Intended for use by occupational therapists, three ratings are derived: functional limitations of person, mobility aid use, and environmental barriers. Ratings guide treatment planning to enhance home safety, minimize environmental barriers, and enhance accessibility in homes. Useful for both clinical and research purposes but does require training in use of system.
International Association of Certified Home Inspectors – Home Safety for the Elderly	https://www.nachi.org/elderlysafety.htm	Recommendations and in-depth checklists for the home safety of older consumers. Comprehensive listing of Yes/No questions and tips per area of the home.
National Institute on Aging: Home Safety and Alzheimer's Disease	https://www.nia.nih.gov/health/home-safety-and-alzheimers-disease	Tips offered to alter the home environment and give persons with dementia more freedom of movement and safe independence. Includes tips concerning home modification as well as specifically addressing dangers derived from sensory deficits possible for a person with dementia.
NC State—A Housing Safety Checklist for Older People	https://content.ces.ncsu.edu/housing-safety-checklist-for-older-people	Room-by-room safety checklist, as well as general safety information and a section for how to select and hire a reputable contractor should work need to be done on the home.

(Continued)

TABLE 8-1 (Continued)

Tool or resource	Where to obtain	Description
Occupational Therapy Geriatric Group/ University at Buffalo Home Safety Self-Assessment Tool	http://sphhp.buffalo.edu/ content/sphhp/rehabilitation-science/research-and-facilities/ funded-research/aging/home-safety-self-assessment-tool/ _jcr_content/par/ download_526197706/file.res/ HSSAT-v.5-1-12-17.pdf	A booklet created to disseminate information regarding how to prevent falls with an evidence base of studies conducted through the Department of Rehabilitation at the University at Buffalo. Consists of 7 major sections covering the self-assessment to "how to" and an action log.
Safety Assessment of Function and the Environment for Rehabilitation (SAFER)	Oliver, Blathwayt, Brackley, & Tamaki (1993)	The SAFER Tool was developed by four clinical therapists to fill a need to identify problems that could endanger the lives of seniors or force them to move into institutions. The four page assessment covers 128 items or functions divided into 15 areas of possible concern such as living situation, mobility, kitchen, eating, fire hazards, dressing, bathroom, medication, communication, general items/security, and wandering. Administered by clinical therapists specializing in geriatrics.
Safety Assessment Scale	de Courval et al. (2006)	Provides health care workers with a structured and validated tool to assist with evaluating the risks for accidents for people with dementia living in the community. The assessment focuses not only on environmental factors but also behaviors in the home which may put an individual at risk. A short-form version can be used as a screening tool

(Continued)

TABLE 8-1 (Continued)

Tool or resource	Where to obtain	Description
		to identify level of risk for many different types of accidents, and a long form can be used to guide intervention.
Taking Action to Prevent Falls: A Home Environmental Assessment	http://www.stopfalls.org/files/ProgramExpansion-HomeAssessmentTool.pdf	Room-by-room assessment of potential environmental hazards that pose risk for a fall. For use by service providers.
US Consumer Product Safety Commission—Safety for Older Consumers Home Safety Checklist	https://www.cpsc.gov/PageFiles/122038/701.pdf	Checklist designed to help assess the homes of older people for hazards. Contains sections with "top 10" safety tips, preparing for emergencies, as well as room-by-room checklists.
Westmead Home Safety Assessment	Clemson, Fitzgerald, & Heard (1999)	Provides a systematic and extensive detailed four-page list of potential hazards in and about the home. There are 72 hazard categories within each area of the home. Although the tool can be used to evaluate people with cognitive impairment, the WeHSA was not developed specifically for them.

As shown, these home environmental assessments may differ as to their measured characteristics, response formats, and sources from which ratings are derived. Assessments are either descriptive in which specific features are identified and described, evaluative in which measured dimensions represent desirable attributes, or a combination. Examples of measured dimensions are physical characteristics (lighting, space); affordance of daily activities (accessibility, prosthetic aids); support of orientation (way-finding). None, however, assess the home for home repair needs that may be interfering with daily life and safe functioning.

ENVIRONMENTAL MODIFICATIONS

Based on an assessment of a home, various modifications can be made to enhance its safety and optimize its support of daily functioning. The fundamental purpose of an assistive device or home modification is to compensate for the changes in cognition and function and to support retained abilities. Families are often highly adaptive and can derive their own solutions to common home hazards. However, still, consultation with a specialist, either a home modification expert or occupational therapist, can assure that the modifications which are made are appropriate and safe. The most frequently employed adaptations found in homes are listed in Box 8-3 (Gitlin et al., 2014).

Few studies have examined assistive technologies and home modifications and what persons living with dementia and/or their family

---

Box 8-3

Common Home Modifications for Safety and Optimization of Function

- Clear pathways in home to facilitate wayfinding
- Good lighting throughout the home
- Clutter-free rooms
- Adaptive equipment in bathroom (grab bars, raised toilet seats)
- First floor access to bathroom and bedroom
- Sturdy, supportive chairs with arm rests
- Medications, knives, cleaning supplies, and other hazardous household materials organized and stored out of sight
- Sturdy railings on interior and exterior staircases
- Dead bolts on all interior and exterior doors
- Bedside commode near bed for nighttime use
- Removal of weapons (safe storage with key)
- Safety locks on cabinets
- Safe storage of dangerous fluids
- Enlarged clock
- Calendars
- Enlarged telephone
- Use of signage on cabinets, drawers
- Medication dispenser
- Dead bolt locks on exit doors

members find of value (O'Keefe, 2017). Much more research in this area is needed to map type of device with cognitive abilities, personal preferences, and cognitive and physical needs. One study of 272 families enrolled in a home intervention to address behavioral symptoms, found that 63 (46.3%) of 136 familes randomized to the treatment arm received one or more assistive devices. A total of 197 devices (three per dyad) were issued of which 87.6% were reported by caregivers as in use at 4 months after receiving training in their use. Caregivers reported that overall devices were somewhat to very helpful. Devices ranged in cost from US $4.80 to US $282.93 with an average cost per dyad of US $152.52(SD = US $102.70) which included the device, its ordering, delivery, and installation (Gitlin, Winter, & Dennis, 2010).

When implementing a modification in the home, consideration must be given to whether it is a rental, and what is permissible or feasible, its implications for others in the household. For example, placing a stair glide in the home may not work if the person is obese or if young children also live in the household.

As such, modifying the home to support both family caregivers and persons living with dementia as well as other members of a household is a potential care tool or therapeutic modality. Assessing the home as well for home repair needs, we would argue, must be part of a new approach to comprehensive dementia care. A hazardous home or poor living condition can threaten the health and well-being of its inhabitants.

Box 8-4 lists key principles when modifying a home environment to support daily functioning.

Box 8-4
Principles for Home Environmental Changes

- Slowly simplify environment—too many changes can be disorienting
- Simplify the environment with disease progression
- Balance safety with autonomy and personal control
- Consider how environmental change affects all household members
- Assure any modifications fit cultural values and preferences of households
- Offer families choices among devices, environmental recommendations
- Provide instruction in use of assistive devices or home modification

> **Box 8-5**
> **Possible Triggers for Relocation to Nursing Home**
>
> - Family members do not live close
> - Complex medical conditions unable to be managed at home
> - Family situation does not enable continued caregiving
> - Caregivers overwhelmed or have own health problems
> - Care needs lead to physical strain
> - Financial strain on family
> - A fall precipitating increased care
> - Behavioral symptoms including wandering
> - Person is a danger to self or others
> - Home environment in need of too much repair or physical layout does not support care needs

WHEN TO STAY PUT AND WHEN TO LEAVE?

Deciding whether to stay put or leave is difficult and the decision may be influenced by multiple factors. Typically, there is not one particular factor or event that leads to relocation but rather a combination of conditions that conspire making staying at home a potential danger to the person living with dementia and/or their family members and no longer possible. Potential key triggers are listed in Box 8-5, although they may not be limited by these.

UNINTENDED NEGATIVE CONSEQUENCES OF STAYING HOME

Staying home may not be right for everyone, and there can be a number of unintended consequences that are negative for both the person living with dementia as well as their family members. One issue is that families report increasing difficulty venturing outside of the home, going on outings, visiting with friends and family, and hence, greater social isolation with disease progression. In this case, technology may be a partial solution. A computer-based program that linked older adults to others found significant decreases in social isolation. Although not tested with dementia caregivers, this represents a potentially promising approach for dementia care too (Czaja et al., 2015). Another unintended negative consequence is increasing social isolation and lack of meaningful activity for the person with dementia. In this case, connecting with community services such as adult day, volunteer services providing in-home companionship, or obtaining guidance from an occupational therapist for tailoring activities (see Chapter 4, Making Life Better for Individuals Living With Dementia, regarding the New Ways for Better Days Program; Gitlin et al., 2009) may offset this concern.

Yet another negative consequence may be that it is not possible for the person living with dementia or caregiver to keep up with home repairs and housekeeping, making it increasingly uncomfortable and unsafe to remain at home. Some area agencies on aging offer home repair services; some communities may be part of the village movement providing vetted handyman and volunteers who may be helpful to address this issue.

CONCLUSION

In this chapter, we have focused on the home as a micro environment with therapeutic potential to maintain a "good life." As the immediate context in which daily life transpires, the home has the potential to support individuals regardless of etiology and disease stage. As an individuated physical space imbued with meaning, history, values, and preferences, the home can also serve as an organizational framework for comprehensive dementia care to deliver coordination along with specific strategies, programs to address changing needs from time of diagnosis to end of life. There are many compelling reasons for dementia care to switch from clinic to home. Dr. Lyketsos explains how we can move forward with having the home as the epicenter of comprehensive dementia care.

A Conversation With Dr. Constantine (Kostas) Lyketsos, MD, MHS

1. *Why is the home an important consideration in dementia care?* This and related questions were taken up by a national Consensus Panel of Experts convened at Johns Hopkins with support from the BrightFocus Foundation (BFF-CPE). The primary report of this panel is in Samus et al., Alzheimer and Dementia (2018). Several converging societal trends point to the home as the nexus for dementia care. Foremost amongst these is the desire of people living with dementia and families to remain at home as long as possible. While the prevalence of dementia will increase in the coming decades, there is uncertainty about "curative treatments" anytime soon. Notably, emerging treatments may prolong dementia duration thus increasing the number of people needing care. Other important considerations are that people living with dementia have social, environmental, emotional,

safety and support care needs that go beyond medical care and services. Meeting such needs must be accomplished without increasing, hopefully by reducing, health care costs, while at the same time improving quality of life. This will require a shift to providing long-term care in the home especially given a mismatch between institutional care supply and need for long term care services, and because the shrinking pool of family caregivers will not likely match the numbers of people who will require care.

2. *How can the home serve as a nexus of care coordination and implementation of strategies to support quality of life of individuals living with dementia?* Providing dementia care in the home emphasizes a holistic, integrated approach, while meeting a wider range of needs for people living with dementia and their caregivers. This is particularly true regarding needs such as fall- and wander-risk management, challenging behaviors, medication administration and adherence, nutrition and hydration, and other home safety issues that are not easily addressed in office-based primary care. Further, home-based dementia care (HBDC) provides an opportunity for innovation in the development and implementation of novel care strategies, incorporating emerging technologies to provide wrap-around care with the home as a natural conduit. Already, there have been widespread but uncoordinated efforts to develop evidence in support of interventions, programs, strategies or approaches some of which are very promising. Home-based dementia care can bridge medical, personal and social care, with other types of community supports such as faith-based organizations and informal social supports (e.g. neighbors, friends, community members). Finally, focusing on the home will likely lead to cost and resource savings by reducing nursing home expenditures, as well as acute and emergency care costs.

3. *What would it take policy wise to make the home central to dementia care?* The BFF-CPE has made the following recommendations (Samus et al., 2018):
   1. "Home-based dementia care should be considered the nexus of new long-term care models.
   2. New payment models are needed to stimulate, reward, and support home care practices.
   3. A skilled new workforce spanning long term care needs to be developed and equipped.
   4. New technologies to promote best practices must be tested, integrated and deployed.
   5. More effective development of value, understanding of competing local priorities and adaption, and improved communication about home-based care are needed."

KEY POINTS

- The home is where most people with dementia live.
- It can contribute to or serve as a barrier to quality of life.
- Evaluating the home for its safety and ways to optimize function should be an important treatment goal and part of comprehensive dementia care.
- There are helpful tools for evaluating home environments, yet only a few are specific to persons living with dementia.
- Asking for and obtaining a home evaluation and specific assistive devices or home modifications from an occupational therapist is key to the effective use of the home environment as a therapeutic modality in dementia care.

What Can be Done Now

- Conduct home assessments at each disease stage or with change in function to evaluate a person's safety and to identify the types of adaptations that can better support daily function
- Consult with an occupational therapist to determine the just right fit of the home with the person's physical and cognitive capacities as well as their preferred treatment preferences
- Simplify the environment - remove clutter or unnecessary objects that may be confusing
- Make simple, to no to low cost modifications to enhance activity engagement such as installing grab bars, non-skid bath mat, rails, raised toilet seat, adequate lighting
- Attend to home repairs, particularly those issues which place a person at risk for injury (e.g., loose rails, steep steps, broken tiles, ripped carpets, poor air circulation)

References

AARP Research. (2016). *2016 Member Opinion Survey Initial Impressions/Insights*. Retrieved from http://www.aarp.org/content/dam/aarp/research/surveys_statistics/politics/2016%20mos/2016-initial-summary-ext.pdf.

Black, B. S., Johnston, D., Rabins, P. V., Morrison, A., Lyketsos, C., & Samus, Q. M. (2013). Unmet needs of community-residing persons with dementia and their informal caregivers: Findings from the maximizing independence at home study. *Journal of the American Geriatrics Society, 61*(12), 2087–2095. Available from https://doi.org/10.1111/jgs.12549.

Callahan, C. M. (2017). Alzheimer's disease: Individuals, dyads, communities, and costs. *Journal of the American Geriatrics Society, 65*(5), 892–895. Available from https://doi.org/10.1111/jgs.14808.

REFERENCES

Calkins, M. (2011). *Evidence-based design for dementia: Findings from the past five years. Long-Term Living, 3.* Retrieved from http://ezproxy.lib.swin.edu.au/login?url = http://go.galegroup.com/ps/i.do?id = GALE%7CA254105938&v = 2.1&u = swinburne1&it = r&p = AONE&sw = w&asid = ceb12668c715f46db811ed65f059ec1b.

Carpenter, J. G. (2017). Hospital palliative care teams and post-acute care in nursing facilities: An integrative review. *Research in Gerontological Nursing, 10*(1), 25–34. Available from https://doi.org/10.3928/19404921-20161209-02.

Clemson, L., Fitzgerald, H. M., & Heard, R. (1999). Content validity of an assessment tool to identify home fall hazards: The Westmead Home Safety Assessment. *British Journal of Occupational Therapy, 62*(4), 171–179.

Czaja, S. J., Boot, W. R., Charness, N., Rogers, A. W., Sharit, J., Fisk, A. D., ... Nair, S. N. (2015). The personalized reminder information and social management system (PRISM) trial: Rationale, methods and baseline characteristics. *Contemporary Clinical Trials, 40*, 35–46. Available from https://doi.org/10.1016/j.cct.2014.11.004.

Davos, S., Byers, S., Nay, R., & Koch, S. (2009). Guiding design of dementia friendly environments in residential care settings: Considering the living experiences. *Dementia, 8*(2), 185–203. Available from https://doi.org/10.1177/1471301209103250.

de Courval, L. P., Gélinas, I., Gauthier, S., Gayton, D., Liu, L., Rossignol, M., & Dastoor, D. (2006). Reliability and validity of the safety assessment scale for people with dementia living at home. *Canadian Journal of Occupational Therapy, 73*(2), 67–75. Available from http://doi.org/10.1177/000841740607300201.

Fausset, C. B., Kelly, A. J., Rogers, W. A., & Fisk, A. D. (2011). Challenges to aging in place: Understanding home maintenance difficulties. *Journal of Housing for the Elderly, 25*(2), 125–141. Available from https://doi.org/10.1080/02763893.2011.571105.

Gitlin, L., & Piersol, C. (2014). *Make the home safe. A caregiver's guide to dementia: Using activities and other strategies to prevent, reduce and manage behavioral symptoms* (pp. 27–34). Philadelphia: Camino Books, Inc.

Gitlin, L. N., & Corcoran, M. (2000). Making homes safer: Environmental adaptations for people with dementia. *Alzheimer's Care Quarterly, 1*(1), 50–58.

Gitlin, L. N. (2017). Reflections on a professional journey to making home life better for older adults and families. *Annual Review of Gerontology and Geriatrics, 38*(1), 89–108. Available from https://doi.org/10.1891/0198-8794.38.89.

Gitlin, L. N. (1998). Testing home modification interventions: Issues of theory, measurement, design, and implementation. *Annual Review of Gerontology and Geriatrics, 18*(1), 190–246.

Gitlin, L. N. (2003). Conducting research on home environments: Lessons learned and new directions. *The Gerontologist, 43*(5), 628–637. Available from https://doi.org/10.1093/geront/43.5.628.

Gitlin, L. N. (2007). The impact of housing on quality of life: Does the home environment matter now and into the future? In H.-W. Wahl, C. Tesch-Romer, & A. Hoff (Eds.), *New dynamics in old age: Individual, environmental, and societal perspectives* (pp. 105–125). Amityville, New York: Baywood Publishing Company, Inc.

Gitlin, L. N., Hodgson, N., & Choi, S. (2016). Home-based interventions targeting persons with dementia: What is the evidence and where do we go from here? In M. Boltz, & J. Galvin (Eds.), *Dementia Care: An Evidence-Based Approach* (pp. 167–188). Switzerland: Springer International Publishing. Available from https://doi.org/10.1007/978-3-319-18377-0_11.

Gitlin, L. N., Hodgson, N., Piersol, C. V., Hess, E., & Hauck, W. W. (2014). Correlates of quality of life for individuals with dementia living at home: The role of home environment, caregiver, and patient-related characteristics. *The American Journal of Geriatric Psychiatry, 22*(6), 587–597. Available from https://doi.org/10.1016/j.jagp.2012.11.005.

Gitlin, L. N., Schinfeld, S., Winter, L., Corcoran, M., Boyce, A. A., & Hauck, W. (2002). Evaluating home environments of persons with dementia: Interrater reliability and validity of the Home Environmental Assessment Protocol (HEAP). *Disability and Rehabilitation*, 24(1–3), 59–71. Available from https://doi.org/10.1080/09638280110066325.

Gitlin, L. N., Winter, L., & Dennis, M. P. (2010). Assistive devices to help manage behavioral symptoms of dementia: What do caregivers use and find helpful? Special issue in honor of Dr. Fozzard. *Gerontechnology*, 9(3), 408–414. Available from https://doi.org/10.4017/gt.2010.09.03.006.00, PMCID: PMC4241973.

Gitlin, L. N., Winter, L., Vause Earland, T., Adel Herge, E., Chernett, N. L., Piersol, C. V., & Burke, J. P. (2009). The tailored activity program to reduce behavioral symptoms in individuals with dementia: Feasibility, acceptability, and replication potential. *The Gerontologist*, 49(3), 428–439. Available from https://doi.org/10.1093/geront/gnp087.

Golant, S. M. (2003). Political and organizational barriers to satisfying low-income U. S. seniors' need for affordable rental housing with supportive services. *Journal of Aging & Social Policy*, 15(4), 21–48. Available from https://doi.org/10.1300/J031v15n04_02.

Hodgson, N. A., Black, B. S., Johnston, D., Lyketsos, C. G., & Samus, Q. M. (2014). Comparison of unmet care needs across the dementia trajectory findings from the MIND at home study. *Journal of Geriatrics and Palliative Care*, 2(2).

Johnson, M., Cusick, A., & Chang, S. (2001). Home-Screen: A short scale to measure fall risk in the home. *Public Health Nursing*, 18(3), 169–177. Available from http:/doi.org/10.1046/j.1525-1446.2001.00169.x.

Kelly, A. J., Fausset, C. B., Rogers, W., & Fisk, A. D. (2014). Responding to home maintenance challenge scenarios. *Journal of Applied Gerontology*, 33(8), 1018–1042. Available from https://doi.org/10.1177/0733464812456631.

Lawton, M. P., & Simon, B. (1968). The ecology of social relationships in housing for the elderly. *The Gerontologist*, 8(2), 108–115. Available from https://doi.org/10.1093/geront/8.2.108.

Lawton, M. P. (1982). Competence, environmental press, and the adaptation of older people. In M. P. Lawton, P. G. Windley, & T. O. Byerts (Eds.), *Aging and the environment*. New York: Springer.

Lawton, M. P. (1999). Environmental taxonomy: Generalizations from research with older adults. In S. L. Friedman, & T. D. Wachs (Eds.), *Measuring environment across the life span*. Washington, DC: American Psychological Association.

Leff, B., Burton, L., Mader, S. L., Naughton, B., Burl, J., Inouye, S. K., & Burton, J. R. (2005). Hospital at home: Feasibility and outcomes of a program to provide hospital-level care at home for acutely ill older patients. *Annals of Internal Medicine*, 143(11), 798–808.

Mackenzie, L., Byles, J., & Higginbotham, N. (2002). Reliability of the Home Falls and Accidents Screening Tool (HOME FAST) for identifying older people at increased risk of falls. *Disability and Rehabilitation*, 24(5), 266–274. Available from https://doi.org/10.1080/09638280110087089.

National Academies of Sciences, Engineering, and Medicine. (2016). *Families caring for an aging America*. Washington, DC: National Academies Press.

National Research Council. (2011). *Health care comes home: The human factors*. Committee on the Role of Human Factors in Home Health Care, Board on Human-Systems Integration, Division of Behavioral and Social Sciences and Education. Washington, DC: The National Academies Press.

O'Keefe, J. (2017). The use of assistive technology to reduce caregiver burden, Issue Brief, Prepared for the Research Summit on Dementia Care: Building Evidence for Services and Supports, for R. Khillan, Office of the Assistant Secretary for Planning and Evaluation.

Oliver, R., Blathwayt, J., Brackley, C., & Tamaki, T. (1993). Development of the safety assessment of function and the environment for rehabilitation (SAFER) tool. *Canadian Journal of Occupational Therapy, 60*(2), 78−82. Available from http://doi.org/10.1177/000841749306000204.

Samus, Q., Black, B., Bovenkamp, D., Buckley, M., Callahan, C., Davis, K., ... Lyketsos, C. G. (2018). Home is where the future is: The BrightFocus Foundation consensus panel on dementia care. *Alzheimer's & Dementia, 14*(1), 104−114. Available from http://dx.doi.org/10.1016/j.jalz.2017.10.006.

Struyk, R. J., & Katsura, H. M. (1988). Aging at home: How the elderly adjust their housing without moving. *Journal of Housing for the Elderly, Vol. 4*, 192, No. 2.

Szanton, S. L., Roth, J., Nkimbeng, M., Savage, J., & Klimmek, R. (2014). Improving unsafe environments to support aging independence with limited resources. *Nursing Clinics of North America, 49*(2), 133−145. Available from https://doi.org/10.1016/j.cnur.2014.02.002.

van Hoof, J., Kort, H. S. M., van Waarde, H., & Blom, M. M. (2010). Environmental interventions and the design of homes for older adults with dementia: An overview. *American Journal of Alzheimer's Disease & Other Dementiasr, 25*(3), 202−232. Available from https://doi.org/10.1177/1533317509358885.

Wahl, H.-W. & Gitlin, L.N. (in press). Linking the socio-physical environment to successful aging: From basic research to intervention to implementation science considerations. In R. Fernandez-Ballesteros, J.-M. Robine, & Benetos, A. (Eds.), *The Cambridge Handbook of Successful Aging*. London: Cambridge Press.

Wiles, J. L., Leibing, A., Guberman, N., Reeve, J., & Allen, R. E. S. (2012). The meaning of "Aging in Place" to older people. *The Gerontologist, 52*(3), 357−366. Available from https://doi.org/10.1093/geront/gnr098.

Further Reading

Amjad, H., Wong, S. K., Roth, D. L., Huang, J., Black, B. S., Johnston, D., & Samus, Q. M. (2018). Health services utilization in older adults with dementia receiving care coordination: The maximizing independence (MIND) at home trial. *Journal of American Geriatric Society, 53*(1), 556−579.

Ortman, J. M., Velkoff, V. A., & Hogan, H. (2014). An aging nation: The older population in the United States. *Economics and Statistics Administration, US Department of Commerce, 1964*, 1−28. Available from https://doi.org/10.1016/j.jaging.2004.02.002.

Rowe, M. A., Farias, J., & Boltz, M. (2016). *Dementia Care: An Evidence-Based Approach* (pp. 215−230). Switzerland: Springer International. Available from https://doi.org10.1007/978-3-319-18377-0.

CHAPTER 9

Living in the Community

You are not alone, we are your neighbors, we care about you, and we want to help. **George Vradenburg, founder of USAgainstAlzheimer's.**

Case Snapshot

Ms. H is eighty-four years old, and living with vascular dementia in York, United Kingdom. She lives alone in her two-bedroom first-floor flat, located in a community with people of all ages. While York is still in the process of becoming entirely dementia friendly, Ms. H is thankful for the resources available to her which make her day-to-day activities doable. She still goes to the local supermarket she's grown familiar with over the years. Because of York's abundant and consistent public transportation, she feels comfortable taking a bus to her stop, and a taxi home. Ms. H has built relationships with employees here who are consistently kind and helpful, so she always knows where to go for assistance. This is the case for her in many parts of town. She felt that dementia had prevented her from some areas of community involvement—she had been a nurse with a passion for adult education, and was involved with her block's management committee. However, Ms. H is still social and goes out with her friends, as they've chosen cafes and restaurants with patient and understanding staff. York is a city with the infrastructural and compassionate foundations for being dementia friendly. Though Ms. H loves her beautiful home and her TV soap operas, she has the freedom and security to go out in her community as well.

Dementia can have a devastating impact on the social lives of people with dementia. The diagnosis brings with it not only the impact on personal and family life but also a change in how the larger community in which individuals reside responds to them (Wilcock et al., 2016). In this chapter we extend our lens to consider how community-level factors impact the needs of individuals living with dementia and their families. We define community broadly as, "a group of people with diverse characteristics who are linked by social ties, share common perspectives, and engage in joint action in geographical locations or settings" (MacQueen et al., 2001). We also discuss the "dementia-friendly" community movement as one important approach to integrate families living with dementia in the community and offer examples from across the globe.

About 70% of all individuals living with dementia reside in communities, rather than in assisted living facilities or in nursing homes. Yet less than half, about 45%, of individuals living with dementia feel that they are a part of their community (Kane & Cook, 2013). As we have discussed in earlier chapters, most individuals living in the community with dementia reside with family or friends for care and support, although approximately 20% of individuals with dementia live alone (Miranda-Castillo, Woods, & Orrell, 2010). When asked to identify the leading barriers to participating in community life, individuals with dementia reported the following (Alzheimer's Australia, 2014):

- 57% indicated that they are afraid of becoming lost or unable to find their way,
- 48% said that they have difficulty communicating with others, and
- 25% said that people in their community seem uneasy around them.

THE NEED FOR SECURITY AND BELONGING

Regardless of the type of home or community (urban, rural, row home, duplex, and so forth), individuals living in the community with dementia need to feel safe, secure, and that they belong (van der Roest et al., 2009). Nevertheless, feeling safe, secure, and connected is not the case for most with 90% of persons living in the community with dementia having unmet safety needs, particularly for fall and wander risk management (Amjad, Roth, Samus, Yasar, & Wolff, 2016). This also includes driving safety and safe management of guns and tools in the home (Black et al., 2013). As discussed in Chapter 2, Lived Experiences of Individuals With Dementia (about the individual), and Chapter 8, The Physical Home Environment: A Neglected Therapeutic Context, (about the home environment), the need for safety transcends disease etiology and stage and is the most prominent documented unmet need for community residing persons with dementia.

Most people living with dementia in the community also express feeling isolated and lonely (Herron & Rosenberg, 2017; Lehmann, Black, Shore, Kasper, & Rabins, 2010). One of our most fundamental, basic needs as humans is to feel a sense of security and belonging—the sense that we feel connected and accepted by others and that we have meaningful and purposeful roles. Despite their need for belonging, many individuals with dementia feel that they cannot or do not know how to contribute to their local community (Box 8-1). Because of these barriers, two thirds of people with dementia do not feel they can make a meaningful contribution to their communities (Kane & Cook, 2013). Prior studies have also found high unmet needs for daytime social activities (Mirando-Castillo, Woods, Galboda, et al., 2010; Wancata, Krautgartner, Berner, et al., 2005).

Despite wanting to do more, individuals living with dementia feel restricted by their condition and hold low expectations about being able to contribute. Using a large population-based survey, the National Health and Aging Trends Study (NHATS), a study of older adults with no dementia ($n = 5269$), possible dementia ($n = 893$), or probable dementia ($n = 518$) found that activity and participation with others was critical for all three cognitive groups. However, compared to cognitively healthy individuals, those with possible and probable dementia were less likely to indicate activities were important and engage in valued activities ($Ps < 0.0001$). Difficulty with transportation was cited as a limiting factor for going out for enjoyment for a greater percentage of those with cognitive impairment than those without impairment (Parisi, Roberts, Szanton, Hodgson, & Gitlin, 2015). This study showed that regardless of cognitive level, older adults highly value activities. Nevertheless, actual participation in valued activities appears to decrease with greater impairment in cognitive and physical health and with transportation challenges. Box 9-1 lists the leading barriers to community involvement.

Collectively, the evidence suggests that there is an urgent need for broader thinking about community-based strategies that can effectively address these basic human needs common to all persons, and to support people living with dementia to continue to live well and be involved in those activities that are preferred and give enjoyment that may have been part of daily life prior to a diagnosis. For individuals with dementia to live safely and comfortably and connected in their community for as long as possible, new ways of organizing community supports is an imperative.

> **Box 9-1**
> **Leading Barriers to Community Involvement for Persons With Dementia**
>
> - Lack of support from others to carry out preferred activities
> - Lack of appropriate activities for people with dementia to do
> - Lack of confidence
> - Worry about becoming confused
> - Worry about getting lost
> - Mobility issues
> - Physical health issues
> - Lack of transportation

DEMENTIA-FRIENDLY COMMUNITIES

What is "dementia friendly"? Imagine a community in which individuals with dementia could reside and feel fully integrated, accepted, and without sensing or being stigmatized for having cognitive impairments. A "dementia-friendly" community considers the role of the neighborhood environment in integrating people with dementia into their community (Fleming, Bennett, Preece, & Phillipson, 2017). A dementia-friendly community is one in which a person living with dementia is empowered to have high aspirations, feel confident, and can contribute and participate in activities that are meaningful to them (Crampton, Dean, & Eley, 2012). The dementia-friendly philosophy is about ensuring that people with dementia are empowered to live well, and exert choice and control in their lives. Importantly, it recognizes the impact that dementia has on relationships and people's confidence to engage in daily tasks and activities. Dementia-friendly communities can have a profound impact on a person's quality of life, affecting not only the individual but also their family caregivers. There is increasing evidence that dementia-friendly communities can support the health and well-being and quality of life of individuals with dementia and their families (Alzheimer's Disease International, 2016; Lin, 2017).

> The rationale for creating dementia-friendly communities comes from the voices and experiences of people living with and affected by the condition.

Box 9-2
Priorities of Individuals With Dementia in Creating Dementia-Friendly Communities

- Accessible social services
- Reliable transportation
- Navigable environments
- Dementia-specific care

Developing a dementia-friendly community starts with a community assessing the following questions: What are the needs of the people with dementia living in our community? How can we go about mobilizing resources to help them; and specifically, help them with transportation, access to businesses, access to support services? How can we help them access medical management and education needed to manage their diseases along with other needs such as home repairs, support as the disease progresses? Surveys of individuals with dementia identified priorities in creating dementia-friendly communities listed in Box 9-2 (Burton & Mitchell, 2006).

Dementia-friendly communities have several key attributes. The first indication of a dementia-friendly community is that there are purposefully organized activities that meet the needs of people with dementia and that are geared towards their abilities. Many respondents to the survey mentioned above indicated that increasing *access to social activities and services* was essential to creating dementia-friendly communities. Easily accessible and comprehensive information about available services and support was also highlighted as a strategy that would help people with dementia access appropriate supports and activity groups within their community. One common need expressed by people living with dementia is that they would like more support and services to allow them to do the things that they still can do in their community. Examples include volunteer activities, social activities that they previously enjoyed, and participation in religious organizations or other community groups and ability to conduct their daily business without fear of stigmatization. This all means that people in the community, including police and firemen, and those who work in the local businesses in the community, have some kind of awareness of what dementia is and are able to respond appropriately to people with dementia.

The second critical attribute is the need for reliable and accessible transportation that individuals with dementia can go safely by various transportation mechanisms. *Reliable transportation* options were identified as essential to ongoing involvement in the community for people with dementia. Often the need for access to services translates into the need for improved transportation options to community organizations and resources. People with dementia need to give up their driver's license at some point following diagnosis (Musselwhite, 2011). Often this creates a crisis as it means a significant loss of independence and control. With access to appropriate community transportation, individuals can continue to engage in activities they were involved in before losing their license. This includes the need for improved ways of negotiating and accessing the transportation system.

Another factor that is indicative of a dementia-friendly community is a *navigable physical environment* and includes attention to way finding, appropriate signage, and the use of open space (Brorsson, Ohman, Lundberg, & Nygard, 2011; Duggan, Blackman, Martyr, & Van Schaik, 2008) More specifically, dementia-friendly physical environments include the use of appropriate signage, lighting, and colors. Individuals with dementia need information that is easily understandable and accessible. Some survey participants (35%) explained that changes to community physical environments would improve their ability to access and interact within their community (Alzheimer's Australia, 2014). For example, minimizing noise where possible, less reflective surfaces such as glass and better maps, signage, and directional cues.

The last but not least aspect of a dementia-friendly community is the availability of dementia specific resources including access to early diagnosis, as well as support following a diagnostic workup including support for the family caregivers. Not surprisingly, people with dementia identified access to dementia-specific health and care services as a priority need. This includes access to a timely diagnosis, support and services after diagnosis, access to respite, affordable assistance with housework and gardening, and opportunities for flexible support within the home (Noel, Kaluzynski, & Templeton, 2017).

"Dementia friendly" is a term gaining increasing popularity worldwide. Other terms are also being introduced in the United States when referring to community-level strategies to improve dementia care. For example, the term "dementia capable" is used to reflect an integration of dementia resources. "Dementia aware" is a term promoting an inclusive society for individuals with dementia and their families. "Dementia ready" refers to the preparedness of a care setting to accommodate people with dementia. Table 9-1 defines each of these terms and their common usage.

TABLE 9-1 Dementia Friendly/Capable/Ready/Aware

Term	Definition	Citation
Dementia friendly	A *dementia-friendly* community is one based on inclusion, where a person living with dementia feels empowered to play an active role in their community and is able to participate in the day-to-day activities we take for granted. The emphasis is on what the person can do, rather than what they can no longer do. In general, this term is applied to communities. A dementia-friendly community is a place where individuals with dementia: • are able to live good lives, • have the ability to live as independently as possible, • continue to be a part of their communities, • are met with understanding, and • are given support where and when as necessary. Individuals with dementia describe a dementia-friendly community as one that enables them to: • find their way around and be safe, • access local facilities they are used to and where they are known, and • maintain their social networks so they feel they continue to belong. The idea of dementia-friendly businesses exists as well, but again falls more in line with making the businesses themselves as accessible to people with dementia as possible.	http://www.ageuk.org.uk/brandpartnerglobal/norfolkvpp/documents/events/idn515%20dfc%20training%20leaflet%20heth%20awb.pdf https://www.fightdementia.org.au/about-us/campaigns/dementia-friendly-communities http://www.bbc.co.uk/news/mobile/uk-england-devon-16603642 Lin & Lewis—Dementia Friendly, Dementia Capable, and Dementia Positive: Concepts to Prepare for the Future; 2015

(*Continued*)

TABLE 9-1 (Continued)

Term	Definition	Citation
Dementia capable	There are at least two meanings to the term *"dementia capable."* It can refer to something that people with dementia are able to do/enjoy (similar to "dementia friendly"). It can also be interpreted as an ability (a combination of staff knowledge, skills, and competency as well as available programs and services) to fulfill the needs of people with dementia and their caregivers. In the US national dementia plan and relevant documents, the term "dementia capable" refers to the latter. Dementia capable is a concept unique to the United States. There is no mention of this term in other country's documents. Regardless, this concept guides the creation of nationwide dementia-capable workforces, services, and programs. In contrast to the focus on the environment in the concept of dementia friendly, the usage of the term dementia capable centers around the language and philosophy of care.	Lin & Lewis—Dementia Friendly, Dementia Capable, and Dementia Positive: Concepts to Prepare for the Future; 2015 http://www.investigage.com/2015/06/01/from-dementia-capable-to-dementia-positive/
Dementia ready	*Dementia ready* refers to a level of preparedness to accommodate people with dementia in a particular setting. For instance, a "dementia-readiness inventory" assesses the availability of dementia-ready features of certain environmental areas (e.g., dementia-ready colors, flooring, way-finding signs and furniture; dementia-ready lighting, sound management, and small group activity environments). Dementia ready also indicates a preemptive readiness before signs of dementia or diagnoses are made and this way precedes "Dementia capable." One could presumably be dementia ready and, once dementia symptoms appear, become dementia capable.	Watchman—Why Wait for Dementia?; 2003 https://books.google.com/books?id=r4qfAwAAQBAJ&pg=PA249&lpg=PA249&dq=%22dementia+ready%22&source=bl&ots=aC5zKkw5Ql&sig=f3Vxhg-TsjIoaG3MRQXeb6TZ87Q&hl=en&sa=X&ved=0ahUKEwiLtpSWuNrOAhUHziYKHSCwDco Q6AEILzAE#v=onepage&q=%22dementia%20 ready%22&f=false http://www.free-alzheimers-support.com/wordpress/5-ways-to-be-dementia-ready-during-most-holidays/

Dementia aware	*Dementia aware* signifies the addressing of negative attitudes and stigma towards people living with dementia through an understanding of the disease. The focus is on providing education and knowledge. This term typically refers to businesses. The "Purple Angel" logo was originally created to help hospital staff identify patients with dementia by giving them a purple wristband. The specific term "dementia aware" does not seem to be widely used, at least in a formal manner as in the case of "capable" and "friendly." Dementia awareness is often used or mentioned as part of dementia-friendly or -capable initiatives and, as mentioned above, seems to indicate knowledge and education.	http://www.purpleangel-global.com/ http://www.bbc.com/news/uk-england-devon-22960804 http://teepasnow.com/events/online-training-course-becoming-dementia/ https://www.nursingtimes.net/every-week-needs-to-be-dementia-aware-for-nurses/5058877.blog

Examples of Dementia-Friendly Programs

The specific characteristics of a dementia-friendly community vary by the community's resources and cultural values. Efforts can range from city or state wide initiatives to small, culturally based, neighborhood activities. An example of the latter includes a neighborhood program that co-occurs during "The Longest Day" event sponsored in the United States by the Alzheimer's Association to honor persons with dementia. In New York City's neighborhood of Korea town, residents participate by making Korean lucky pouches called jumoni. These pouches are one traditional way of recognizing and honoring the traditions of the elders in the community living with dementia.

Another example of a dementia-friendly community is from Santiago Chile, in the municipality called Peñalolén. Here, the community developed an adult day center named Kintun embedded in the senior center for all older adults regardless of cognitive or physical impairments. This senior center is also located within a larger community center that the entire community uses (children, young adults, and older adults) such that people living with dementia and their families become integrated within the community at large. This geographic arrangement normalizes the activities and experiences of persons with dementia and enables them to feel connected to their community (Gajardo et al., 2017).

Memory cafes are yet another example of dementia-friendly initiatives common in the United Kingdom and the Netherlands and gaining a presence throughout Europe, Australia, and the United States. Memory cafes are described as welcoming and gathering places for individuals with memory impairments or dementia and their caregivers. Most provide activities designed to prevent boredom or to promote relaxation. Typically, memory cafes are hosted and/or facilitated by health and human service professionals to provide guidance and respond to questions or requests for resources. They take place in a wide range of venues including coffee houses, galleries/museums, community centers, and conference centers. Watertown, Wisconsin, in the United States, is home to several memory cafes. In addition, the town's shops and businesses have a display of a decal that indicates that their employees are specifically trained to recognize and assist people with dementia.

Bruges, Belgium, is an international leader in championing the role of cities to be dementia friendly, and their approach has been adopted in cities in Germany and France. Businesses that have adopted dementia-friendly practices are connoted by placing the logo of a knotted red handkerchief signifying "dementievriendelijk Brugge" (e.g., dementia-friendly Burges) in their windows or other business materials. Bruges also has established a database that allows emergency responders to quickly react when individuals with cognitive impairment are missing. In the past, it might have taken many hours to locate an individual's address or the common places a person with dementia may have frequented. Burges also promotes meaningful activities for persons with dementia. One of the most common is the town choir, specifically developed for individuals with dementia. Also, the city has conducted dementia training for staff in different shops, so that the staff can recognize individuals with cognitive impairment and work with them in their shop settings.

Another recognized dementia-friendly initiative is the Village concept launched in the Netherlands. Here the long-term care setting has been designed to resemble a village or town square community in which individuals with dementia reside in previously. For example, the shops look like traditional supermarkets or other traditional business settings, but they are specifically designed for the individuals with dementia that reside within that "village."

Regardless of the scale or scope of the program, the key to developing a dementia-friendly moment is to engage multiple community partners, or stakeholders, in the planning and implementation process (Box 9-3).

Often the most significant challenge in initiating a dementia-friendly community is in achieving stakeholder involvement. Key is establishing networks and including people representative of the local community, involving people affected by dementia, and gaining commitment from

---

Box 9-3

Examples of Community Partners for Dementia

- Businesses that support customers with dementia
- Health care systems that promotes timely diagnosis and specialist care and support
- Specialized residential options for persons with memory loss
- Dementia-aware legal and financial planning
- Dementia-informed emergency responders
- Engaged communities of faith
- Accessible transportation and public spaces
- Understanding neighbors and community members

organizations. Earlier dementia-friendly initiatives have developed a set of strategies for achieving stakeholder involvement and include (1) a sustainable approach; (2) spreading the word; and (3) sharing of ideas. By highlighting these challenges and the approaches that have been used within communities to overcome them, the beginning foundation for the creation of dementia-friendly, community-based initiatives has been established (Barclay, Barclay, Mastery, Miller, & Paone, 2015; Heward, Innes, Cutler, & Hambidge, 2017).

From this chapter, an expansive vision emerges as to specific ways to transform dementia care at the community level. This involves addressing the needs of individuals living with dementia in the community with a particular focus on security and belonging. Of importance is that this is all achievable now with a coalition of local forces which has energy and passion.

KEY POINTS

- Individuals with dementia living in the community have a desire to contribute.
- The voice of people living with dementia is essential to the design and execution of dementia-friendly initiatives.
- Dementia-friendly initiatives can take many forms from small neighborhood projects, to city-wide programs with multiple community partners, to larger state or country wide initiatives that are part of a national dementia plan.

What Can be Done Now

- Identify and form a collaborative involving key organizations, business, corporations, families, individuals with dementia and community leaders willing to work towards creating a dementia friendly community.
- Consult with local police, fire stations, city health departments to determine their dementia awareness.
- Meet with public transportation leaders to determine how to partner.
- Link with local health and human service professionals and colleges to involve faculty and students to develop dementia education for communities.

References

Alzheimer's Australia. (2014). *Living with dementia in the community: Challenges & opportunities.* Scullin. Retrieved from https://www.dementia.org.au/sites/default/files/DementiaFriendlySurvey_Final_web.pdf.

Alzheimer's Disease International. (2016). *Dementia friendly communities.* London. Retrieved from https://www.alz.co.uk/adi/pdf/dfc-principles.pdf.

Amjad, H., Roth, D. L., Samus, Q. M., Yasar, S., & Wolff, J. L. (2016). Potentially unsafe activities and living conditions of older adults with dementia. *Journal of the American Geriatrics Society, 64*(6), 1223–1232. Available from https://doi.org/10.1111/jgs.14164.

Barclay, T. R., Barclay, M., Mastery, O., Miller, E. F., & Paone, D. (2015). Building dementia-friendly communities: A collective action approach. *Alzheimer's & Dementia, 11*(7), P578–P579. Available from https://doi.org/10.1016/j.jalz.2015.06.763.

Black, B. S., Johnston, D., Rabins, P. V., Morrison, A., Lyketsos, C., & Samus, Q. M. (2013). Unmet needs of community-residing persons with dementia and their informal caregivers: Findings from the maximizing independence at home study. *Journal of the American Geriatrics Society, 61*(12), 2087–2095. Available from https://doi.org/10.1111/jgs.12549.

Brorsson, A., Ohman, A., Lundberg, S., & Nygard, L. (2011). Accessibility in public space as perceived by people with Alzheimer's disease. *Dementia, 10*(4), 587–602. Available from https://doi.org/10.1177/1471301211415314.

Burton, E., & Mitchell, L. (2006). *Inclusive urban design: Street for life.* Amsterdam: Elsevier.

Crampton, J., Dean, J., & Eley, R. (2012). *Creating a dementia-friendly York.* York: Joseph Rowntree Foundation.

Duggan, S., Blackman, T., Martyr, A., & Van Schaik, P. (2008). The impact of early dementia on outdoor life: A 'shrinking world'? *Dementia, 7*(2), 191–204. Available from https://doi.org/10.1177/1471301208091158.

Fleming, R., Bennett, K., Preece, T., & Phillipson, L. (2017). The development and testing of the dementia friendly communities' environment assessment tool (DFC EAT). *International Psychogeriatrics, 29*(2), 303–311. Available from https://doi.org/10.1017/S1041610216001678.

Gajardo, J., Aravena, J. M., Budinich, M., Larraín, A., Fuentes, P., & Gitlin, L. N. (2017). The Kintun program for families with dementia: From novel experiment to national policy (innovative practice). *Dementia (London, England).* Available from https://doi.org/10.1177/1471301217721863, 1471301217721863.

Herron, R. V., & Rosenberg, M. W. (2017). "Not there yet": Examining community support from the perspective of people with dementia and their partners in care. *Social Science & Medicine, 173,* 81–87. Available from https://doi.org/10.1016/j.socscimed.2016.11.041.

Heward, M., Innes, A., Cutler, C., & Hambidge, S. (2017). Dementia-friendly communities: Challenges and strategies for achieving stakeholder involvement. *Health & Social Care in the Community, 25*(3), 858–867. Available from https://doi.org/10.1111/hsc.12371.

Kane, M., & Cook, L. (2013). *Dementia 2013: The hidden voice of loneliness.* London: Alzheimer's Society.

Lehmann, S. W., Black, B. S., Shore, A., Kasper, J., & Rabins, P. V. (2010). Living alone with dementia: Lack of awareness adds to functional and cognitive vulnerabilities. *International Psychogeriatrics, 22*(5), 778–784. Available from https://doi.org/10.1017/S1041610209991529.

Liu, S.-Y. (2017). "Dementia-friendly communities" and being dementia friendly in healthcare settings. *Current Opinion in Psychiatry, 30*(2), 145–150. Available from https://doi.org/10.1097/YCO.0000000000000304.

MacQueen, K. M., McLellan, E., Metzger, D. S., Kegeles, S., Strauss, R. P., Scotti, R., ... Trotter, R. T. (2001). What is community? An evidence-based definition for participatory public health. *American Journal of Public Health, 91*(12), 1929–1938.

Miranda-Castillo, C., Woods, B., Galboda, K., Oomman, S., Olojugba, C., & Orrell, M. (2010). Unmet needs, quality of life and support networks of people with dementia living at home. *Health and Quality of Life Outcomes, 8*(1), 132. Available from https://doi.org/10.1186/1477-7525-8-132.

Miranda-Castillo, C., Woods, B., & Orrell, M. (2010). People with dementia living alone: What are their needs and what kind of support are they receiving? *International Psychogeriatrics, 22*(4), 607–617. Available from https://doi.org/10.1017/S104161021000013X.

Musselwhite, C. (2011). The importance of driving for older people and how the pain of driving cessation can be reduced. *Journal of Dementia and Mental Health, 15*(3), 22–26.

Noel, M. A., Kaluzynski, T. S., & Templeton, V. H. (2017). Quality dementia care. *Journal of Applied Gerontology, 36*(2), 195–212. Available from https://doi.org/10.1177/0733464815589986.

Parisi, J. M., Roberts, L., Szanton, S. L., Hodgson, N. A., & Gitlin, L. N. (2015). Valued activities among individuals with and without cognitive impairments: Findings from the National Health and Aging Trends Study. *The Gerontologist, 57,* 309–318. Available from https://doi.org/10.1093/geront/gnv144.

van der Roest, H. G., Meiland, F. J. M., Comijs, H. C., Derksen, E., Jansen, A. P. D., van Hout, H. P. J., ... Dröes, R.-M. (2009). What do community-dwelling people with dementia need? A survey of those who are known to care and welfare services. *International Psychogeriatrics, 21*(5), 949. Available from https://doi.org/10.1017/S1041610209990147.

Wancata, J., Krautgartner, M., Berner, J., Alexandrowicz, R., Unger, A., Kaiser, G., ... Weiss, M. (2005). The Carers' Needs Assessment for Dementia (CNA-D): Development, validity and reliability. *International Psychogeriatrics, 17*(3), 393–406. Available from https://doi.org/10.1017/S1041610205001699P.

Wilcock, J., Jain, P., Griffin, M., Thuné-Boyle, I., Lefford, F., Rapp, D., & Iliffe, S. (2016). Diagnosis and management of dementia in family practice. *Aging & Mental Health, 20*(4), 362–369. Available from https://doi.org/10.1080/13607863.2015.1011082.

PART IV

ABOUT SOCIAL SYSTEMS AND POLICIES

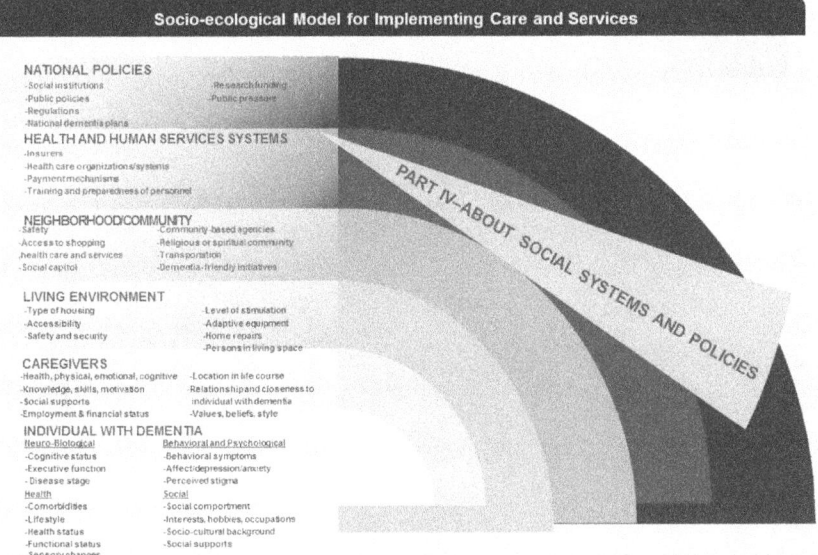

Part IV starts off by examining the clinical health and social service practices and environment (see Chapter 10: Services and Settings of Care). Then we move to a more macro-level domain of our social–ecological model, specifically, global actions and national plans (see Chapter 11: Global Efforts and National Plans). We start with a broad strokes understanding of noteworthy global activities and then drill down to the scope and role of national plans. We explore essential questions concerning the content of such plans, the elements in common across nations and their potential and real impact. We also compare national plans, identify their common elements, and show how some countries are changing the landscape of dementia care.

Then in Chapter 12, Transforming Dementia Care, we highlight key transformative actions at each social–ecological level as a way to pull together immediate actions that could change and move us toward comprehensive dementia care. While we do not specify particular legislation, social policy actions, we map out the underlying principles for taking actions.

CHAPTER 10

Services and Settings of Care

> *We must teach ourselves to see places where elders live as habitats for human beings rather than facilities for the frail and elderly.* **Dr. Bill Thomas, author, geriatrician and founder of the Eden Alternative.**

Individuals living with dementia may access care across a variety of health and social service care settings through which they receive needed services and supports. Most of these services function in silos that are more organization or program-focused than person and family-focused. Consequently, most persons living with dementia and their family caregivers face a dizzying array of services with different funding streams, locations, and payment structures that they need to figure out and coordinate on their own. These multiple services each have different eligibility criteria, coverage limitations, and typically require multiple appointments that are a challenge to navigate. Individuals and their family caregivers are often confused as to where they can turn to and for which types of services and information, and feel that they are left to their own devices in terms of finding the type of care and supportive services they may need.

In an ideal situation, once a person has received a diagnosis of dementia, he or she would receive effective coordination of ongoing and seamless health and social care services, as these are vital for achieving quality of life or the "good life". Unfortunately, this is not the typical experience, especially in the United States.

Case Scenario: Mrs. O.

Mrs. O, age 77 had been diagnosed with early-stage dementia but was otherwise in good health. Her symptoms had been mild, and she lived at home with her husband. One morning she had an episode that put her in danger; thinking her husband was an intruder, she ran to their neighbors' home. The neighbors contacted the police, who suggested she be taken to the hospital. Once in the Emergency room, Mrs. O became agitated and combative. The care team and family went back and forth with care options; her doctor was unsure whether to hospitalize her. Eventually, Mrs. O was admitted for treatment but she remained confused and combative and was given medications for sedation, which increased her confusion. With no further plans, her husband waited to see what the doctors would suggest for her care. Her children were afraid that having their mother return home might not be feasible as it was becoming increasingly difficult for Mr. O to manage. However, the family were unsure where she could receive the best care. Ms. O was ultimately moved to a nursing home close to her former residence but her experience was not easy. The new environment was generally challenging and confusing, and Mrs. O often tried to enter other residents' rooms. She was resistant to care and easily agitated. One week after her admission to the nursing home, Mrs. O fell out of bed and fractured her hip. She was transferred back to the hospital where her family faced more uncertainty about where she would receive the best care.

The case of Mrs. O describes the fragmented system of services that many individuals living with dementia and their families encounter. Rather than a coordinated network between service providers and settings of care, most individuals with dementia and their families must navigate a broken or nonexistent network in their community. This fragmented care results in higher rates of poor outcomes for persons with dementia such as hospital-acquired complications, morbidity, mortality, and excess health care expenditures (Kable, Chenoweth, Pond, & Hullick, 2015; Phelan, Borson, Grothaus, Balch, & Larson, 2012). Persons living with dementia, in comparison to those without dementia, have greater odds of having potentially avoidable hospitalizations for chronic conditions such as diabetes and hypertension (Lin, Fillit, Cohen, & Neumann, 2013). Most individuals living with dementia in the United States (89.2%) have at least one or more hospital stays and 54% have at least one stay in a nursing home in the past year (Callahan et al., 2015). In addition, nearly 20% of nursing home residents with dementia experience one or more changes in settings of care and experience an average of 1.6 transitions across multiple settings of care in the last 90 days of life (Gozalo et al., 2011).

> A better-coordinated, more integrated network of services and supports is needed that will enable individuals living with dementia, and their family members, to live well throughout the disease trajectory

In this chapter, we review the range of common settings and services of care that are available to individuals living with dementia and their families across the disease trajectory. We discuss "person- and family-centered" care as the framework for coordinating care and describe the physical and programmatic features that characterize "person- and family-centered" care and services. We then summarize several evidence-based care models that exemplify a coordinated, person-/family-centered approach to dementia care.

WHAT IS PERSON- AND FAMILY-CENTERED CARE?

Person- and family-centered care is an essential element in dementia care, whether at home, at an adult day service program, in the hospital or living in a long-term care setting (Brooker, 2004). Person-centered services refers to the actual provision of care and support based on individual preferences, values, lifestyle choices and needs, and the belief that there can be a partnership between the provider of care and the recipient of care to ensure respect for the individual person's preferences and personal dignity (Koren, 2010). This approach must include the family member(s) when they are available and part of the network of care of individuals.

Since the person living with dementia is the common link between services and settings, a person- and family-centered framework is the optimal model of care for guiding dementia care (Brooker, 2004). Given that most people prefer to live in their own homes and communities, aging in place is a common, person- and family-centered goal for most individuals living with dementia. Nevertheless, as an individual's and family's needs change across the dementia trajectory so to their needs for services and supports (Fig. 10-1).

In the earlier stages of disease, community-based services (including the home, outpatient care, support services) are the most appropriate. As the disease transitions to more advanced stages, institutionally based settings (hospitals, nursing homes) may be required. Table 10-1 summarizes the most common services and settings available for persons with dementia.

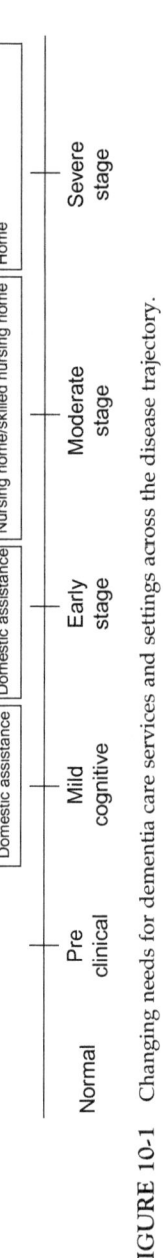

FIGURE 10-1 Changing needs for dementia care services and settings across the disease trajectory.

TABLE 10-1 Common Settings of Care

Service	Setting Location	Description of services provided
Home help/personal care	Community	Companionship and basic domestic or household tasks such as house cleaning, meal preparation and shopping, washing, and ironing.
Memory clinic	Community	Identifies, investigates, diagnoses, and treats individuals with memory problems including dementia.
Caregiver support	Community	Includes in-person support groups and online resources for family caregivers. Often serves as the starting point for caregiver education and support.
Home healthcare	Community	Medically prescribed, skilled care provided by a licensed health professional (e.g., nurse, occupational therapist, or physical therapist).
Day care	Community	Socialization and planned activities provided in a safe environment. Transportation and meals are often provided.
Medical/primary care	Community	Refers to the first point of contact and principle point of contact with a healthcare practitioner (e.g., doctor or nurse practitioner) for basic rather than specialized care.
Transportation support	Community	Enables individuals who are no longer able to drive safely the ability to gain access to other community services, activities, and resources. Examples include public transit, taxi or car share service, special transportation services, or medication, grocery or meal delivery.
Respite	Community or institution	Short-term relief program provided by skilled care professional to assume caregiver responsibilities for a predetermined amount of time.
Hospice	Community or institution	End-of-life care provided by a team of specially trained providers, including doctors, nurses, home health aides, social workers, counselors, clergy, and volunteers. Includes medical care to alleviate symptoms and pain (including medications and medical equipment), counseling about the emotional and spiritual impact of the end-of-life, respite care to allow caregivers relief, and grief support for the family.

(Continued)

TABLE 10-1 (Continued)

Service	Setting Location	Description of services provided
Specialist services	Community or institution	Secondary care services used to address complex health care needs, such as comorbid illnesses that cannot solely be met through primary care services.
Residential care/nursing homes/skilled nursing	Institution	Provides skilled or unskilled nursing care for individuals with disabilities including dementia. Provides continuous, 24-hour/day care and long-term medical treatment. Services address issues such as nutrition, care planning, recreation, spirituality, nursing, and medical care.
Assisted living	Institution	Congregated residential settings that coordinate personal services, 24-hour/day supervision, and health-related services.
Memory care	Institution	Provides intensive, long-term medical care for individuals with moderate to advanced stage dementia conditions in a fully staffed and monitored facility. Supervised care includes meals, activities, personal assistance, medication management, and health management for residents and is staffed 24 hours/day
Acute care	Institution	Level of care and services where a person with dementia receives brief and active treatment for a severe injury or episode of illness, an urgent medical condition, or during recovery from surgery.

SERVICE NEEDS ACROSS THE DEMENTIA TRAJECTORY

Mild-stage dementia: Person- and family-centered services for individuals with mild-cognitive impairment—when problems with memory, thinking, and concentration first begin to appear—are most often community based. The focus of services provided in the mild stage is to assist people to remain living in their home and community, help with understanding the diagnosis, and supporting the family's information needs and plan for the future. These services typically include assistance with understanding the disease, providing support for simple daily routines, and educating individuals and family members with information on resources. These include a comprehensive assessment, of individual and caregiver needs and structured counseling and education programs and education. Additional resources may include grocery and meal delivery services, transportation services, and legal and financial planning services.

Early-stage dementia: At this stage, those with dementia may be unable to recall their own address or phone number but still remember significant details about themselves and their family and still require no assistance eating or using the toilet. The availability of daily recreation, socialization, and stimulation is especially valuable for enhancing person-centered care. Given the increasing structure, consistency, support, and personal assistance required by a person, and the increased burden placed upon caregivers to provide the vast majority of this support, adult day care is an optimal person-centered setting. Compared with nonusers of adult-day services, caregivers of individuals with early-stage dementia adult-day service experience have been shown to have fewer behaviors, fewer conflicts with caregivers, and lower levels of caregiver depression and worry (Dziegielewski & Ricks, 2001; Gaugler et al. 2003a; Gaugler *et al.* 2003b; Schacke & Zank, 2006; Zarit, Stephens, Townsend, & Greene, 1998). Other supports and services that may be helpful to individuals with early-stage dementia include transportation services and personal care.

Moderate-stage dementia: In this stage, memory continues to worsen, personality changes may take place, and individuals need significant help with daily activities. The person may lose awareness of recent experiences as well as their surroundings, distinguish familiar and unfamiliar faces but have trouble remembering the name of a spouse or caregiver, need help dressing properly, experience behavioral changes such as suspiciousness or repetitive behavior, and tend to wander or become lost. Family caregivers may find it difficult to manage their family member with dementia at home without significant support. In this stage, many additional services may be required. Residential care such as assisted living may be the most appropriate and effective way of meeting someone's needs and providing a service of choice when community supports are insufficient (Hyde, Perez, & Forester, 2007). Respite care is another service that is necessary in the moderate stage of dementia. Respite care refers to the temporary provision of care for a person living with dementia to afford family carers' opportunities time off from their care responsibilities. It can take place in a variety of settings including the home of the person with dementia, and day-care center or in a residential setting. Respite care may also vary in duration—ranging from a few hours to a several weeks—and may involve daytime-only care or overnight care.

Severe or late-stage dementia: In the final stage of this disease, individuals lose the ability to respond to the environment, to carry on a conversation and, eventually, to control movement. Individuals need help with much of their daily personal care, including eating, bathing, and toileting. Muscles become weaker, and reflexes such as swallowing become impaired. Nursing homes may be the most appropriate setting and the safest and wisest choice for some adults with advanced dementia and for their family caregiver since many persons with late-stage dementia require 24-hour skilled nursing care. Attention to comfort, dignity, and honoring a person's end-of-life wishes become the focus of late-stage dementia care, and a palliative care philosophy is essential. Timely referral to hospice care is an important consideration.

BEST PRACTICES IN SETTING DESIGN AND PROGRAMMING

Regardless of the setting of care, a person- and family-centered approach can be greatly enhanced by designing environments that respond to the needs of people with dementia (Lin, 2017) A stronger emphasis on design features in the environment that enhance the dignity and privacy of individual residents and promote care practices that improve quality of life and quality of care for individuals with dementia and their caregivers is essential to this effort (Calkins, 1988; Cohen & Weisman, 1991; McCormack et al., 2010; Rijnaard et al., 2016). A summary of these best practices is outlined in Box 10-1.

Beyond the physical environment, attention to the structure of programs available within a setting is also an important consideration

---

Box 10-1

Principles Underpinning Best Practice in Dementia Care Settings:

- Compensate for disability
- Maximize independence
- Enhance self-esteem and confidence
- Demonstrate care for staff
- Be orientating, predictable, and understandable
- Reflect a balance of safety and autonomy-reinforced personal identity
- Allow control of stimuli
- Involve the caregiver

(Thurman, Harrison, Blozis, Dionne-Vahalik, & Mead, 2017). For example, structured routines that can be implemented across a variety of settings including assisted living, nursing home, and hospital settings can significantly improve the quality of life and health outcomes for people with dementia (Tilly & Reed, 2008). Examples of person-centered programming could include attention to nutrition and feeding such as allowing individuals control of the eating process and eating while listening to music have resulted in people consuming more food and reducing anxiety. Similar strategies for bathing, dressing, sleeping, and other daily living functions demonstrate that a pleasant environment and supports that promote a "person-centered" approach all contribute to improved quality of life. More person-centered communication strategies that directly involve family caregivers have also been shown to improve care for people with dementia in dementia care setting by identifying the person's strengths, goals, preferences, service needs, and desired outcomes (Lepore, Ferrell, & Wiener, 2017).

> The future of dementia cares services should be person- and family-centered not system-centered.

EXAMPLES OF PERSON-CENTERED SERVICE MODELS

While there is growing recognition of the benefits of a person- and family-centered approach to dementia care services and settings, few programs are available to meet these needs. There is a significant body of research indicating that different models for embedding care managers, or a team approach to service delivery, can have significant positive impacts upon the individual and caregiver, delay institutionalization and improve the quality of life for both the person and the caregiver. In the section below we summarize several evidence-based, person-centered models of care that have demonstrated benefits on important outcomes.

Care Management Models

A care management model is one approach in which an assigned case manager facilitates needs assessment, oversees the development of a care plan, coordinates the delivery of services, and monitors outcomes to support individuals with dementia in their homes. In the United States, very few people with dementia have access to a case manager or even a key worker to directly represent their interests as consumers and citizens. The MIND at Home intervention involves 18 months of care management designed to link persons living with dementia and their caregivers to community-based agencies, medical and mental health care providers, and community resources (Samus et al., 2014). MIND at Home is delivered by an interprofessional team who conducts comprehensive in-home dementia-related needs assessments and provides individualized plans to establish goals of care and implementation. The team uses six basic care strategies: resource referrals, attention to environmental safety, dementia care education, behavior management skills training, informal counseling, and problem solving, as well as on-going monitoring, assessment, and planning for emergent needs. Results from the MIND at Home trial support that a home-based dementia care coordination supports staying home a longer time and longer survival time (Samus et al., 2014). More recent results demonstrated that MIND at Home participants had increased use of dementia-related outpatient medical care and nonmedical supportive community services, a combination that may have helped participants remain at home longer (Amjad et al., 2017).

Care Coordination

Research suggests that embedding case managers into primary care settings can ease the burden on the physician and ensure better use of community resources for persons with dementia. The Aging Brain Medical Home is a care coordination model in which individuals with dementia receive 1 year of care management by an interdisciplinary team led by an advanced practice nurse working with the individual's family caregiver and integrated within primary care. Results of this collaborative care study resulted in significant improvement in the quality of care and in behavioral and psychological symptoms of dementia among primary care patients and their caregivers (Callahan et al., 2006).

Transitional Care

Transitional care—the planning and implementation of a move between care settings—offers an opportunity to focus on person- and family-centered care (Hirschman, & Hodgson, 2018). The Transitional Care Model consisted of visits by the advanced practice nurse in the hospital and at home to discuss goals for care and establish the care plan; a collaborative visit with the older adult, caregiver, and at least one of their physicians; telephone calls and advanced practice nurse availability 7 days a week for education and support (Hirschman, Shaid, McCauley, Pauly, & Naylor, 2015). Individuals with memory problems who received the Transitional Care Model had lower rates of rehospitalization and death than those who did not receive this care model (McCauley, Bradway, Hirschman, & Naylor, 2014).

Program of All-Inclusive Care for the Elderly

Established in 1971 and expanded with federal demonstration funding from 1987 to 1997, Program of All-Inclusive Care for the Elderly (PACE) is a fully integrated system that provides acute and long-term care services coordinated by and organized around an adult day health center. PACE offers adult day health center services integrated with geriatric primary care health, social, and respite services, woven together in a case management system (Chatterji, Burstein, Kidder, & White, 1998). Although not exclusively a dementia care program, approximately 50% of PACE participants having been diagnosed with dementia. The goal of the program is to maintain frail older individuals in the community for as long as possible. The program targets individuals who are eligible for Medicare and Medicaid.

The PACE model has been shown to be an effective person- and family-centered collaborative approach to dementia care (Abt Associates Inc., 1998). Researchers have emphasized the highly personalized service delivery and high individual and family satisfaction (Kane, Illston, & Miller, 1992) Participation in PACE has been associated with a decrease in hospital use, reduced institutionalization, balanced with substantial increases in utilization of outpatient medical care as well as home-based support (Senin, Cherubini, & Mecocci, 2003)

CONCLUSIONS

Integrated and coordinated settings and services are needed to meet the changing needs of people living with dementia and their caregivers (Gilmore-Bykovskyi, Roberts, King, Kennelty, & Kind, 2016). There is growing recognition that investments in home- and community-based services will yield significant returns (Borson et al., 2016). Importantly, achieving high-quality services for people with dementia and their caregivers requires person-centered strategies that acknowledge and individual's unique strengths and needs and enable individuals and families to make informed decisions about service needs. Communities and healthcare systems are seeking ways to become "dementia-friendly," and service providers are using a wide array of evidence-based and new innovative practices to support people with dementia and their caregivers by advancing the development of more person-centered services and settings that will help society meet the needs of current and future needs of individuals living with dementia.

What Can Be Done Now

Recommendations for Optimizing Person-Centered Services and Settings

1. Prepare and educate persons living with dementia and their family caregivers about common care settings and likely transitions across settings, such as home to hospital or skilled nursing facility, nursing home to emergency department; within care settings, such as from an emergency department to an intensive care unit; or from one team of clinicians or care providers to another.
2. Ensure coordination of care by facilitating communication of information between, across and within settings using standardized ways to share medical records and advance care-planning forms between individuals, caregivers and providers.
3. Evaluate the preferences and goals of the person living with dementia along the continuum of transitions in care, and revisit preferences and goals for care, including advance directives and social and living situation.
4. Create strong interprofessional collaborative team environments and utilize care managers or care advocates to support the person living with dementia and their family as they move across setting.
5. Use evidence-based, person- and family-centered models of service delivery to promote quality of life and minimize the likelihood of poor outcomes.

References

Abt Associates Inc. (1998). *Evaluation of the Program of All-Inclusive Care for the Elderly (PACE): Factors contributing to care management and decision-making in the PACE model.* Cambridge. Retrieved from http://www.abtassociates.com/reports/19986221714721.pdf.

Amjad, H., Wong, S. K., Roth, D. L., Huang, J., Willink, A., Black, B. S., & Samus, Q. M. (2017). Health services utilization in older adults with dementia receiving care coordination: The MIND at Home Trial. *Health Services Research., 53*(1), 556–579. Available from https://doi.org/10.1111/1475-6773.12647.

Borson, S., Boustani, M. A., Buckwalter, K. C., Burgio, L. D., Chodosh, J., Fortinsky, R. H., ... Geiger, A. (2016). Report on milestones for care and support under the U.S. national plan to address Alzheimer's disease. *Alzheimer's & Dementia, 12*(3), 334–369. Available from https://doi.org/10.1016/j.jalz.2016.01.005.

REFERENCES

Brooker, D. J. (2004). What is person-centered care in dementia?. *Reviews in Clinical Gerontology, 13*(3), 215–222.

Callahan, C. M., Boustani, M. A., Unverzagt, F. W., Austrom, M. G., Damush, T. M., Perkins, A. J., ... Hendrie, H. C. (2006). Effectiveness of collaborative care for older adults with Alzheimer disease in primary care. *JAMA, 295*(18), 2148. Available from https://doi.org/10.1001/jama.295.18.2148.

Callahan, C. M., Tu, W., Unroe, K. T., LaMantia, M. A., Stump, T. E., & Clark, D. O. (2015). Transitions in care in a nationally representative sample of older Americans with dementia. *Journal of the American Geriatrics Society, 63*(8), 1495–1502. Available from https://doi.org/10.1111/jgs.13540.

Calkins, M. P. (1988). *Design for dementia: Planning environments for the elderly and the confused*. Owing Mills, MD: National Health Publishing.

Chatterji, P., Burstein, N., Kidder, D., & White, A. (1998). *Evaluation of the Program of All-inclusive Care for the Elderly (PACE). The impact of PACE on participant outcomes*. Baltimore: US Health Care Financing Administration, Contract No. 500-96-0003/TO4.

Cohen, U., & Weisman, G. D. (1991). *Holding on to home: Designing environments for people with dementia*. Baltimore, MD: Johns Hopkins University Press.

Dziegielewski, S. F., & Ricks, J. L. (2001). Adult day programs for elderly who are mentally impaired and the measurement of caregiver satisfaction. *Activities, Adaptation & Aging, 24*(4), 51–64. Available from https://doi.org/10.1300/J016v24n04_05.

Gaugler, J. E., Jarrott, S. E., Zarit, S. H., Stephens, M.-A. P., Townsend, A., & Greene, R. (2003a). Adult day service use and reductions in caregiving hours: Effects on stress and psychological well-being for dementia caregivers. *International Journal of Geriatric Psychiatry, 18*(1), 55–62. Available from https://doi.org/10.1002/gps.772.

Gaugler, J. E., Jarrott, S. E., Zarit, S. H., Stephens, M.-A. P., Townsend, A., & Greene, R. (2003b). Respite for dementia caregivers: The effects of adult day service use on caregiving hours and care demands. *International Psychogeriatrics, 15*(1), 37–58. Available from https://doi.org/10.1017/S1041610203008743.

Gilmore-Bykovskyi, A. L., Roberts, T. J., King, B. J., Kennelty, K. A., & Kind, A. J. H. (2016). Transitions from hospitals to skilled nursing facilities for persons with dementia: A challenging convergence of patient and system-level needs. *The Gerontologist, 57*(5), 867–879. Available from https://doi.org/10.1093/geront/gnw085.

Gozalo, P., Teno, J. M., Mitchell, S. L., Skinner, J., Bynum, J., Tyler, D., & Mor, V. (2011). End-of-life transitions among nursing home residents with cognitive issues. *New England Journal of Medicine, 365*(13), 1212–1221. Available from https://doi.org/10.1056/NEJMsa1100347.

Hirschman, K. B., & Hodgson, N. (2018). Evidence-based interventions for transitions in care for individuals living with dementia. *The Gerontologist, 58*, S129–S140.

Hirschman, K. B., Shaid, E., McCauley, K., Pauly, M. V., & Naylor, M. D. (2015). Continuity of care: The transitional care model. *Online Journal of Issues in Nursing, 20*(3), 1. Available from https://doi.org/10.3912/OJIN.Vol20No03Man01.

Hyde, J., Perez, R., & Forester, B. (2007). Dementia and assisted living. *The Gerontologist, 47*(suppl 1), 51–67. Available from https://doi.org/10.1093/geront/47.Supplement_1.51.

Kable, A., Chenoweth, L., Pond, D., & Hullick, C. (2015). Health professional perspectives on systems failures in transitional care for patients with dementia and their carers: A qualitative descriptive study. *BMC Health Services Research, 15*(1), 567. Available from https://doi.org/10.1186/s12913-015-1227-z.

Kane, R. L., Illston, L. H., & Miller, N. A. (1992). Qualitative analysis of the Program of All-inclusive Care for the Elderly (PACE). *The Gerontologist, 32*(6), 771–780. Available from https://doi.org/10.1093/geront/32.6.771.

Koren, M. J. (2010). Person-centered care for nursing home residents: The culture-change movement. *Health Affairs, 29*(2), 312–317. Available from https://doi.org/10.1377/hlthaff.2009.0966.

Lepore, M., Ferrell, A., & Wiener, J. (2017). *Living arrangements of people with Alzheimer's disease and related dementias: Implications for services and supports*. Washington DC: National Alzheimer's Project Act. Retrieved from https://pdfs.semanticscholar.org/77e3/7974d41d5d225079a354b594c39685f0b163.pdf.

Lin, P.-J., Fillit, H. M., Cohen, J. T., & Neumann, P. J. (2013). Potentially avoidable hospitalizations among Medicare beneficiaries with Alzheimer's disease and related disorders. *Alzheimer's & Dementia, 9*(1), 30–38. Available from https://doi.org/10.1016/j.jalz.2012.11.002.

Lin, S.-Y. (2017). "Dementia-friendly communities" and being dementia friendly in healthcare settings. *Current Opinion in Psychiatry, 30*(2), 145–150. Available from https://doi.org/10.1097/YCO.0000000000000304.

McCauley, K., Bradway, C., Hirschman, K. B., & Naylor, M. D. (2014). Translating evidence based interventions for acutely ill cognitively impaired older adults: Lessons from "real-world" applications. *American Journal of Nursing, 114*(10), 44–52.

McCormack, B., Dewing, J., Breslin, L., Coyne-Nevin, A., Kennedy, K., Manning, M., ... Slater, P. (2010). Developing person-centred practice: Nursing outcomes arising from changes to the care environment in residential settings for older people. *International Journal of Older People Nursing, 5*(2), 93–107. Available from https://doi.org/10.1111/j.1748-3743.2010.00216.x.

Phelan, E. A., Borson, S., Grothaus, L., Balch, S., & Larson, E. B. (2012). Association of incident dementia with hospitalizations. *JAMA, 307*(2), 165. Available from https://doi.org/10.1001/jama.2011.1964.

Rijnaard, M. D., van Hoof, J., Janssen, B. M., Verbeek, H., Pocornie, W., Eijkelenboom, A., ... Wouters, E. J. M. (2016). The factors influencing the sense of home in nursing homes: A systematic review from the perspective of residents. *Journal of Aging Research, 2016*, 1–16. Available from https://doi.org/10.1155/2016/6143645.

Samus, Q. M., Johnston, D., Black, B. S., Hess, E., Lyman, C., Vavilikolanu, A., ... Lyketsos, C. G. (2014). A multidimensional home-based care coordination intervention for elders with memory disorders: The Maximizing Independence at Home (MIND) pilot randomized trial. *The American Journal of Geriatric Psychiatry, 22*(4), 398–414. Available from https://doi.org/10.1016/j.jagp.2013.12.175.

Schacke, C., & Zank, S. R. (2006). Measuring the effectiveness of adult day care as a facility to support family caregivers of dementia patients. *Journal of Applied Gerontology, 25*(1), 65–81. Available from https://doi.org/10.1177/0733464805284195.

Senin, U., Cherubini, A., & Mecocci, P. (2003). [Impact of population aging on the social and the health care system: Need for a new model of long-term care]. *Annali Italiani Di Medicina Interna: Organo Ufficiale Della Societa Italiana Di Medicina Interna, 18*(1), 6–15.

Tilly, J., & Reed, P. (2008). Intervention research on caring for people with dementia in assisted living and nursing homes. *Alzheimer's Care Today, 9*(1), 24–32. Available from https://doi.org/10.1097/01.ALCAT.0000309012.39716.78.

Thurman, W., Harrison, T. C., Blozis, S. A., Dionne-Vahalik, M., & Mead, S. (2017). A capabilities approach to environmental impact on nursing home resident quality of life. *Research in Gerontological Nursing, 10*(4), 162–170. Available from https://doi.org/10.3928/19404921-20170621-03.

Zarit, S. H., Stephens, M. A. P., Townsend, A., & Greene, R. (1998). Stress reduction for family caregivers: Effects of adult day care use. *The Journals of Gerontology Series B: Psychological Sciences and Social Sciences, 53B*(5), S267–S277. Available from https://doi.org/10.1093/geronb/53B.5.S267.

CHAPTER 11

Global Efforts and National Plans

All of us can assist future generations in the hand-off of a cure for Alzheimer's disease with a greater collective understanding of the disease, more resources, and a worldwide commitment... My hope is that we all listen more. **Greg O'Brien, Preface from, "On Pluto: Inside the Mind of Alzheimer's" Codfish Press, 2014.**

We reach this chapter with a collective understanding that while advances are being made there is currently no cure for dementia, and pharmacological treatments can at best only slow progression very temporarily, yet still with side effects for many individuals. The burdens imposed by dementia on persons, their families and friends, and communities are extraordinary. While evidence-based programs are available to improve the quality of life of persons living with dementia and reduce the burden on caregivers, few individuals or their families receive these essential services and supports. Moreover, the projected demand for future services and supports for the growing population of persons living with dementia will soon outstrip the current capacity of every country. It is therefore imperative that countries prepare for this escalating crisis by developing strategies to address the unmet and quality of life needs of their citizens with dementia and their caregivers. In this chapter, we broaden our lens fully to consider the global impact of dementia. We present examples of national strategies that select countries have developed to address this global burden.

Imagine what could be possible if a collective commitment and dedication from the public and private sectors of society, the scientific community, the medical community, and government was realized. The first essential step in this process would need to be an acknowledgment—rather than a denial of—the true scale and scope of the global burden of dementia.

> The lack of awareness and understanding of dementia in most countries results in barriers to diagnosis and care, stigmatization, and tremendous burden to caregivers, families and societies physically, psychologically and economically.

DEMENTIA BY THE NUMBERS GLOBALLY

In 2017, dementia affected over 47 million people worldwide, and that number is estimated to increase to 75 million in 2030, and 132 million by 2050 (Prince, et al., 2016). Nearly 10 million people develop dementia each year globally, which translates into one case every 3 seconds (Rizzi, Rosset, Roriz-Cruz, 2014). Dementia occurrence rates vary from country to country, due in part to differences in diagnosing and reporting methods. Alzheimer's Disease International (ADI) estimates that between 2013 and 2050, the rates of dementia diagnosis are predicted to increase by 90% in Europe, 226% in Asia, 248% in America, and 345% in Africa (Prince, Guerchet, & Prina, 2015). In some countries, the projected dementia rates are almost 10% higher than was originally anticipated and in others that rate of underestimation is 50% higher than what was originally anticipated (e.g., Columbia). In the United States, dementia is the only major disease category projected to increase by 65% or more. This projection is due in large part to better identification of persons with dementia and to the improved preventative treatment and management strategies for other common chronic conditions such as stroke, heart disease, HIV, and cancer.

GLOBAL DISEASE BURDEN

Improvements in treating chronic conditions such as heart disease have been credited with some hopeful news in some countries including England, Netherlands, Sweden, Denmark, and the United States. Studies suggest that the age-specific risk of dementia has actually decreased in these high-income countries over the last 25 years, possibly due to increasing levels of education and improvements in lifestyle, including nutrition and aggressive treatments of cardiovascular risk factors that increase the risk of cognitive decline (for example, hypertension, hypercholesterolemia, and diabetes) (Schrijvers et al., 2012). In addition, education has been associated with decreased dementia risk suggesting that environmental factors can have a powerful role (Langa, 2015). Whether these optimistic trends in high-income countries will continue in the face of rising levels of obesity and diabetes and persistent health and educational disparities is unknown, and it is also unclear whether there has been a similar or opposite trend in low- and middle-income countries (Chan et al., 2013; Wu et al., 2016).

It is also important to note that these optimistic trends do not hold up across all racial and ethnic groups, particularly in the United States. African Americans and Latinos have higher rates of dementia at each age group, and these rates are expected to increase. Less is known about other racial and ethnic minority groups in the United States (Mehta & Yeo, 2017). It remains unclear how these disparities in dementia rates and trends are related to known social determinants of health such as education level, occupations, income, health behaviors, and access to health care (Mayeda, Glymour, Quesenberry, & Whitmer, 2016).

Regardless, the global disease burden of dementia is shouldered mostly by low- and middle-income countries as higher rates of dementia are seen in those resource poor countries compared to high-income countries (Prince et al., 2016). Nearly 60% of people with dementia live in low- or middle-income countries and over 70% of all new cases of dementia are expected to occur in these countries (Wortmann, 2012). As a consequence, in high-income countries the rates of dementia are predicted to remain stable, while in low- and middle-income countries these rates are expected to increase exponentially as shown in Fig. 11-1 (Wortmann, 2012).

While these sheer numbers are staggering, they do little to capture the global impact of dementia in terms of the financial burden these estimates place on society (Hurd, Martorell, Delavande, Mullen, & Langa, 2013). The direct cost of care for persons living with dementia is

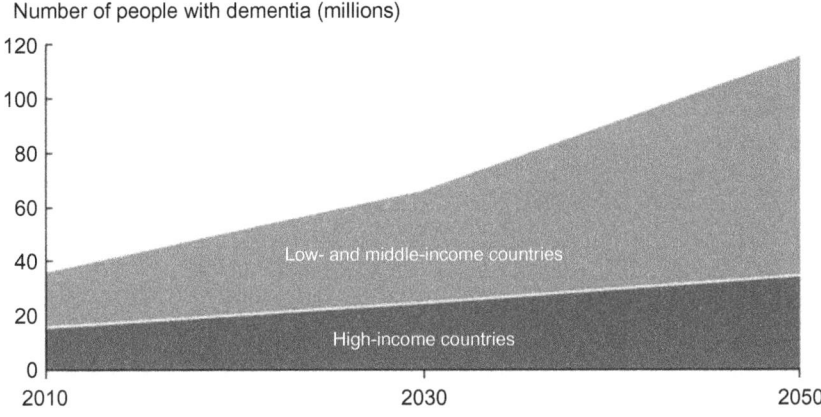

FIGURE 11-1 Comparison of number of people in low-, middle-, and high-income countries with dementia. Source: *Prince, M., Wimo, A., Guerchet, M., Ali, G.C., Wu, Y.T., & Prina, M. (2015). World Alzheimer report 2015. The global impact of dementia. London: Alzheimer's Disease International.*

estimated to be $213 billion dollars per year in North America, $210 billion dollars per year in Western Europe, and $82 billion in the Asia Pacific (Wortmann, 2012). In 2010, the worldwide global cost was estimated to be $604 billion dollars (Wimo, Jönsson, Bond, Prince, & Winblad, 2013). This figure equated to around 1% of the aggregated world gross domestic product (GDP), indicating a particularly significant global socioeconomic impact for one illness. Updated estimates, completed in 2017, increased by 35% compared to a 2010 report, and these more recent estimates report the global societal economic cost of dementia as high as $818—a number similar in magnitude to the GDP of countries like Indonesia, the Netherlands, and Turkey—the 16th–18th largest economies in the world (Wimo et al., 2017). As a point of comparison, these global costs are larger than the market values of companies such as Apple (US $742 billion), Google (US $368 billion), and Exxon (US $357 billion). Most concerning is that the global economic burden from dementia is predicted to rise to 2 trillion dollars by 2030 (Wimo et al., 2017).

NATIONAL PLANS AND THEIR IMPACT

While it is seems obvious to state that the global burden of dementia is devastating, only within the last decade has it been recognized as a global public health priority (Rees, 2017). In 2008, French President Nicolas Sarkozy launched a National Plan for Alzheimer's. In 2011, United States President Barack Obama signed the National Alzheimer's Project Act into law directing new efforts to improve the treatment and prevention of dementia. In 2012, the World Health Organization (WHO) and ADI WHO jointly released an extensive report, "Dementia: A Public Health Priority" in order to articulate a public health approach and to advocate for action at international and national levels (Wortmann, 2012). This was followed in 2013 by the first G8 Dementia Summit, held in London in recognition of the growing global impact of dementia and to begin to coordinate efforts for international collaboration and data sharing (Wimo et al., 2013). More recently, in 2015, the first Ministerial Conference on Global Action Against Dementia was held by the WHO (Prince et al., 2015). Eighty countries signed the call to action to improve the quality of life for persons living with dementia.

> Dementia requires an "all-in" approach that includes sustained action and coordination across multiple levels and with all stakeholders at the international, national, regional and local level

As a result of these international efforts a number of countries have undertaken the development of national plans or strategies. These initiatives are important advancements for their ability to shape policy and to impact resource allocation for societies. National plans also help to prioritize and redirect both health and healthcare initiatives. There is evidence that national strategies have a direct influence on the care that persons with dementia receive (Edvardsson, Sandman, & Borell, 2014).

At the time this chapter was written, 37 countries had initiated national plans or strategies (Table 11-1). There are three basic elements common across existing national dementia plans, although most plans vary with regard to their features and level of complexity and detail provided. As shown in Fig. 11-2, the first basic element contained in all national plans to date is an emphasis on the need to raise public awareness and education about dementia in an attempt to mitigate the stigma and fear.

A second element in most national plans is the emphasis on improving early symptom recognition and the identification and treatment of persons with dementia. This includes an emphasis on the need for earlier diagnosis and more accessible treatment in their country such as providing centers for diagnoses or treatment in community care settings or memory care settings.

A third common element present in most national plans is the recognition of the need for training a healthcare workforce in core competencies in dementia care. Examples of two national plans that are focused primarily on these three elements are the national plans of Australia (https://agedcare.health.gov.au/sites/g/files/net1426/f/documents/09_2015/national-framework-for-action-on-dementia-2015-2019.pdf) and the Republic of South Korea (https://www.alz.co.uk/plans/republic-of-korea). In both of these national plans, the focus is on early detection, helping educate the public on common signs indicating possible dementia, and training providers on screening for those cognitive changes.

Of all the national plans to date, Scotland is often identified as one of the most sophisticated (http://www.gov.scot/Resource/Doc/324377/0104420.pdf). Framed initially as a basic bill of rights for people with dementia and their families, the plan was grounded on standards of care from which they have been building an infrastructure for and evaluating services. The first and fundamental premise of this plan is that people with dementia have the right to a diagnosis. The second premise is that people with dementia have the right to be regarded as a unique individual and to be treated with dignity and respect. The third premise is that people with dementia have the right to access a range of treatment and supports as the disease progresses. The forth premise is that people with dementia have the right to be as independent as possible and be included in their community. The fifth premise is that people

TABLE 11-1 Thirty-Seven National Dementia Plans

Country	Year created	Year updated	Key contact/author	Has it been used to shape care yet?
France	2001	2008	http://www.alzheimer-europe.org/Policy-in-Practice2/National-Dementia-Strategies/France https://www.alz.co.uk/sites/default/files/plans/Alzheimer-Plan-2008-2012-France-ENG.pdf http://www.alzheimer-europe.org/Policy-in-Practice2/National-Dementia-Strategies/France#fragment3 http://www.alzheimer-europe.org/Policy-in-Practice2/Country-comparisons/2013-National-policies-covering-the-care-and-support-of-people-with-dementia-and-their-carers/France	Earlier diagnosis due to increased research and biomarkers. Care card for those with dementia so that in the event of emergency, the person's information, as well as "golden rules" for caring for them is on their person. Training programs for caregivers significantly increased. Medical care for persons with dementia reimbursed at 100%. Nursing homes must create individual care plans for each patient. Increased respite care for persons with dementia.
Australia	2006	2015	https://agedcare.health.gov.au/sites/g/files/net1426/f/documents/09_2015/national-framework-for-action-on-dementia-2015-2019.pdf http://journalofdementiacare.com/public-health-interventions-dementia/ https://www.fightdementia.org.au/files/20101105_Nat_SUB_CommentsLAMAEval.pdf	Increased training for early dementia diagnosis for healthcare professionals. Improved training and budget allocations for residential care facilities for persons with dementia. Financial supplement added to Home Care Packages specifically for the presence of dementia in the home. Focus on community engagement due to specific community-based grants. Development of three research centers dedicated solely to dementia.
South Korea	2006	2011	https://www.alz.co.uk/sites/default/files/national-alzheimer-and-dementia-plans.pdf http://alzheimerstoday.elsevier.com/Content/PDF/Countrywide_strategic_plans_on_Alzheimers_disease.pdf	Increased eligibility for long-term care insurance. This includes access to day centers and hospice care. Dementia Center dedicated in each of the four main regional hospitals.

	2007	https://www.bupa.com/~/media/files/site-specific-files/our%20purpose/healthy%20ageing%20and%20dementia/improving%20dementia%20care/improving%20dementia%20care%20english.pdf https://www.alz.co.uk/plans/republic-of-korea	Training set in place specifically for dementia specialists.
Norway	2015	http://www.alzheimer-europe.org/Policy-in-Practice2/National-Dementia-Strategies/Norway#fragment3 http://www.alzheimer-europe.org/content/download/72536/452004/file/Norway%20Dementia%20Plan%202007-2015.pdf http://www.alzheimer-europe.org/content/download/126620/791302/file/Norway%20dementia%20plan%202020%20-%20regular%20version.pdf	Some increase in daily access to daily activities for persons with dementia but not as much as they wanted to see. Association formed of only persons living with dementia to "be involved in decisions about their care."
The Netherlands	2008 2013	https://www.alz.co.uk/sites/default/files/plans/netherlands.pdf http://www.alzheimer-europe.org/content/download/72431/451392/file/Dutch%20Dementia%20Strategy%20(June%202008).pdf https://www.government.nl/binaries/government/documents/publications/2015/07/07/the-delta-plan-on-dementia/dementia-nl-parliament-2015-appendix-2.pdf https://www.centreforpublicimpact.org/case-study/tackling-dementia-netherlands-national-strategy/	Efforts to take on diagnosis processes of early onset dementia and those who have suffered for a while independently. Increased transfer of ideas between regions—joined cooperation and regional networks. More professional support reported by informal caregivers. Research improvements, specifically in cognitive training, behavioral problems, and quality of life. Increased availability of case management.
England	2009 2012	http://www.alzheimer-europe.org/Policy-in-Practice2/National-Dementia-Strategies/United-Kingdom-England http://www.alzheimer-europe.org/content/download/72402/451250/file/PM's%20challenge%20on%20dementia%202012.pdf http://www.alzheimer-europe.org/content/download/72406/451266/file/PM's%20challenge%20on%20dementia%202012%20-%20Progress%20report%20May%202014.pdf	Increased awareness through distribution of flyers and information to those 65 years and older receiving a National Health Service Health Check in. Dementia Choices website launched by NHS with resources for persons with dementia and their families, including information and dementia newsletters that help form a community.

(Continued)

TABLE 11-1 (Continued)

Country	Year created	Year updated	Key contact/author	Has it been used to shape care yet?
				Rewards instituted to practices who complete timely diagnosis and care plans for persons with dementia. Individualized care plans provided for all persons diagnosed with dementia. Four times increase in the number of people being assessed by memory clinics. Dementia Commissioning for Quality and Innovation expanded to include data collection and support for carers.
Denmark	2010	2016	http://www.alzheimer-europe.org/Policy-in-Practice2/National-Dementia-Strategies/Denmark#fragment1 http://www.alzheimer-europe.org/Policy-in-Practice2/National-Dementia-Strategies/Denmark#fragment3 https://www.unece.org/fileadmin/DAM/pau/age/country_rpts/2017/DNK_-_National_Report.pdf	Increased access to nursing homes, as well as legislation to restructure them as needed specifically for persons with dementia. Municipalities offering independent living training programs for persons with dementia. (Reablement process). All elderly people qualify for annual home visits that screen for dementia. Increased respite care and financial compensation for carers.
Scotland	2010	2013 (2017 in progress)	http://www.gov.scot/Resource/Doc/324377/0104420.pdf http://www.alzheimer-europe.org/content/download/45036/292583/file/Scottish%20National%20Dementia%20Strategy%202013.pdf https://www.fightdementia.org.au/files/20111410_Paper_25_low_v2.pdf http://www.alzheimer-europe.org/Policy-in-Practice2/National-Dementia-Strategies/United-Kingdom-Scotland#fragment3 http://www.gov.scot/Topics/Health/Policy/Dementia	Focus on updating Dementia Register, increase in number of persons diagnosed with dementia as a result. Implemented training for hospital staff and home care staff for early diagnosis. Greater focus on postdiagnostic support. Forum created for input from all Dementia stakeholders. Funding and training allocated for specialized dementia nurses.

Northern Ireland	2011	NA	http://www.alzheimer-europe.org/content/download/35067/235411/file/Northern%20Ireland%20dementia%20strategy%20-%20full%20text%20version.pdf http://www.alzheimer-europe.org/Policy-in-Practice2/National-Dementia-Strategies/United-Kingdom-Northern-Ireland https://www.alzheimers.org.uk/download/downloads/id/2320/dementia_2014_opportunity_for_change_-_northern_ireland_summary.pdf https://www.alzheimers.org.uk/info/20090/national_policies/48/dementia_strategy_for_northern_ireland	Dementia-Friendly Communities Programs, including a Dementia Friends initiative, in place. Increased research for dementia. Legislation in place to give persons with dementia more autonomy over health decisions, encouraging caregivers/healthcare professionals to respect their decisions.
Wales	2011	(2017-Drafted)	http://www.alzheimer-europe.org/content/download/20741/152710/file/National%20Dementia%20Vision%20for%20Wales.pdf https://consultations.gov.wales/sites/default/files/consultation_doc_files/170109dementia-consultationen.pdf	Implemented Dementia Supportive Communities and Dementia Friends campaigns. Increased diagnosis rates via specialized training. More budgeting allocations for memory assessment services. Accessible national dementia helpline/Website. Additional dementia training in healthcare settings, as well as increased occupational therapy support workers hired for persons with dementia.
Finland	2012	NA	http://www.alzheimer-europe.org/Policy-in-Practice2/National-Dementia-Strategies/Finland https://www.alz.co.uk/dementia-plans/national-plans https://www.julkari.fi/bitstream/handle/10024/126202/Reports_2013_9_Memory_verkko.pdf	NA
The United States	2012	2016	https://www.alz.co.uk/plans/usa https://aspe.hhs.gov/system/files/pdf/205581/NatlPlan2016.pdf	Increase and expansion of research efforts surrounding dementia, including quality of life, biomarkers, clinical trials, etc. Improved educational resources for healthcare staff regarding family/caregiver support. More funding for services to persons with dementia in all types of living

(*Continued*)

TABLE 11-1 (Continued)

Country	Year created	Year updated	Key contact/author	Has it been used to shape care yet?
				conditions (alone, with a carer, assisted living community, etc.) Variety of behavioral and symptom management trainings available to caregivers.
Japan	2012	2015	http://alzheimerstoday.elsevier.com/Content/PDF/How_should_a_national_dementia_policy_interact_with_the_public_health_and_social-care_systems.pdf http://accj.paradigm.co.jp/documents/2015WP_ENG_CHPT23.pdf http://www.who.int/mental_health/neurology/dementia/Member_State_Japan.pdf?ua=1	"Dementia Supporters" training available for not only caregivers and healthcare professionals but anyone who wants to show support and be educated on the subject. Specific long-term care system added to Universal Health Coverage. Increased research, specifically in risk reduction and early detection.
Israel	2013	NA	https://www.health.gov.il/English/Topics/SeniorHealth/DEMENTIA/Pages/National_program.aspx http://www.alzheimer-europe.org/content/download/117195/734185/file/Israel%20national%20dementia%20strategy%202013.pdf https://academic.oup.com/innovateage/article/1/suppl_1/1320/3902075/THE-ISRAELI-NATIONAL-DEMENTIA-PLAN-INCREASING	Increased public awareness, as well as professional. More education for healthcare leaders surrounding primary care, specifically quality of life, and end of life.
Luxembourg	2013	2015	http://www.alzheimer-europe.org/Policy-in-Practice2/National-Dementia-Strategies/Luxembourg#fragment1	Introduction of subplan program for dementia prevention, which is personalized care targeted at those with early diagnosis.
Taiwan	2013	NA	https://www.alz.co.uk/sites/default/files/plans/taiwan-dementia-policy.pdf	NA
Switzerland	2014	NA	http://www.alzheimer-europe.org/content/download/72425/451359/file/Swiss%20national%20dementia%20strategy%202014%20-%20summary.pdf https://www.bag.admin.ch/bag/en/home/themen/strategien-politik/nationale-gesundheitsstrategien/nationale-demenzstrategie-2014-2017.html http://www.sociopolitical-observatory.eu/uploads/tx_aebgppublications/2016-04_WP_National_dementia_strategies_MM.pdf	Higher dementia awareness in the public via the web, posters, television, etc.

Costa Rica	2014	NA	(Spanish, with year) http://www.conapam.go.cr/mantenimiento/Plan%20Nacional%20Alzheimer.pdf http://journal.frontiersin.org/article/10.3389/fnagi.2017.00221/full	Increased presence of memory centers. Implemented trainings for caregivers. Coverage of medications associated with dementia through social security.
Cuba	2014	NA	http://www.medicc.org/medicreview/index.php?issue=41&id=560&a=vahtml (Mostly Spanish)https://www.alz.co.uk/sites/default/files/conf2014/OC024.pdf http://www.scielosp.org/scielo.php?script=sci_arttext&pid=S1555-79602015000100014 https://www.alz.co.uk/sites/default/files/plans/cuba-english.pdf	Inclusion of dementia screening in early check-ups for older adults. Increase in nursing homes and adult day centers. Family education for those related to/caring for persons with dementia: "caregivers' schools." Increased research and funding for dementia studies
Mexico	2014	NA	https://www.alz.co.uk/sites/default/files/plans/mexico-english.pdf (PDF translated to English in 2016)	NA
Italy	2014	NA	http://www.scielosp.org/pdf/aiss/v51n4/v51n4a02.pdf http://www.alzheimer-europe.org/Policy-in-Practice2/National-Dementia-Strategies/Italy#fragment2	Access to services improved due to online map of services for persons with dementia. Strengthened network of services for earlier diagnosis and continuity of care. Increased dementia training and assessment of healthcare workers and social workers. Monitoring well-being of caregivers as well as persons with dementia. National and regional campaigns for dementia awareness.
Greece	2014	NA	http://eurocarers.org/Greece-Greek-Dementia-Action-Plan http://www.alzheimer-europe.org/Policy-in-Practice2/National-Dementia-Strategies/Greece#fragment1 https://www.alz.co.uk/sites/default/files/plans/greece-national-plan-2016.pdf	National dementia registry in process. Financial aid for persons with dementia and their families, based on a newly developed rating system for

(Continued)

TABLE 11-1 (Continued)

Country	Year created	Year updated	Key contact/author	Has it been used to shape care yet?
				the level of impact dementia has on different families. Six memory clinics established in hospitals, and sixteen adult day care centers in various cities. Increase in hospice care.
Ireland	2014	NA	http://www.alzheimer-europe.org/Policy-in-Practice2/National-Dementia-Strategies/Ireland http://www.alzheimer-europe.org/content/download/83878/518299/file/Irish%20National%20Dementia%20Strategy%202014.pdf	Increase in research for quality of life and dementia-friendly healthcare facilities.
Malta	2015	NA	http://www.alzheimer-europe.org/Policy-in-Practice2/National-Dementia-Strategies/Malta http://www.alzheimer-europe.org/content/download/87486/559443/file/Malta%20National%20Dementia%20Strategy%202015-2023.pdf	NA
Indonesia	2015	NA	https://www.alz.co.uk/sites/default/files/plans/Indonesia.pdf	NA
Puerto Rico	2015	NA	http://act.alz.org/site/DocServer/PR_State_Plan_English_Summary__2015_.pdf?docID=50230	NA
Czech Republic	2016	NA	http://www.alzheimer-europe.org/Policy-in-Practice2/National-Dementia-Strategies/Czech-Republic	NA
Spain	2016	NA	http://www.alzheimer-europe.org/Policy-in-Practice2/National-Dementia-Strategies/Spain	NA
Slovenia	2016	NA	http://www.alzheimer-europe.org/Policy-in-Practice2/National-Dementia-Strategies/Slovenia	NA
Argentina	2016	NA	https://www.alz.co.uk/news/national-plan-launched-in-argentina	NA
Canada	2017	NA	https://www.alz.co.uk/news/canada-becomes-30th-country-to-launch-national-dementia-strategy	NA
Chile	2017	NA	https://www.alz.co.uk/news/chilean-government-adopts-national-plan-on-dementia	NA
Bulgaria	In progress	NA	http://www.alzheimer-europe.org/Policy-in-Practice2/National-Dementia-Strategies/Bulgaria https://www.alz.co.uk/sites/default/files/plans/bulgaria-english.pdf	**Progress:** 2014—Bulgarian government reviewed a draft for a national dementia strategy

Country	Status		Links	Progress
Germany	In progress	NA	http://www.alzheimer-europe.org/Policy-in-Practice2/National-Dementia-Strategies/Germany https://globaldementiaframework.wordpress.com/leadership/ http://www.alzheimer-europe.org/News/Policy-watch/Thursday-10-December-2015-Dementia-Strategy-for-state-of-Saarland-is-launched	2015—Alzheimer's Bulgaria released a report on national policies and practices in providing health and social services to people with dementia **Progress:** 2013—German state of Bavaria published its own sub-national dementia plan. 2014—German government established "Alliance for People with Dementia" to be the initial foundation of a future national plan. It is made up of coordinating federal agencies and public organizations. 2015—German state of Saarland published its own sub-national dementia plan.
India	In progress	NA	http://alzheimerstoday.elsevier.com/Content/PDF/Countrywide_strategic_plans_on_Alzheimers_disease.pdf http://ardsi.org/downloads/main%20report.pdf http://alzheimerstoday.elsevier.com/Content/PDF/Countrywide_strategic_plans_on_Alzheimers_disease.pdf	**Progress:** 2010—Alzheimer's and Related Disorders Society of India released extensive Dementia India Report, with a call for national action.
Portugal	In progress	NA	http://www.alzheimer-europe.org/Policy-in-Practice2/National-Dementia-Strategies/Portugal	**Progress:** 2010—Alzheimer Portugal proposes a national plan. 2013—National plan submitted to Ministry of Health. 2015—Alzheimer Portugal writes the Prime Minister to encourage prioritization and forward movement of the plan.
Uruguay	In progress	NA	https://www.alz.co.uk/sites/default/files/plans/uruguay%20-%20eng.pdf	**Progress:** 2016—National dementia plan drafted by The Uruguayan Association of Alzheimer and Similar Diseases.

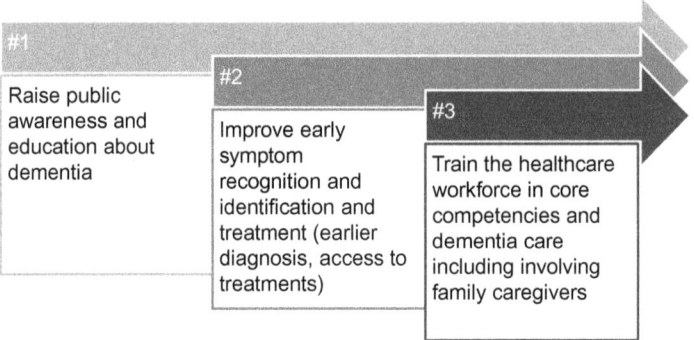

FIGURE 11.2 Three common elements of national plans.

with dementia have the right to have caregivers who are well supported and educated about dementia. The sixth and final premise is that people with dementia have the right to end-of-life care that respects their unique wishes. These critical assumptions are not explicitly stated in other plans and have directly shaped how Scotland has designed its outreach to and services for families.

Additional elements of some national plans include the need for dementia friendly community efforts such as those discussed in Chapter 9, Living in the Community, but also can include the creation of online communities for access to services.

Many plans also focus on the need for ongoing research, often with an emphasis on discovering a cure to the disease, treatments to delay disease progression, and to derive better diagnostic indicators. Less attention has been given to research on the social impact of dementia and supportive care and services for individuals living with dementia and their caregivers. For example, the plans of both the United States (https://aspe.hhs.gov/national-alzheimers-project-act) and the United Kingdom (https://www.gov.uk/government/uploads/system/uploads/attachment_data/file/168221/dh_094052.pdf) address the need for clinical care quality and efficiency and need for additional research with an emphasis on a plan on preventing and effectively treating Alzheimer's disease. Both plans also include the need to enhance public awareness and engagement and improve data in order to track progress towards each of these goals. The level of complexity and detail varies greatly across plans and is continually refined in revisions (see Table 11.1). Some plans detail the need to improve quality of life of individuals with dementia and emphasize care in the home. Others target institutional care programs and include tackling the complexity of transitioning from one care setting to the other, and care coordination across care systems. The most complex elements of national dementia plans include monitoring the impact of all

> **Box 11-1**
> **Missing Pieces in National Plans**
>
> - End-stage disease and end-of-life care
> - Support of family caregivers
> - Family-centered dementia care services
> - Implementation of evidence-based programs
> - Preparation of an interprofessional care team
> - Some plans refer to Alzheimer's disease but include other forms of dementia making the language confusing and the possibility of policies being restricted to one form of dementia

these different elements on people with dementia, their quality of life, and their family caregivers.

GAPS IN GLOBAL EFFORTS

While the development of national plans is positive, there are important gaps in these efforts. Box 11-1 lists the missing pieces in most plans that need attention.

Very few plans, with the exception of France (https://www.alz.co.uk/sites/default/files/plans/Alzheimer-Plan-2008-2012-France-ENG.pdf) and Scotland (http://www.gov.scot/Resource/Doc/324377/0104420.pdf), have given attention to the end-stage disease or to end-of-life care.

Despite the progress that has been made in developing national plans, most give little attention to the needs of family caregivers. As the 2013 World Alzheimer's Report indicated,

> Caregiver multi-component interventions that comprise education, training, support and respite, maintain caregiver mood and morale and reduce caregiver strain. Nevertheless, we are aware of no governments that have invested in this intervention to scale a provision throughout the dementia care system, and hence, coverage is minimal. *Prince, Prina, & Guerchet (2013)*

Thus, missing from most plans is a philosophy of dementia care as family-centered or one that considers the impact of the diagnosis on the larger sphere of influence beyond the person with dementia to include family and friends who serve as caregivers.

Another common missing element is a research agenda that addresses the evidence–practice gap (Gitlin, Marx, Stanley, & Hodgson, 2015). Research evidence should underpin the recommendations and actions included in any global dementia efforts, and national plans should address important shared concerns about translating what is already known into action. Future revisions of national plans should recommend strategies to require multidisciplinary collaborations across basic sciences, health services, health systems, and health policy research in order to address this research–practice gap.

> Dementia poses one of the greatest societal challenges for the 21st century and global commitment is needed to generate strategies, policies, services and supports for individuals living with dementia and their caregivers.

In the 2012 WHO and ADI report, a six-stage "Acceptance of Dementia" model was presented including: Stage 1: Ignoring the problem; Stage 2: Some awareness; Stage 3: Building dementia infrastructure; Stage 4: Advocacy efforts; Stage 5: Policies and dementia plans or strategies; and Stage 6: Normalization. Our review of global initiatives shows that while some countries are moving towards Stage 5, most countries in the world are still struggling in Stage 2 reflecting "some awareness" (e.g., Chen et al., 2017).

As recently as May 2017 a global action plan on the public health response to dementia was approved at the World Health Organization (2016). The goal of this plan, similar to the goal of this book, is to minimize impact of dementia and improve quality of life on individuals, families, societies, and countries. It envisions a world in which people can live well with or without dementia, and receive the supports they need to fulfill their potential with dignity, respect, and equality. This global initiative is expected to facilitate governments, policy-makers, and other stakeholders to address the impact of dementia as an increasing threat to global health. One key recommendation from this plan is that 75% of countries will have developed or updated national strategies, policies, plans, or frameworks for dementia by 2025—an ambitious but essential goal. Our next charge is to move into action the recommendations that arise from global and national plans. This will require a coordinated response—one that involves all stakeholders—with engagement at the government level and from all relevant public and private sectors of our society.

KEY POINTS

- National dementia plans are important because they help shape national policy, healthcare services, and resource development.

- Future plans and plan revisions need to consider family-centered approaches for people living with dementia and their caregivers, and the need to move existing evidence-based programs into routine care.
- Dementia poses one of the greatest societal challenges for the 21st century, and global commitment is needed to generate strategies, policies, services, and supports for individuals living with dementia and their caregivers.

Conversation With Dr. James Pickett, Head of Research, Alzheimer's Society, United Kingdom

The first dementia strategy for England was published in 2009 entitled "Living well with dementia - a national strategy". It set out a vision for transforming dementia services with the aim of achieving better awareness of dementia, early diagnosis and high quality treatment at whatever stage of the illness and in whatever setting. This was then superseded by a Prime Ministers challenge on Dementia in 2012, which ran from 2012-2015 and then renewed with a Challenge on Dementia running to 2020. The current challenge on dementia covers four key themes - Risk Reduction, Health and Care Delivery (including Workforce training and development), Dementia Awareness (and social action), Research. Whilst this Challenge for the UK, Scotland has held separate dementia strategies since 2010, and Wales has recently published Dementia Friendly Wales 2017-2022.

1. *What do you see as the importance of having a national plan on dementia?*

   Having a dementia strategy has put dementia on the map. It has allowed has to map out ambitions for the longer term, and be able to hold their delivery to account. The strategy has given us the ability to ability to review and measure and set real outcomes for the future.

   We have also seen some improvements during the strategy period. The number of people with a diagnosis has increased over this period from around 40% to 66%, prescription of antipsychotics has reduced, and the number of people prescribed a dementia medication has increased.

   What is harder to measure, but is almost certainly changed is an increase in awareness of dementia. Both in the public and amongst professionals. Dementia training has been rolled out across the UK workforce. The Alzheimer's Society has helped to make 2.2 million dementia friends, who have undertaken an information session about dementia and committed to social action. We have hundreds of areas that have declared themselves dementia friendly.

2. *How has a National plan changed policy and/or service delivery in your country?*
Investment in research has also grown substantially over this period from around £40 million a year in 2009 to over £100 m today. This includes a new flagship Dementia research institute to focus on etiology of disease, and investment in social care research. However, investment in research in dementia still lags far behind that invested in cancer.

3. *What do you see as the policy needs in your country moving forward to assure comprehensive person and family centered and directed dementia care?*
Having a strategy and requirement for measurement has highlighted the strong variation across the country, and in particular, the stark social economic factors that are in involved in dementia care outcomes. Future strategies must seek to address inequalities that exist in the current system. Strategies do date have yet to address the fragmented system which people with dementia have to navigate to get care and support. Embracing an agenda that integrates health care, social care and other community-based services will be important in the future. Given the pace of policy change in dementia, innovative initiatives have been rolled out often without full evaluation of their impact, and as we collect better and more information about initiatives that work it will provide the opportunity to focus on the thing that are most effective.

References

Chan, K. Y., Wang, W., Wu, J. J., Liu, L., Theodoratou, E., Car, J., & Rudan, I. (2013). Epidemiology of Alzheimer's disease and other forms of dementia in China, 1990–2010: A systematic review and analysis. *The Lancet*, *381*(9882), 2016–2023. Available from https://doi.org/10.1016/S0140-6736.(13)60221-4.

Chen, Z., Yang, X., Song, Y., Song, B., Zhang, Y., Liu, J., & Yu, J. (2017). Challenges of dementia care in China. *Geriatrics*, *2*(1), 7. Available from https://doi.org/10.3390/geriatrics2010007.

Edvardsson, D., Sandman, P. O., & Borell, L. (2014). Implementing national guidelines for person-centered care of people with dementia in residential aged care: Effects on perceived person-centeredness, staff strain, and stress of conscience. *International Psychogeriatrics*, *26*(7), 1171–1179. Available from https://doi.org/10.1017/S1041610214000258.

Gitlin, L. N., Marx, K., Stanley, I. H., & Hodgson, N. (2015). Translating evidence-based dementia caregiving interventions into practice: State-of-the-science and next steps. *Gerontologist*, *55*(2), 210–226. Available from https://doi.org/10.1093/geront/gnu123.

Hurd, M. D., Martorell, P., Delavande, A., Mullen, K. J., & Langa, K. M. (2013). Monetary costs of dementia in the United States. *New England Journal of Medicine, 368*(14), 1326–1334. Available from https://doi.org/10.1056/NEJMsa1204629.
Langa, K. M. (2015). Is the risk of Alzheimer's disease and dementia declining? *Alzheimer's Research & Therapy, 7*(1), 34. Available from https://doi.org/10.1186/s13195-015-0118-1.
Mayeda, E. R., Glymour, M. M., Quesenberry, C. P., & Whitmer, R. A. (2016). Inequalities in dementia incidence between six racial and ethnic groups over 14 years. *Alzheimer's & Dementia, 12*(3), 216–224. Available from https://doi.org/10.1016/j.jalz.2015.12.007.
Mehta, K. M., & Yeo, G. W. (2017). Systematic review of dementia prevalence and incidence in United States race/ethnic populations. *Alzheimer's & Dementia: The Journal of the Alzheimer's Association, 13*(1), 72–83. Available from https://doi.org/10.1016/j.jalz.2016.06.236.
Prince, M., Ali, G.-C., Guerchet, M., Prina, A. M., Albanese, E., & Wu, Y.-T. (2016). Recent global trends in the prevalence and incidence of dementia, and survival with dementia. *Alzheimer's Research & Therapy, 8*(1), 23. Available from https://doi.org/10.1186/s13195-016-0188-8.
Prince, M., Guerchet, M., & Prina, M. (2015). *The epidemiology and impact of dementia: Current state and future trends.* Geneva: World Health Organization.
Prince, M., Prina, M., & Guerchet, M. (2013). *World Alzheimer report 2013: Journey of caring.* London: Alzheimer's Disease International.
Prince, M., Wimo, A., Guerchet, M., Ali, G. C., Wu, Y. T., & Prina, M. (2015). *World Alzheimer report 2015: The global impact of dementia.* London: Alzheimer's Disease International.
Rees, G. (2017). Global action on dementia. *Australian Journal of Dementia Care, 6*(4), 7–9.
Rizzi, L., Rosset, I., & Roriz-Cruz, M. (2014). Global epidemiology of dementia: Alzheimer's and vascular types. *BioMed Research International, 2014*, 1–8. Available from https://doi.org/10.1155/2014/908915.
Schrijvers, E. M. C., Verhaaren, B. F. J., Koudstaal, P. J., Hofman, A., Ikram, M. A., & Breteler, M. M. B. (2012). Is dementia incidence declining? Trends in dementia incidence since 1990 in the Rotterdam Study. *Neurology, 78*(19), 1456–1463. Available from https://doi.org/10.1212/WNL.0b013e3182553be6.
Wimo, A., Guerchet, M., Ali, G.-C., Wu, Y.-T., Prina, A. M., Winblad, B., & Prince, M. (2017). The worldwide costs of dementia 2015 and comparisons with 2010. *Alzheimer's & Dementia, 13*(1), 1–7. Available from https://doi.org/10.1016/j.jalz.2016.07.150.
Wimo, A., Jönsson, L., Bond, J., Prince, M., & Winblad, B. (2013). The worldwide economic impact of dementia 2010. *Alzheimer's & Dementia, 9*(1), 1–11.e3. Available from https://doi.org/10.1016/j.jalz.2012.11.006.
World Health Organization. (2016). *WHO global action plan on the public health response to dementia 2017–2025.* Retrieved from http://www.who.int/mental_health/neurology/dementia/zero_draft_dementia_action_plan_5_09_16.pdf.
Wortmann, M. (2012). Dementia: A global health priority—Highlights from an ADI and World Health Organization report. *Alzheimer's Research & Therapy, 4*(40). Available from https://doi.org/10.1186/alzrt143.
Wu, Y.-T., Fratiglioni, L., Matthews, F. E., Lobo, A., Breteler, M. M. B., Skoog, I., & Brayne, C. (2016). Dementia in Western Europe: Epidemiological evidence and implications for policy making. *The Lancet Neurology, 15*(1), 116–124. Available from https://doi.org/10.1016/S1474-4422(15)00092-7.

Further Reading

Alzheimer's Association. (2014). *2014 Alzheimer's disease facts & figures.* Retrieved from https://www.alz.org/downloads/facts_figures_2014.pdf.

CHAPTER 12

Transforming Dementia Care

> *Although an intensely personal issue, family caregiving has become an urgent public policy issue, linked to important social, health, and economic goals.* **National Academies of Sciences, Engineering, and Medicine, Families Caring for an Aging Society, 2017.**
>
> *I don't yet see a lot of health systems coordinating with their local Meals on Wheels, or their local senior center, or local food bank, or personal care services. All those services of social stuff that social workers know about, but that doctors and most health care providers don't know how to tell people to access, including me.* **Clinician as reported in Institute for Healthcare Improvement/National Patient Safety Foundation, Cambridge and Boston, MA, 2017.**
>
> *Family caregivers and the person they're caring for are intertwined like a double helix. We're completely intertwined, so what happens to me happens to [my spouse], and what happens to [my spouse] happens to me.* **Family caregiver as reported in Institute for Healthcare Improvement/National Patient Safety Foundation, Cambridge and Boston, MA, 2017.**

MOVEMENT TOWARDS A SOCIAL–MEDICAL COMPREHENSIVE DEMENTIA CARE MODEL

Each of these quotes highlights the key areas in which dementia care needs to be transformed and how each of the levels of our social ecological model are implicated and intertwined with the other. As dementia and hence dementia care is complex, there will not be a single solution for any one family, health system, or country; rather there must be "many ways to many," in order to reflect, accommodate, and be integrated with local needs, values, resources, infrastructures, and policies (Mccannon, Massoud, & Alyesh, 2016).

In this close to final chapter, we consider transformative actions that need to occur at each level of our social ecological model in order to support or result in comprehensive dementia care. We argue that we must address issues on multiple fronts and somewhat simultaneously in order to make a real difference to real people, communities, and society. Our social ecological model calls upon and reflects the possibility for multiple and iterative actions, practices, and policies in order to obtain and assure continuance in transformation. In this regard, the lines on our model are porous and not necessarily temporally ordered; hence, layers are interactive as we have tried to illustrate throughout this book and embrace meaningful actions that need to occur independently, in concert, and in an integrated fashion.

In each previous chapter, we have offered varied points, recommendations and covered a lot of ground. Here in this chapter, we highlight a few areas for transformation—what we consider to be the principal areas—those that take primacy or priority at each layer of our model in order to achieve a "good life" for persons living with dementia and caregivers (Lawton, 1994). This chapter helps to pave the way for taking direct action, as well (see Chapter 13: Developing and Implementing an Action Plan). It also serves as a high-level summary of major points in previous chapters but somewhat differently than what we offer in Chapter 14, Putting it all Together: Synthesis and Future Directions, to reach the goal of comprehensive dementia care for individuals/families and over the elongated time frame from diagnosis to end of life. We neither propose specific policies nor legislation; rather we offer an overarching framework and within that framework core actions that we consider transformative. How our framework and actions are particularized we believe will depend upon a variety of factors including any one actor's location in dementia care (e.g., the affected individual vs family member vs health provider vs lobbyist vs payor vs researcher, and so forth), the socio-political and organizational context including values, resources, and needs.

In thinking about transformation at each level of our model, the question arises as to where to begin. We could start with the top layer involving change in social policy and social structure, we could start with the bottom—the individual level, or we could start somewhere in between. One could argue that a top-down, social structural transformation will drive all other sectors and thus it would be best to start there. We agree in part and this may be particularly true in the context of the United States in which fragmented health systems and antiquated payment models dominate and drive health and social care delivery. Making impact at that level requires a political will and broad coalitions and social trends that push dementia care forward. However, even if change was made at this high level which involved a restructuring of delivery and payment models, this would still not be sufficient. Furthermore, despite the imperative of policy/restructuring changes, actions can and must still be taken at all other levels of our model including at the local community, social agency, and/or individual/family level; in other words, we want to emphasize the synergies and connections among levels and urge for change from individuals, families, communities, as well as society at large. Hence, we have decided to start with the individual who is the centerpiece or the heart of the matter.

INDIVIDUAL LEVEL

> When thousands of patients rise up, refuse to be stigmatized, discuss their symptoms and participate in research, science benefits. A new test for Alzheimer's could help to create that movement, but let's not wait. Twenty-five percent to 50 percent of us will show signs of Alzheimer's by the age of 85. When it comes to dementia, we all should consider ourselves vulnerable. No matter what genes you carry, your odds of developing cognitive problems increase as you age. In other words, welcome to the club: If you plan to live a long time, then you, too, belong to the high-risk group. Now what are you going to do about it?
> P. Kennedy, Sunday Review NY Times "What if You Knew" November 17, 2017.

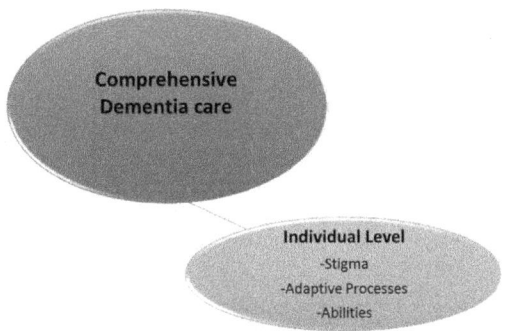

At the individual level, we suggest three areas for which research, practice, and policy would help to transform dementia care (see Part I,

About the Person Living With Dementia). These are understanding and addressing stigma, adaptive processes, and abilities. As to stigma, of importance is understanding through research the elements of diagnosis and living with dementia that are stigmatizing to individuals (perceived stigma) and how individuals confront structural stigma in their interactions with and access to communities, health providers, and health and care systems, and other resources (Riley, Burgener, & Buckwalter, 2014). Secondly, understanding adaptive processes—specifically, psychosocial and compensatory strategies—that individuals adapt to maintain ego integrity, remain connected, and have control over everyday events is critical for informing approaches to supporting people. Finally, within this social ecological level, identifying remaining or preserved abilities at each disease stage would support advancing care approaches emanating from a positive, strength-based framework. This will entail developing new measures to assess what a person can do (versus current cognitive and physical tests which focus on identifying deficit areas) that can be used in research and clinically and which would form the heart of an assessment in comprehensive dementia care, as well as policies that destigmatize dementia and support payment models for strength-based care (D'Alton, Hunter, Whitehouse, Brayne, & George, 2014). Underlying these three areas is a critical assumption—we must move towards a strength-based and inclusive framework for comprehensive dementia care.

CAREGIVERS

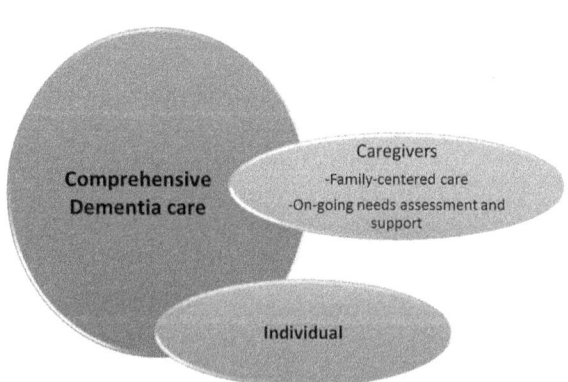

As we consider transforming dementia care from the perspective of caregivers, the most critical element here is moving from a person-based to a family-based centered model of care and providing on-going need assessments and support (see Part II: About the Caregiver). As to the first element, this would reflect transformation at all subsequent levels of our social ecological model. For example, to be family-centered would entail having mechanisms in place in clinical and social care settings to identify a care partner, recognize care partners in electronic medical records, conduct assessments of need and risk, and develop a plan of action. Research is needed to identify the best practices for identifying care partners as many families do not self-identify or use the label of "caregiver." Furthermore, research is needed to identify parsimonious assessment approaches that address family needs for each disease stage. This will entail educating and preparing a workforce for family-centered care by identifying specific competencies, how to assess new competencies, how to work on an interprofessional team, and where in the education of different health and human service professionals these new competencies should be introduced. As the workforce also serves as carers in dementia care, attending to their needs for education, support, knowledge, and skills about dementia care strategies is an imperative (Surr et al., 2017).

LIVING ENVIRONMENT

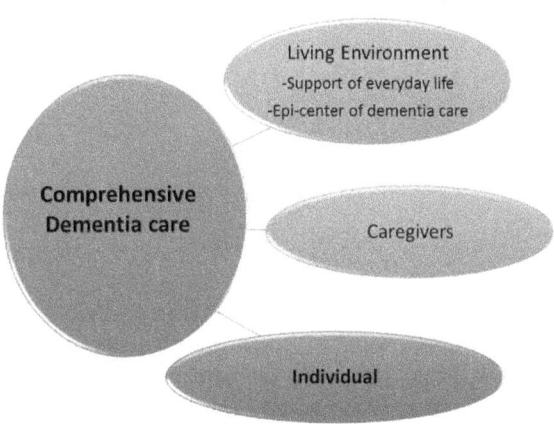

We now broaden our lens to the immediate living environment of individuals and caregivers and consider in particular, the home (see Part III: About Living Environments). While home could be any residential setting, the goal of individuals and families is to remain in their familiar residence and community. We suggest that a transformative step at this level is viewing the home as an immediate/proximal therapeutic environment as well as an epicenter for coordinating all dementia care from diagnosis to end of life. We have the evidence-based strategies that could be integrated into a comprehensive dementia care system where the home is the central organizing location. For this to be accomplished, there must be strategies to address the existing system level barriers to providing support at home (Donnelly, Humphries, Hickey, & Doyle, 2017). In this regard, technology will be imperative. Different technologies will need to deliver and reinforce care strategies, monitor safety and health, and connect different health and human service providers.

NEIGHBORHOOD AND COMMUNITY

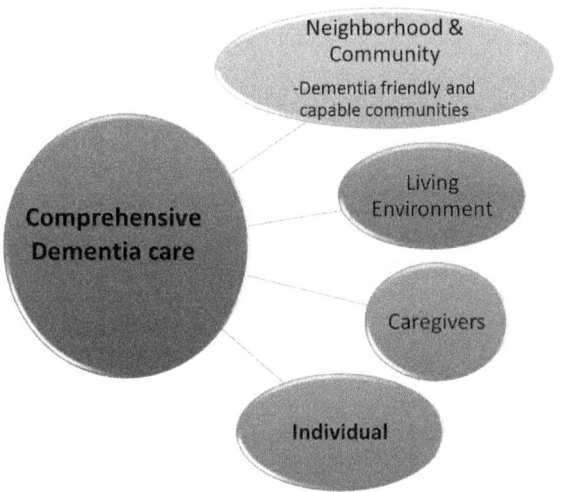

Next up is the neighborhood and community. The essential element here is transformation to dementia-friendly and capable communities (see Part III: About Living Environments). These principles, defined and discussed in Chapter 9, Living in the Community, are designed to enable full integration of individuals living with dementia and their caregivers in everyday community life, reduce stigma, and provide community members including restaurateurs, police, community leaders, and others the knowledge and skills to support individuals in their community with cognitive disorders (Lin, 2017).

HEALTH AND HUMAN SERVICES

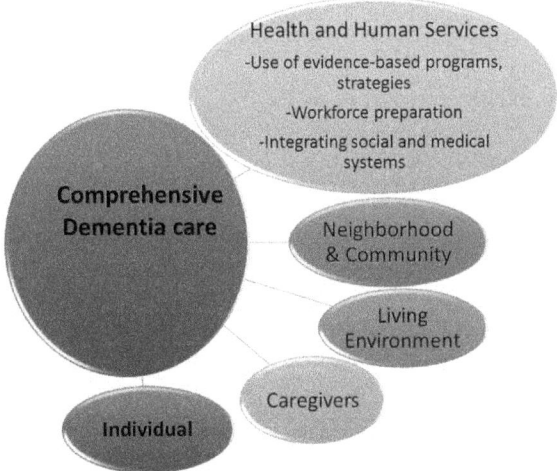

Three key and interrelated transformative actions at this level of our social ecological model include integrating existing evidence-based strategies, programs, practices within systems of care, adequately preparing an interprofessional workforce, and linking social and medical care/services in a seamless system of care (see Part IV: About Social Systems and Policies). Infusing existing services with evidence is not as easy as it may appear (Gitlin, Marx, Stanley, & Hodgson, 2015). In the United States, there have been many barriers to implementation including payment mechanisms and financial models, inadequate workforce preparation and availability, dissemination challenges as there is not a single payer system for diffusion, and a sole focus on cure and prevention at the expense of individuals and families living with dementia.

Strategies for Implementing Evidence

Although more research is necessary, there is sufficient evidence to move forward and implement programs/services/strategies in all delivery settings to support families now (Broda et al., 2017; Friss Feinberg, 2017). We identify here five possible models for bringing evidence to families and which agencies, clinics, and health and human service professionals can consider. Approaches for augmenting existing services with an evidence-based program are listed in Box 12-1.

> **Box 12-1**
> **Five Strategies for Implementing Evidence for Dementia Care**
>
> - Implement a program in a clinical or service setting keeping all components
> - Adapt an existing program to local needs
> - Layer and integrate different programs/strategies within a practice setting
> - Use select components of programs (evidence-informed)
> - Develop a "minimum viable product" for delivery based on the evidence (evidence-informed)

One approach is to implement an evidence-based program in a service setting as it was tested. This would entail implementing all of its components as originally tested within a particular context and maintaining fidelity. While small adaptations may be possible in this context, discussion with the developer to determine what can and cannot be modified to assure fidelity and effectiveness would be necessary (Washington et al., 2014; Zarit, Lee, Barrineau, Whitlatch, & Femia, 2013). The extent to which a particular program can be modified without affecting outcomes found from its original test is controversial and still dependent upon counsel from the original investigative team.

The CDC provides a helpful guideline as to what aspects of an evidence-based program may be adapted without disturbing fidelity and what changes may jeopardize the effectiveness of a program (https://preventyouthhiv.org/content/promoting-evidence-based-approaches-adaptation-guidelines). For example, translating a program into a different language or replacing materials with more culturally appropriate ones would be acceptable (a green light), whereas shortening the program, removing a treatment component, or changing its focus would alter the program too much and not be acceptable (a red light), requiring additional rigorous evaluation.

The challenges associated with integrating a proven intervention as is into a delivery setting are manifold. These include but are not limited to the need to (1) budget for training, (2) possibly hire new staff to deliver the program, (3) identify financial support for implementing and sustaining the program, and (4) identify mechanisms for assuring fidelity. Furthermore, programs evaluated outside of service delivery contexts typically include more homogenous samples of caregivers than that encountered by service providers, often require lengthy training time in its delivery and by specially trained interventionists who may not be available. Other challenges include that the length of the program (e.g., 10 sessions in the case of COPE) may not fit the service delivery context in which perhaps only three to four sessions can reasonably be delivered.

Another approach is to adapt a program for delivery in a particular context. This has been the case for the REACH II initiative which initially involved 12 sessions and use of an expensive videoconferencing computer/telephone support mechanism to provide education. Adaptations to the REACH II intervention for delivery in the Veterans Administration health systems have involved removing the technology component, providing information previously delivered via the technology through written materials, and shortening sessions to four (Nichols, Martindale-Adams, Burns, Zuber, & Graney, 2016). These types of adaptations require systematic evaluation to assure benefits are still derived. In the case of REACH II, benefits have been shown for its shortened versions (Burgio et al., 2009; Nichols, Martindale-Adams, Burns, Graney, & Zuber, 2011; Nichols et al., 2016; Stevens, Smith, Trickett, & McGhee, 2012).

Another approach is to layer, link, and integrate different evidence-based programs to maximize reach and outcomes. As any one tested approach, program, or service may not suffice given the range of changing needs and preferences of diverse families, offering several different programs may be an important approach (Abma, Pittens, Visse, Elberse, & Broerse, 2015). For example, whereas one caregiver may want to access information via the web, another may prefer to meet with other caregivers in a group; yet others may need more hands-on assistance learning different techniques (e.g., safe bathing practices or transfers from bed to chair). Thus, offering families a range of possible programs and/or sequencing programs to maximize support could be beneficial. For example, families could start with the Savvy Caregiver program (telephone, group, or online) to obtain foundational knowledge. For those needing more personalized support, this could be followed by providing REACH II, which provides face-to-face home-based support. For those needing more counseling and help also resolving family conflict, participation in the New York Family Caregiver Support Program would be important (Mittelman et al., 1993). Finally, for those families who are managing complex behavioral and functional changes, the COPE program could be introduced (Gitlin, Winter, Dennis, Hodgson, & Hauck, 2010). While offering more than one evidence-based program may be complex from an organizational and financial perspective, it is clear that one particular tested intervention will not suffice as it cannot address all needs of all persons at all disease stages.

Yet another approach to infusing evidence into care and services for individuals and families is to use an evidence-informed approach. This involves reading the literature and building a service based on the best evidence available but taking some liberties as to how it is implemented. For example, it may not be possible to implement all 10 sessions of the COPE program. However, adopting its principles of family-centeredness, tailoring, behavioral activation, problem-solving, or using its assessment approach and providing families with specific strategies may be effective, although evaluating benefits to families would be important to achieve (Gitlin, Cigliana, Cigliana, & Pappa, 2017).

Disaggregating evidence-based programs and offering only select protocols: Related to the above, one approach is to disaggregate evidence-based programs into their specific protocols and introduce select protocols. For example, REACH II, COPE, ADS Plus, and other interventions introduce caregivers to a problem-solving approach to address common care challenges. Similarly, REACH II, COPE, ADS Plus use similar stress reduction techniques. These are stand-alone protocols with evidence for their effectiveness that can be systematically integrated into existing services with families (Belle et al., 2006; Gitlin, Reever, Dennis, Mathieu, & Hauck, 2006; Nichols et al., 2016).

Still another related approach is to identify what is referred to in the business and start-up worlds as the "minimum viable product" that would have value to family caregivers (Silva, Calado, Silva, & Nascimento, 2013). This entails identifying the key components of evidence-based programs that all families need and offering these elements. This might include the following components: on-going education, stress reduction techniques, how to be an advocate, talk to health professionals and coordinate care, how to communicate effectively and engage people living with dementia in daily routines and meaningful activity, advance care planning, financial and legal advice, and ways to take care of self.

Strategies for Selecting Evidence for Implementation

Unfortunately, to date, there is not a single repository of tested and proven programs for individuals and caregivers that service providers, health and human service professionals, or administrators can consult in order to learn about and identify a program that may be right for a particular care/service context. Rather, we are all basically left on our own to cull through the literature to identify a program or its components to adapt and offer in a particular setting. One way to think about identifying a program is to adapt a simple-stepped approach that we outline in Fig. 12-1.

This figure suggests that the first step is to clearly define the targeted population. For example, it is important to consider the specific needs that individuals and families in a particular community being served

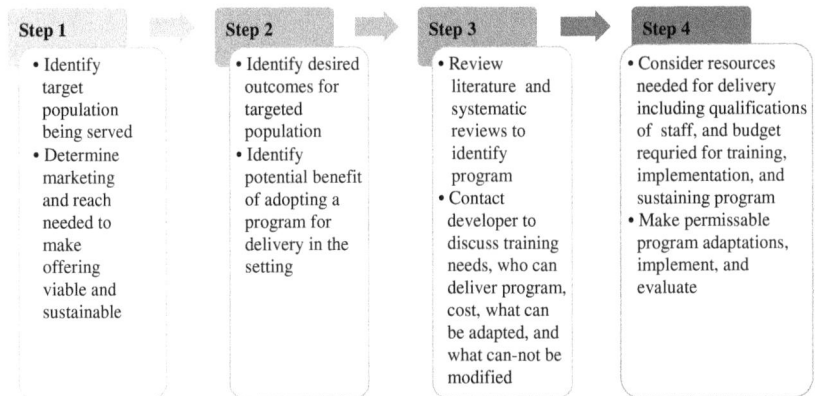

FIGURE 12-1 Selecting an evidence-based program for implementation in a service setting.

may have such as the need for generalized knowledge about the disease, or alternately an agency may be working with very overwhelmed and depressed caregivers. Determining who the target population is and how a program will be marketed in order to reach those who could benefit from the particular program are critical inputs needed for selecting the right program. Secondly, the desired outcomes or potential benefits that caregivers and agency personnel seek should be considered; it could be to improve general knowledge, confidence in being a caregiver, and reducing depression and/or distress with particular aspects of care. Next, in Step 3, it is helpful to determine the range of programs that have been tested to determine if there may be a match with the target population, its needs, and the desired outcomes. Finally, in Step 4 it is important to consider the resources needed to implement the chosen programs. Examples of resources include the costs associated with training in the program, how many staff may need to be trained, whether current staff have the requisite knowledge and skills to offer the program or whether new staff would have to be hired, and whether the program would replace existing services or augment existing services and if the latter, what is its added value.

In the United States, there are different ways of moving the evidence forward and embedding it in different health and social service systems. This may include implementing the tested program within an existing payment system such as the Veterans Administration (Nichols et al., 2016), Medicaid Waiver and community-based programs (Fortinsky et al., 2016), home care (Gitlin et al., 2017), adult day services (Gitlin et al., 2006), or other aging-related services, through support of foundations and private pay (Bass et al., 2013; Gitlin et al., 2017). However, this places the onus of diffusion on research teams which may not be knowledgeable or have the resources to engage in the very time-consuming and expensive efforts required for scaling up for and enabling widespread implementation. The challenge remains how best to effectively diffuse the evidence so that families and individuals can benefit.

SOCIAL POLICY

Social Policy
- Comprehensive payment models
- Employer-based efforts
- Legislative efforts

Comprehensive Dementia care
- Health and Human Services
- Neighborhood & Community
- Living Environment
- Caregivers
- Individual

At this level of the model (see Part V: Taking Action), key transformative actions focus on developing payment models for comprehensive dementia care, evolving employer-based innovative efforts that support employed family caregivers, and a range of legislative efforts that promote recognition and integration of family caregivers in medical records, hospital intake and discharge and in other care settings. In the United States in particular, a reimbursement model that supports the use of evidence-based strategies, family-centered approaches, care coordination, and care management is essential. These structural changes must occur for all other transformations to occur. Box 12-2 identifies fundamental principles for advancing policies.

Any system for dementia care must address issues related to stigma and disparities in prevalence and access to care (Mayeda, Glymour, Quesenberry, & Whitmer, 2016). Also, any system for dementia care, whether home as epicenter or elsewhere, must promote continuous access to assessment and reassessment as the disease progresses and with changes in cognition, function, behavioral symptoms, medical issues,

> **Box 12-2**
> **Principles for Advancing Policies to Support Persons Living With Dementia and Families**

- Integrate and coordinate social and medical services.
- Flexible, nimble system of care recognizing that one size does not fit all.
- Sensitivity to nomenclature and recognition that individuals and their families live with different forms of dementia.
- Care coordination and management of dementia and comorbidities is needed across disease trajectory.
- Person- and family-centered and directed care is heart of all medical and social services. It is important to see the whole person and their family behind the disease.
- Information and services provided when, where, and how families need and want different forms of support.

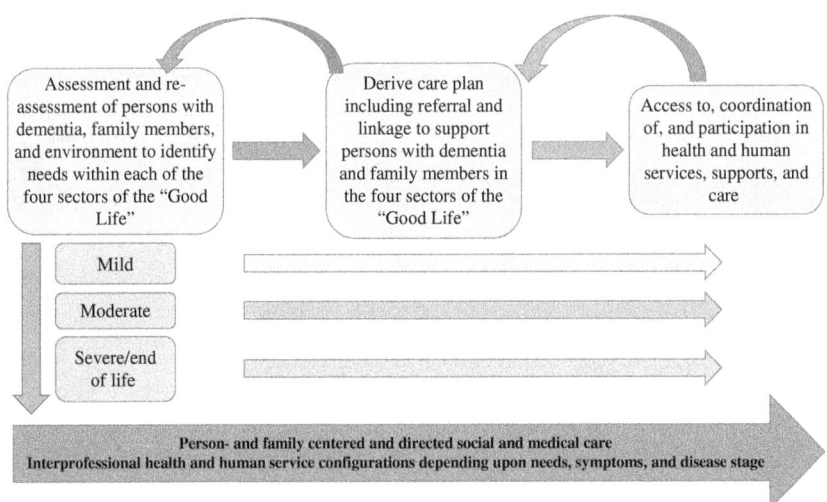

FIGURE 12-2   With diagnosis, then what? Moving towards comprehensive dementia care.

or caregiver needs (Callahan et al., 2014). In Fig. 12-2, we graphically display some of the key elements of a flexible, nimble system of care encapsulated by an interprofessional team and supported by technologies supporting coordination and communications. As we suggest (see Dr. Lyketsos' commentary in Chapter 8: The Physical Home Environment: A Neglected Therapeutic Context), the epicenter of such a care delivery system could be the home.

PUTTING IT ALL TOGETHER

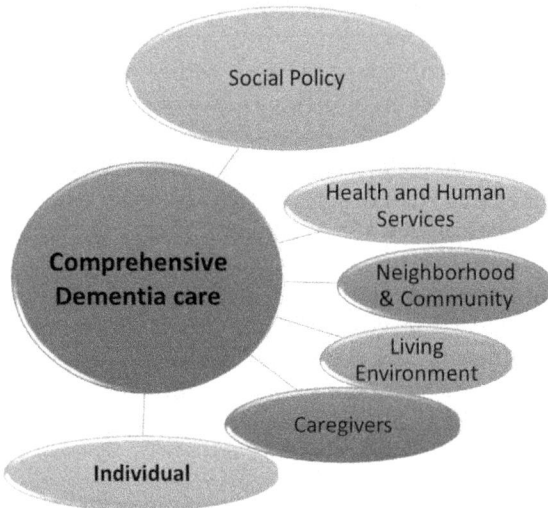

Our model suggests interconnectivity such that a change in one level is necessarily connected to another and leads to or is modified as a consequence of actions in another layer. While we recognize the importance of top-down change, we also encourage individual action—the complexity of dementia care can be distilled by individuals who take immediate action in their own life sphere as well as simultaneously working at a policy level for bigger changes.

CONCLUSION

In this chapter, we summarize key points raised in previous chapters that compose a transformative approach. We emphasize that we must obtain a better understanding of the lived experience in order to destigmatize dementia, recognize dementia care and caregiving as a public policy issue that societies must attend to, link social and medical care systems to provide comprehensive dementia care, and extend dementia care from being person-centered to person- and family-centered and directed. We argue that transformation is critical at every level of our social ecological model and must also be based on fundamental principles summarized here and presented throughout this book.

A Conversation With Dr. Jean Garjardo, PhD, OTR/L

1. *What is your vision for a comprehensive dementia care system?* My vision of a comprehensive dementia care system involves multi-sectorial approaches promoting coordination and integration when addressing dementia care. People with dementia and those who support them, government, civil society, private sector, and state sectors to jointly achieve outcomes. Outcomes should not be improvised, as they should result from a plan also jointly developed. Evidence-informed interventions facilitate the pathway towards integrated care, as good practice in dementia care highlights better results from coordinated actions, tailoring goals and therapies, and integrated social and health services.
2. *What are key societal levers that could be pushed to transform dementia care in your country (Chile)?* So far, academy has played a major role in making dementia a public health priority, as several poles of research and dissemination, including biomedical, psychosocial, a clinical, have contributed to inform policy and most importantly, to increase governmental interest and motivation to move forwards in a field that remained unknown and formally unaddressed. I would say the institutional level represented by the health sector (Ministry of Health) has led the road in terms of policy funding, design, and implementation. Advocacy by NGOs (non-government organizations) has been influential as well. I think the participation of civil society, people with dementia and their families, is yet to be pushed. Dementia is still a very stigmatized and taboo condition, so people with dementia are still a hidden population. Also, social affairs should also involve more intensely, as social services and supports are a key component for dementia care. As said before, dementia still is a highly stigmatized condition, and often media promotes inadequate images of people with dementia, ideas that perpetuate a fatal image of dementia separating those who would benefit from diagnosis and support as they assume that nothing can be done for a better life despite of dementia. In a general context of low health literacy in Chilean population, the role of media in community education needs to be improved. In every level, leadership is a key component. Building leaderships to promote dementia awareness and direct policy makers and stake holders.
3. *What do you think could be done now to improve dementia care by health systems and providers within the current care system in your country?* Reinforce that dementia is a public health priority for Chile, guaranteeing access to diagnosis, treatment, and support.

We need training. Health and human services professionals present training needs that are not being satisfied in undergraduate programs. Professionals the technical human force should be provided of foundational elements to be adapted to each country zone, as a country with such contrasts in terms of geography and culture. Understand the need for evidence-based interventions, and evidence-informed policies. We should not put efforts on creating what is already known, but adding layers to what is recommended depending on contextual features. We need more collaboration among professionals, and innovation within a frame of person-centered care. We need to move from "my profession is relevant for dementia" to "dementia is relevant for my profession". For Chile, as any other middle-income country, it is imperative to develop, creatively and based on what we know so far, the strategies that we assume will enhance a better living for those who live with dementia. We are currently implementing our first national dementia plan, starting in very delimitated zones of the country. We need to think bigger. We need the future governments to commit and think long-term.

References

Abma, T. A., Pittens, C. A. C. M., Visse, M., Elberse, J. E., & Broerse, J. E. W. (2015). Patient involvement in research programming and implementation. *Health Expectations*, 18(6), 2449–2464. Available from https://doi.org/10.1111/hex.12213.

Bass, D. M., Judge, K. S., Lynn Snow, A., Wilson, N. L., Morgan, R., Looman, W. J., ... Kunik, M. E. (2013). Caregiver outcomes of partners in dementia care: Effect of a care coordination program for veterans with dementia and their family members and friends. *Journal of the American Geriatrics Society*, 61(8), 1377–1386. Available from https://doi.org/10.1111/jgs.12362.

Belle, S. H., Burgio, L., Burns, R., Coon, D., Czaja, S. J., Gallagher-Thompson, D., ... Zhang, S. (2006). Enhancing the quality of life of dementia caregivers from different ethnic or racial groups: A randomized, controlled trial. *Annals of Internal Medicine*, 145 (10), 727–738.

Broda, A., Bieber, A., Meyer, G., Hopper, L., Joyce, R., Irving, K., ... Stephan, A. (2017). Perspectives of policy and political decision makers on access to formal dementia care: Expert interviews in eight European countries. *BMC Health Services Research*, 17(1), 518. Available from https://doi.org/10.1186/s12913-017-2456-0.

Burgio, L. D., Collins, I. B., Schmid, B., Wharton, T., McCallum, D., & Decoster, J. (2009). Translating the REACH caregiver intervention for use by area agency on aging personnel: The REACH OUT program. *Gerontologist*, 49(1), 103–116. Available from https://doi.org/10.1093/geront/gnp012.

Callahan, C. M., Sachs, G. A., LaMantia, M. A., Unroe, K. T., Arling, G., & Boustani, M. A. (2014). Redesigning systems of care for older adults with Alzheimer's disease. *Health Affairs*, 33(4), 626–632. Available from https://doi.org/10.1377/hlthaff.2013.1260.

D'Alton, S., Hunter, S., Whitehouse, P., Brayne, C., & George, D. (2014). Adapting to dementia in society: A challenge for our lifetimes and a charge for public health. *Journal of Alzheimer's Disease: JAD, 42*(4), 1151–1163. Available from https://doi.org/10.3233/JAD-140213.

Donnelly, N.-A., Humphries, N., Hickey, A., & Doyle, F. (2017). "We don't have the infrastructure to support them at home": How health system inadequacies impact on long-term care admissions of people with dementia. *Health Policy., 21*(12), 1280–1287. Available from https://doi.org/10.1016/j.healthpol.2017.09.020.

Fortinsky, R. H., Gitlin, L. N., Pizzi, L. T., Piersol, C. V., Grady, J., Robison, J. T., & Molony, S. (2016). Translation of the Care of Persons with Dementia in their Environments (COPE) intervention in a publicly-funded home care context: Rationale and research design. *Contemporary Clinical Trials, 49*, 155–165. Available from https://doi.org/10.1016/j.cct.2016.07.006.

Friss Feinberg, L. (2017). *From research to standard practice: Advancing proven programs to support family caregivers of persons living with dementia*. Retrieved from http://www.aarp.org/content/dam/aarp/ppi/2017/08/from-research-to-standard-practice.pdf%0Ahttp://www.aarp.org/content/dam/aarp/ppi/2017/08/from-research-to-standard-practice.pdf.

Gitlin, L. N., Cigliana, J., Cigliana, K., & Pappa, K. (2017). Supporting family caregivers of persons with dementia in the community: Description of the "Memory Care Home Solutions" program and its impacts. *Innovation in Aging, 1*(1). Available from https://doi.org/10.1093/geroni/igx013.

Gitlin, L. N., Marx, K., Stanley, I. H., & Hodgson, N. (2015). Translating evidence-based dementia caregiving interventions into practice: State-of-the-science and next steps. *Gerontologist, 55*(2), 210–226. Available from https://doi.org/10.1093/geront/gnu123.

Gitlin, L. N., Reever, K., Dennis, M. P., Mathieu, E., & Hauck, W. W. (2006). Enhancing quality of life of families who use adult day services: Short- and long-term effects of the Adult Day Services Plus Program. *The Gerontologist, 46*(5), 630–639. Available from https://doi.org/10.1093/geront/46.5.630.

Gitlin, L. N., Winter, L., Dennis, M. P., Hodgson, N., & Hauck, W. W. (2010). A biobehavioral home-based intervention and the well-being of patients with dementia and their caregivers. *JAMA, 304*(9), 983–991. Available from https://doi.org/10.1001/jama.2010.1253.

Lawton, M. P. (1994). Quality of life in Alzheimer disease. *Alzheimer Disease and Associated Disorders, 8*(Suppl 3), 138–150. Available from https://doi.org/7999340.

Lin, S.-Y. (2017). "Dementia-friendly communities" and being dementia friendly in healthcare settings. *Current Opinion in Psychiatry, 30*(2), 145–150. Available from https://doi.org/10.1097/YCO.0000000000000304.

Mayeda, E. R., Glymour, M. M., Quesenberry, C. P., & Whitmer, R. A. (2016). Inequalities in dementia incidence between six racial and ethnic groups over 14 years. *Alzheimer's and Dementia, 12*(3), 216–224. Available from https://doi.org/10.1016/j.jalz.2015.12.007.

Mccannon, J., Massoud, M.R., & Alyesh, A. (2016). Many ways to many. In *Stanford Social Innovation Review*. Retrieved from https://ssir.org/articles/entry/many_ways_to_many.

Mittelman, M. S., Ferris, S. H., Steinberg, G., Shulman, E., Mackell, J. A., Ambinder, A., & Cohen, J. (1993). An intervention that delays institutionalization of Alzheimer's disease patients: Treatment of spouse-caregivers. *The Gerontologist, 33*(6), 730–740. Available from https://doi.org/10.1093/geront/33.6.730.

Nichols, L. O., Martindale-Adams, J., Burns, R., Graney, M. J., & Zuber, J. (2011). Translation of a dementia caregiver support program in a health care system—REACH VA. *Archives of Internal Medicine, 171*(4), 353–359. Available from https://doi.org/10.1001/archinternmed.2010.548.

Nichols, L. O., Martindale-Adams, J., Burns, R., Zuber, J., & Graney, M. J. (2016). REACH VA: Moving from translation to system implementation. *The Gerontologist, 56*(1), 135–144. Available from https://doi.org/10.1093/geront/gnu112.

Riley, R. J., Burgener, S., & Buckwalter, K. C. (2014). Anxiety and stigma in dementia. *Nursing Clinics of North America, 49*(2), 213–231. Available from https://doi.org/10.1016/j.cnur.2014.02.008.

Silva, S. E. P., Calado, R. D., Silva, M. B., & Nascimento, M. A. (2013). Lean startup applied in healthcare: A viable methodology for continuous improvement in the development of new products and services. *IFAC Proceedings Volumes, 46*(24), 295–299. Available from https://doi.org/10.3182/20130911-3-BR-3021.00054.

Stevens, A. B., Smith, E. R., Trickett, L. R., & McGhee, R. (2012). Implementing an evidence-based caregiver intervention within an integrated healthcare system. *Translational Behavioral Medicine, 2*(2), 218–227. Available from https://doi.org/10.1007/s13142-012-0132-9.

Surr, C. A., Gates, C., Irving, D., Oyebode, J., Smith, S. J., Parveen, S., ... Dennison, A. (2017). Effective dementia education and training for the health and social care workforce: A systematic review of the literature. *Review of Educational Research, 87*(5), 966–1002. Available from https://doi.org/10.3102/0034654317723305.

Washington, T., Zimmerman, S., Cagle, J., Reed, D., Cohen, L., Beeber, A. S., & Gwyther, L. P. (2014). Fidelity decision making in social and behavioral research: Alternative measures of dose and other considerations. *Social Work Research, 38*(3), 154–162. Available from https://doi.org/10.1093/swr/svu021.

Zarit, S. H., Lee, J. E., Barrineau, M. J., Whitlatch, C. J., & Femia, E. E. (2013). Fidelity and acceptability of an adaptive intervention for caregivers: An exploratory study. *Aging & Mental Health, 17*(2), 197–206. Available from https://doi.org/10.1080/13607863.2012.717252.

PART V

TAKING ACTION

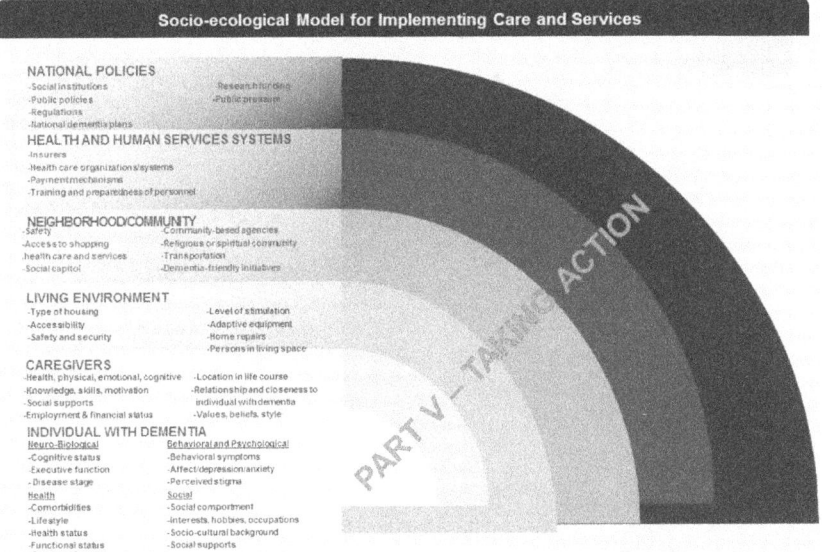

In this final section, Part V, we first provide a structure for readers to develop an action plan to make a difference in their local context (see Chapter 13: Developing and Implementing an Action Plan). An action plan is an important mechanism by which to commit to a behavioral action. We urge action plans to be developed at any level of our social—ecological model to contribute to changes in dementia care and improve the lives of individuals concerned. We invite readers to construct their own personal action plan committing ideas in a simple-to-use template that can also be uploaded and shared on a website.

Then in our final chapter (see Chapter 14: Putting It All Together: Synthesis and Future Directions), we highlight the major points made throughout this book as a way to provide a concise synthesis for easy reference by readers.

CHAPTER 13

Developing and Implementing an Action Plan

A goal without a plan is just a wish. **Antoine de Saint-Exupery.**

We hope that you have come to the end of this book with a greater understanding of the impact of dementia on individuals, families, communities, and societies, and that your understanding is coupled with a firm commitment to improving the lives of persons living with dementia and their family members. In this chapter, we provide a vehicle for you to take what you have learned and put it in action. This chapter is a "call to action." We aim to move your commitment to improving the lives of persons living with dementia and their families into action. Here we provide a mechanism for you to do something about dementia in your environment!

Action planning is a process by which intentions are transformed into goals that can be acted upon, as shown in Fig. 13-1. Engaging in action planning enables individuals to be strategic about and enact the specific steps necessary to make change and implement the plan. Action planning helps individuals realize their intentions. People who form action plans are more likely to act on what they intended more so than those who do not form action plans.

The goal of this chapter is to provide the impetus and tools for you to develop a one-page action plan to address an unmet need of individuals with dementia or their caregivers in your particular situation or environment.

To move from intention to action, there are six fundamental steps as shown in Fig. 13-2.

1. As a first step, identify which level of the socioecological model you want to impact: it could be at the person, family, home or caregiving environment, community, or societal level (see Fig. 13-3).

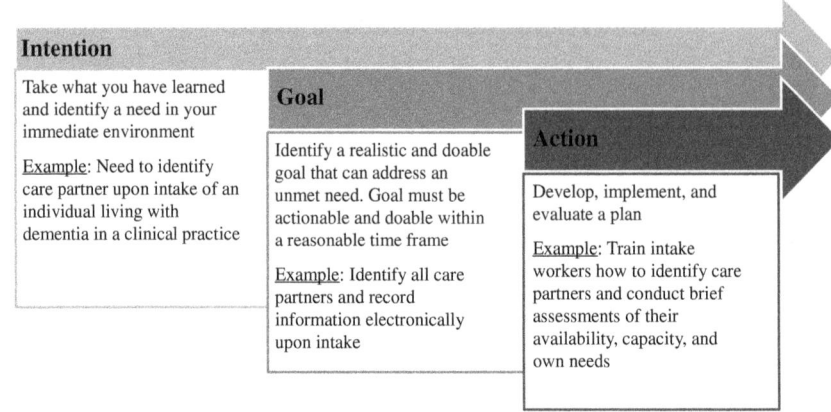

FIGURE 13-1 From intention to action.

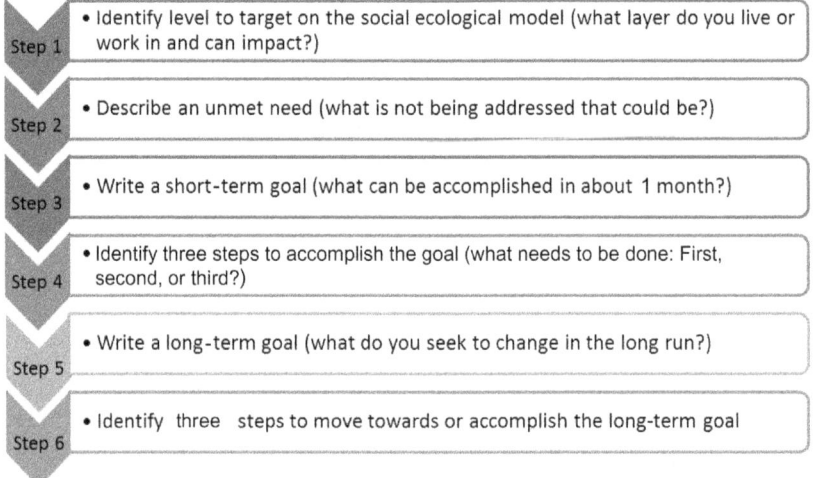

FIGURE 13-2 Six steps in an action plan.

An example might include targeting the community level and addressing the need to raise dementia awareness. This could be accomplished by sharing your care story in a form of a letter to a government representative, local newspaper, or your hospital administrator. You could address the need for better dementia awareness in local business by developing a plan to meet with a local business manager to implement a training program for staff to recognize and effectively help customers with cognitive impairment. Alternatively, you could address the need in your hospital for better

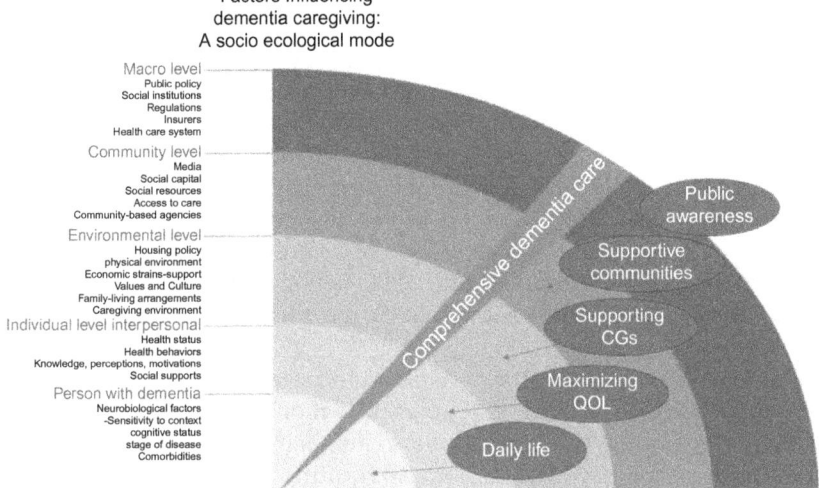

FIGURE 13-3 Action plans mapped to the socioecological model.

assessments of persons with dementia (the health organization/community level).

2. Second, briefly describe one unmet need in the particular level of the socioecological model you seek to target.

   The unmet need I wish to address is:_____.

3. Third, write one short-term goal: "In the next month I will: _____".

   Set a realistic goal that can be accomplished and within a short time frame (within 1 month), but also identify a goal that challenges you, that you want to accomplish and which will make a difference.

4. Fourth, identify up to the three steps that will need to be accomplished to put this goal into action.
   1. _____
   2. _____
   3. _____

5. Now write one long-term goal "In the next year I will: _____".

   This long-term goal is intended to articulate your vision for improving dementia care; it should build on the short-term goal and also serve to inspire you.

6. What are three steps that you need to take to put this long-term goal into action?
   1. _____
   2. _____
   3. _____

In order to spur your thinking to develop a reasonable, inspiring action plan that addresses a local unmet need, we have provided some examples of action plans that were developed and implemented by global participants in our 6-week, massive open online course, "Living with Dementia: Impact on Individuals, Families and Society," through Coursera.[1] The final assignment for this course involved submission of an "action plan," in which learners were asked to generate a brief description of how they intended to use the new knowledge they had acquired in the course to solve a dementia care challenge in their location and practice setting. Overall, 1200 action plans were submitted, with plans targeting different levels of the socioecological perspective (Fig. 13-3).

The leading category of action plans focused on the macro-level of our socioecological model. Examples of action plans in this category included developing public awareness campaigns, using social media as a platform to raise awareness, and advocating with policy makers for payment systems to support caregivers on family leave:

> The goal of my action plan is to reconcile theoretical concepts of intervention and promote individual action plans, profile the role of interdisciplinary teams then embed a relative assignment in a field experience course. *P.L. Bloomington, IL.*

A second category of action plans focused on creating supportive communities. Example action plans in this category were geared towards students' specific community and included training of police officers and firefighters, and developing "dementia-friendly" parks, libraries, or other public spaces:

> The goal of my action plan is to provide educational programs at clubhouses for age 55+ communities, religious institutions, libraries and hospitals to make people more aware of what to look for. Provide outlines for educational programs to the appropriate contact people at local hospitals, libraries, etc. and assess their willingness to allow me to speak or arrange for another speaker on this topic to increase awareness to the members of the community. *O.L., New Delhi, India.*

The third category of action plans included helping family caregivers by initiating support groups, caregiver training programs, and respite programs:

> The goal of my action plan is to manage triggers to reduce use of psychotropic medication and create a panel of experts on dementia care and create educational

---

[1] This course is free and ongoing and can be accessed at: https://www.coursera.org/learn/dementia-care?utm_source = Aging&utm_campaign= 27aad572b7-Dementia_MOOC_2017.5.22%28DontMissOut%29&utm_medium=email&utm_term=0_db254c31c5-27aad572b7-161249021.

materials. Offer seminars to administrators of dementia facilities across a given geographical area. Once the implementation is noted effective by the facilities leaders, collaborate with providers to taper any psychotropic medications as they deem appropriate. Continue to provide the non-pharmacological approach, be it music therapy or companionship (and) ensure ongoing education is provided to families/caregivers. *G.A., Berlin, Germany.*

The fourth category was focused on projects seeking to improve the dignity and quality of life for persons with dementia. Proposed projects included collaborating with theater/music groups, engaging persons with dementia in the arts, developing web-based applications or games:

> The goals of my action plan are to: (1) identify all local key providers of services to people at risk for dementia, including contact information, (2) establish an email list to contact all these providers, and a booklet of contacts for later distribution, (3) establish a web-based online local forum for these providers to post information and events, (4) identify a location in which quarterly meetings for providers could be held., (5) create calendar of dates and email all providers to invite them to a quarterly "roundtable of dementia care" meeting to increase communication and referrals for clients; and (6) establish basic leadership (Chair, Secretary, Treasurer) to insure group continues to meet and grow. *C.L, Nova Scotia, CA.*

The final category of action plans was focused on practical strategies to improve the daily life of individuals with dementia such as daily life such as keeping persons with dementia engaged in meaningful activities, modifying the home environment to promote safety and developing reminder system:

> The goal of my action plan is to create centers that make the link between homes, hospitals, nursing homes and social services on dementia related issues. People with dementia could come for day stays, not only participate in activities or receive individualized care but also to a certain extend get information on the disease (diagnosis, technology for home safety, etc.). This last point would be more useful for families or caregivers who often do not have enough support (the right place, the treatment approach, home settings, quality of live, general information on the disease, etc. *A.D., Owings Mills, MD.*

You should now be ready to implement a part or all of your action plan. Remember that your action plan is not something that is set in stone, but something that you can return to again and again—revising your goals, or the way you might reach them, in response to the learning you will obtain as you start to implement your plan and as your priorities may also change.

To upload your action plan, go to this link: https://sites.nursing.upenn.edu/betterlivingwithdementia/ where you will see the instructions that are summarized in Fig. 13.3. Click on the "Leave a Comment" tab. Here you can tell us about your action plan.

As Margaret Mead reminded us, "Never doubt that a small group of thoughtful, committed citizens can change the world; indeed, it is the only thing that ever has."

CHAPTER 14

Putting It All Together: Synthesis and Future Directions

This book addresses the complex considerations in living with dementia and specifically its implications and impacts on persons themselves, family members, communities, and societies. We highlight the major concerns, the existing evidence, what we know and what we do not know, and areas for which change could happen immediately to make a difference in all persons affected.

Our approach to understanding dementia is transformative in that it goes beyond the molecular, cellular, and neuronal considerations to understand ways in which pathophysiology plays out in particular social ecologies to impact daily lives. We contend that an understanding of the dementia experience cannot just be about the brain. Consideration must be given to the social, environmental, organizational, and political context which occur around the individual living with dementia and their family in order to more fully grasp the magnitude and vicissitudes of this progressive, deteriorating condition and its variegated consequences.

There is sufficient evidence to support our assumptions and approach. For example, a recent yet consistent research finding is that the lack of education is an important risk factor for dementia along with other social determinants such as having low-income, being of minority status (in the United States, for example, dementia differentially impacts individuals who are African American and of Latino heritage and women). Other behavioral and environmental factors such as lifestyle choices have also been identified as reducing risk factors including diet, physical activity, social connectedness, cognitive stimulation, and bilingualism. Untreated depression, hearing loss, and poor sleep have also been implicated as potential risk factors for dementia. Likewise, we show in these chapters how social—ecological factors including perceived and structural stigmata, access or lack thereof to social services and other resources (financial, legal), housing conditions and arrangements, and community and health professional preparedness differentially (positively or negatively) affect the experiences of having dementia and its trajectory and important outcomes including health, well-being and "a good life."

We argue for the importance of an all-encompassing social–ecological approach to frame and capture the multiple and interactive domains and specific factors impacting the lives of individuals affected by dementia and that may also inform the pathways of disease progression. More specifically, a family living in a dementia-friendly community will have different exposures and experiences than a family located in a low-resourced community with little to no access to dementia-appropriate social services and supports. A family using an emergency room in a US hospital in which health providers are not well trained in dementia care will have a very different experience fraught with stress and negative consequences compared to a family for example in Scotland who upon receiving a diagnosis is also assigned a care manager. Similarly, families living in countries with National Plans that have enacted care coordination and other dementia-specific and family-centered services will fare differently than those living in countries without systematic plans enacting dementia care.

Our goal throughout this book is to provide foundational knowledge from a social–ecological perspective in order to move forward with transformative research, service/practice, and education as well as to help guide immediate individual and local actions to improve daily care and supports. We assume an "all in approach"—that is, we seek to provide fundamentals of living with dementia from a new perspective that would be relevant to individuals, family caregivers, health and human service providers, and policy makers—or all stakeholders in dementia.

Here, in our final chapter, we capture our major points in order to provide the reader with a concise synthesis of our principal arguments and the presented evidence. We also suggest that the reader refers back to the introductory chapter as it summarizes the core threads woven throughout this book and reflects what can be referred to as our polemic.

In that opening introductory chapter, we present an overarching theme which we then repeat in subsequent chapters. This overarching theme underscores the unique and important perspective of this book, that is, we desperately need new strategies and models of care in dementia that address in a systematic and organized fashion all factors along our social–ecological framework, and which addresses change over time with disease progression. Intersecting or overlapping with disease progression is the life course. By now we hope the reader grasps the importance of considering when in the life course a person is diagnosed (e.g., early onset versus late in life) as well as when in the life course a family member assumes care responsibilities. Of significance is how these sentinel events—diagnosis and becoming a care partner—intersect with other life developmental roles, responsibilities, tasks, needs, health events, life and employment requirements, and pulls (e.g., caring for young children, completing college, balancing care with employment).

Each chapter following our introductory remarks tackles a particular domain along our social−ecological model, highlighting what we know and what we need to know and emphasizing what can be done now to make life better for all concerned.

In Part I, About the Person Living With Dementia, we focus on the person living with dementia. All four chapters in this section address different but interrelated considerations of how dementia impacts individuals themselves with a diagnosis. We began in Chapter 1, How the Brain Is Affected, with an examination of what is known and not known about pathophysiology and different etiologies. It provides foundational knowledge and where we are at in terms of the science of this condition that continues to allude a complete understanding of its route causes. Recent thinking is that this complex condition may not have a single causative source, but rather a number of factors may converge to create a perfect storm. Of importance is that recent research suggests nine potential factors that pose as risks for dementia but which are modifiable: childhood education, midlife hearing loss, hypertension, and obesity, and late-life smoking, depression, physical inactivity, social isolation, and diabetes. These factors require us to carefully reconsider policy investments and to examine risk reduction efforts and use a life course perspective.

In Chapter 2, Lived Experiences of Individuals With Dementia, we tackle the meaning and implications of a dementia diagnosis for the individual affected. Although research on the experience of dementia from the perspective of the individual is thin, there are clearly social, emotional, cognitive, functional, financial implications that have been documented and are critical to consider. In this chapter, we provide insights as to some of the key challenges that are experienced by individuals including when and how to disclose a diagnosis and to whom, how to cope with changing capabilities, how ego integrity is maintained or the biographical management work associated with receiving a diagnosis of dementia particularly in the early stages of the disease process. The role of stigma and disparities in enveloping quality of life is particularly noteworthy because of their pervasiveness and pernicious consequences.

Next in Chapter 3, Breaking the Cycle of Despair, we describe a particular structural form of stigma we label a "cycle of despair." Upon diagnosis (in the United States), families typically do not receive any information, not even referrals to vetted websites or advocacy groups that provide various forms of support and education. Rather, health professionals typically believe there is no cure. This leads to their conclusion that nothing can be done; hence, families are customarily sent home to manage on their own, setting up a cycle of despair on the part of health providers and families. We argue that this is a structural form of stigma that adds yet another layer of complexity to disease management and which further perpetuates negativity, social isolation, despair, and disease burden. We suggest that this cycle must and can be disrupted. In the United States, at a minimum, families must be offered helpful and accurate information about dementia and referrals and linkages to local resources. In primary care, health professionals have a moral and ethical responsibility to inquire about the well-being of the care partner of patients with dementia and provide support in the form of at least education or referrals.

Chapter 4, Making Life Better for Individuals Living With Dementia, moves the reader along to consider ways to support a good life. We suggest 15 treatment goals that guide dementia care in any care setting (clinical or social service) and that can be acted upon now. We suggest that these goals are relevant at all disease stages and for any etiology and that there is sufficient evidence to make headway in addressing each. We also highlight a few exemplars of approaches and provide a table of suggested actions for reaching each goal. This chapter also highlights the complexities in delivering dementia care: first, all 15 treatment goals must be met; second, goals need to be addressed by different health and human service professionals thus necessitating training all professionals; third, coordination of delivery then becomes essential and the measurement of a successful outcome for each goal and by disease stage and preferences become essential and still need to be developed.

In Part II, About the Caregiver, we broaden our lens to examine the impact of dementia on family members. We begin in Chapter 5, Family Member as Care Partner, by examining the effects on family members from time of diagnosis to end of life and how the experience varies by access to resources and disparities as well as once the role of caregiving is assumed. We discuss how the experience of dementia and caregiving may be very different for a daughter caring for her mother with the diagnosis, who is also working and caring for small children in the home (e.g., the woman in the middle) versus a spouse who may also be experiencing age-related chronic illness and functional challenges.

In Chapter 6, How We Can Support Families, we focus on specific ways to support family caregivers and address their many, changing needs. We emphasize the importance of assessing a family member's abilities, situation, personal health, and care needs in clinical and service settings involving either the person with dementia or the family caregiver themselves. Some existing assessments are brief while others are more comprehensive, but assessment is critical and leads to tailoring a treatment plan and specific strategies supportive of family members' own needs and care preferences.

We argue that simply asking caregivers how they are doing, what they are doing, and if they are taking care of themselves can go a long way in supporting their efforts and reducing excess burden and distress. In turn, when asking these questions, health and human service professionals must be prepared to offer, at the minimum, vetted resources to address concerns indicated by families. As health and social service systems fully rely upon and moreover expect family members to provide quality care, families become the hidden "patients" often tackling complex care challenges without the requisite knowledge, skills, or access to resources to effectively carry out tasks that are expected of them. We also argue that this gap between expectations, abilities, and knowledge and skills can harm persons living with dementia, and that a balance must be achieved between familial and societal responsibilities in long-term care. Noteworthy is that this is an area for which there is much evidence which can guide the most effective ways to support families. Yet, it is also important to recognize the gaps in evidence., For example, we are just now learning about the extent of the financial toll of dementia on families although there are no tested strategies or policies for addressing the extraordinary fiscal burdens.

In Chapter 7, Formal Caregivers: The Role of the Interprofessional Team, we turn our attention to the formal caregiver. We examine in some specificity their concerns, experiences, and stressors in managing dementia in various care settings. We note that in many respects, formal caregivers' concerns and challenges are not unlike those of family caregivers. We also indicate that health and human service professionals— from home health aide to physician—are ill-prepared to effectively engage and support persons with dementia and their family caregivers. This huge education and practice chasm is significant, and efforts must be expended to assure that the current and next generation of providers are adequately informed and prepared in new ways to effectively engage persons living with dementia (particularly in the early stages) to identify their preferred treatment goals and needs as well as their family members to provide dementia care. In the United States, the structure of medical encounters (amount of time allocated to patients, reimbursement, and quality indicators) does not support family-centric dementia care; new configurations will be essential affecting all social−ecological layers such as policy, education/training, health care organization, to the next generation of research geared towards ways of efficiently and effectively identifying treatment goals and their attainment for individuals with diminishing cognitive and functional capacities and family members.

Next, in Part III, About Living Environments, we attend to the essential domain of home and community environments, the next layer of our social–ecological model. We start this section with a discussion of the home (see Chapter 8: The Physical Home Environment: A Neglected Therapeutic Context) as that is the location in which most people with dementia live, age, and die. Here we examine the way in which home environments can support (or not) safety and daily functioning as well as common home modifications that can optimize quality of life for both persons living with dementia and their caregivers. The key point here is that the home is critical for maintaining cognitive and physical function and overall well-being. As such, attending to potential hazards is an important aspect of comprehensive dementia care. Simple and low-cost modifications such as installing grab bars, tub benches, and adequate lighting can go a long way to provide comfort, security, and safety. Also, modifications and simplifying the physical environment can be helpful to family caregivers. Chapter 9, Living in the Community, then examines the community as a location that can support living with dementia. We explore what is meant by dementia-ready and dementia-friendly communities, and provide specific strategies for enabling neighborhoods to be safe environments for people living with dementia and their caregivers, and providing connectivity to civic life. Exemplars from countries such as Chile or the Netherlands, and a few states in the United States, show promising ways of organizing communities to everyone's benefit.

Moving on to Part IV, About Social Systems and Policies, we explore issues related to the Social Systems and Policy levels of our social–ecological framework. We start in Chapter 10, Services and Settings of Care, to explore dementia care environments and service and care including assisted living, nursing homes, and specialized memory units within a facility, highlighting again the role of the physical environment and the cultural environment including quality and training of staff, organization of care, and inclusion of tailored activities as part of daily care. In Chapter 11, Global Efforts and National Plans, we tackle global efforts and the role of national plans in shaping policy and ground level delivery of care. We show that National Plans have promise to make a difference in dementia care but their power to do so varies by country and how health care is organized. In Chapter 12, Transforming Dementia Care, we propose particular approaches that could transform dementia care now, focusing mostly on the United States, yet we maintain that the key points are relevant to most countries. This chapter represents a summation in part of key points developed in previous chapters, suggesting transformation at each level of our social—ecological framework.

In this last section of the book (see Part V: Taking Action), we invite you to take action. Chapter 13, Developing and Implementing an Action Plan, describes various actions that can be taken by individuals, families, communities, health and human service professionals, and society at-large. We also provide a template for creating an action plan to change one's immediate local context and exemplars of action plans generated by individuals worldwide based on our previous lectures.

Overall, this book illustrates the multifaceted and complex transformations that will need to occur within each layer of our social—ecological model to advance comprehensive dementia care and services. Our model serves as a guidepost for all countries. How change is operationalized at each level will depend upon national plans, policies, local health and human service structures, and cultural contexts. Each chapter offers best practices, identified gaps, and has sought to push dementia care forward by indicating what can be done now. We now invite you to take action as we have outlined in the previous chapter!

The final word of this book belongs to the individuals who are living with dementia.

> In the past, sadly, those with dementia felt discounted on many fronts, disregarded, and ignored. There will always be obstacles—countless barriers of misunderstanding, indifference, lack of funding, the dense complexity of Dementia. I am deeply concerned about this. Thus, we must work to overcome these hurdles with persistence, faith, hope, and we must walk together, arms tightly locked—those suffering from dementia and the best medical minds in the world. Collectively, we can beat this! *Greg O'Brien, an investigative journalist, author of "On Pluto: Inside the Mind of Alzheimer's" and a patient-advocate for the Alzheimer's Association. Quoted with permission from his speech to the National Research Summit on Care and Services for Persons with Dementia and Caregivers, October 17, 2017, Washington DC.*

Index

Note: Page numbers followed by "*f*," "*t*," and "*b*" refer to figures, tables, and boxes, respectively.

A
Academy, 261
"Acceptance of Dementia" model, 242
Acetylcholine, 74
Action plan, 267
  from intention to action, 268*f*
  mapped to socioecological model, 269*f*
Activity
  activity/engagement/participation, 82
  principles for using, 84*b*
  remaining engaged in, 40
  as therapeutic agent, 81–85
Adaptive processes, 248–249
ADI. *See* Alzheimer's Disease International (ADI)
ADS Plus programs, 138–139
Adult day care, 219
Age of onset, 33
Age-specific dementia, 33–34
Aging, 33–34
  in place, 215
Aging Brain Medical Home, 222
"All-in" approach, 230
All-inclusive care, 35–36
Alzheimer's Association, 8–10, 59
Alzheimer's disease, 4–5, 35, 45–46
  neurodegenerative process, 5–6
  pathology, 13
Alzheimer's Disease International (ADI), 228
American Academy of Neurology, 67–68
Amyloid-β immunotherapy, 74–75
Anti-amyloid-β therapies, 74–75
Antidepressants medications, 32–33
Antipsychotics
  atypical, 75
  medications, 32–33
Anxiety, 13–15
Appraisal of life, 26
Assessment
  exemplar caregiver, 123*t*
  families support, 121–127
Atypical antipsychotics, 75

B
Basic program, 145–146
Behavioral and psychological symptoms of dementia (BPSD), 88
Behavioral competency, 26
Behavioral symptoms, 15, 36–37, 79–81, 79*f*
Better life for individuals living with dementia, 87–88. *See also* Lived experiences of individuals with dementia; Quality of life
  case example, 65*b*
  conversation with Dr. Helen Kales, 88*b*
  ethical dilemmas providing care and supports, 85–87
  treatment goals, 66–69
    actions for, 69–74
    activity as therapeutic agent, 81–85
    behavioral symptoms, 79–81, 79*f*
    cognitive decline, 77–78
    description and possible assessment approach, plan of action, 70*t*
    functional decline, 78–79
    nonpharmacological options, 75–77
    pharmacological treatment options, 74–75
Biomarkers, 12–13
  role in diagnosis of dementia, 11–13
BPSD. *See* Behavioral and psychological symptoms of dementia (BPSD)
Brain
  biomarkers role in diagnosis, 11–13
    fluid biomarkers, 11–12
    imaging biomarkers, 12–13
  case example, 3*b*
  challenge of diagnosis, 8–11
    benefits of early diagnosis, 10–11

282 INDEX

Brain (*Continued*)
   diagnosis disclosure, 8–10
   changing needs, 15–16
   conversation with Dr. Ester Oh, 18*b*
   etiology, 7
   metabolism, 12
   pathophysiology of dementia, 4–7
     Alzheimer's disease, 4–5
     FTD, 7
     Lewy body dementia, 6–7
     mixed dementia, 5–6
     vascular dementia, 6
   trajectory of dementia, 13–15, 14*f*
Breaking cycle of despair
   case example, 59*b*
   development of system for care and supportive services, 60–61
   paradigm of despair, 57–60
   three buckets of research, 54–57, 55*f*

C

Cardiovascular disease, 54
Cardiovascular risk factors, 54–56, 228–229
Care. *See* Dementia care
Care of Persons with Dementia in their Environments (COPE), 136, 137*b*
   dyads, 136–138
   prescription, 136
Care partner, family member as
   caregivers, 100–103, 101*f*
   caregivers need, 105–106
   consequences of caregiving, 103–105
   family caregivers, 98–100, 99*t*
   future of caregiving, 107
   research implications, 106
   Suzanne and Good Life Model, 97*b*
Caregiver(s), 37–38, 44, 100–103, 101*f*, 145–146, 250–251
   caregiver-centered approach, 115–116
   caregiver-directed approach, 115–116
   interventions, 119
   multi-component interventions, 241
   need, 105–106
Caregiving, 100–101, 104
   consequences, 103–105
   future, 107
CDC, 254
Childhood education, 275
Cholinesterase inhibitors boost, 74
CI. *See* Confidence interval (CI)
Citizenship, 42

Classic social–ecological framework, 38
Clinical trajectory of dementia, 30*f*
Clutter, 177–179
Cognitive decline, 77–78
Cognitive rehabilitation, 77–78
Cognitive Stimulation Therapy (CST), 77
Cognitive training, 77–78
Cognitive–behavioral intervention, 129
Communication disorders, 35–36
Community, 172, 252
   community-based program, 138–139
   community-based services, 215
   living in, 197–198
     barriers to community involvement, 200*b*
     case examples, 197*b*
     community-based strategies, 199
     dementia-friendly communities, 200–208
     need for security and belonging, 198–199
   services, 189–190
Competencies, 163
Comprehensive dementia, 33, 38
   care, 248
   for individuals/families, 248
   system, 261
Computer-based program, 189–190
Confidence interval (CI), 36
Consequentialist framework, 37
COPE. *See* Care of Persons with Dementia in their Environments (COPE)
Costs, 36
CST. *See* Cognitive Stimulation Therapy (CST)
CT scan, 9, 12
Cultural environment, 278–279
Culture, 32–33
Cure, 56
"Cycle of despair", 54, 58*f*, 275–276

D

Daily challenges, 33–43, 34*b*
Daily tips, 140–142
Decision-making, 30
Degenerative brain disease process, 29
Dementia, 3–4, 29–31, 34, 38, 42–43, 197–198, 228, 230, 242, 261–262, 267, 275
   caregivers characteristics, 99
   competencies across all practitioners, 165*b*

diagnosis, 8–9, 11b
  goals of dementia disclosure, 10b
  individuals with, 198
  needs of people with, 28b
  by numbers globally, 228
  still, 261
  trajectory, 13–15, 14f, 218–220
  types, 5b
"Dementia aware", 202, 203t
"Dementia capable", 202, 203t
Dementia care, 213, 217t, 247–248,
    258–259, 274, 276
  best practices in setting design and
    programming, 220–221, 220b
  changing needs for dementia care, 216f
  coordination, 222
  critical drivers of home as epicenter for,
    172–174
  dementia trajectory, 218–220
  home as epicenter for, 190–191
  management models, 221–222
  person-and family-centered care,
    215–217
  person-centered service models,
    221–223
  practical implications for, 43
  program, 42
  strategies for implementing evidence for,
    254b
  transformation
    caregivers, 250–251
    conversation with Dr. Jean Garjardo,
      PhD, OTR/L, 261b
    health and human services,
      253–258
    individual level, 249–250
    living environment, 251–252
    neighborhood and community, 252
    putting it all together, 260
    social policy, 258–259
    social–medical comprehensive
      dementia care model, 247–249
Dementia care and services, 42, 54, 59
  assumptions for developing a system of,
    61b
  development of system for, 60–61
  ethical dilemmas, 85–87
    case scenarios of common challenges,
      85–87
    ethical challenges providing care and
      services, 85b
  research on, 56–57

Dementia impacts and supporting quality
    of life
  caring about care, 32–37
    disease burden imperative, 34–35
    economic imperative, 36–37
    moral imperative, 37
    numbers imperative, 33–34
  challenges, 43–45
  conceptual framework for dementia care,
    38–43
    case example, 40b
    socio-ecological model for
      implementing care and services, 39f
  roadmap, 45–46
"Dementia ready", 202, 203t
Dementia-based competencies, 163
Dementia-friendly communities, 200–208
  examples, 206–208
  priorities of individuals with dementia in
    creating, 201b
"Dementia-friendly", 197–198, 203t
Dementia-specific interprofessional
  competencies, 163t
"Dementievriendelijk Brugge", 206–207
Demography, 173
Deontological/Kantian approach, 37
Depression, 275
Describe, Investigate, Create, and Evaluate
    approach (DICE approach), 79–81,
    88–89, 140
Despair, paradigm of, 57–60
Diabetes, 54–56, 275
Diagnosis of dementia, 8, 10–11, 30
  challenge of, 8–11
  diagnosis-seeking behavior, 17
  diagnostic process, 3
  disclosure, 8–10
DICE approach. See Describe, Investigate,
    Create, and Evaluate approach
    (DICE approach)
Disease burden, 35
  on families, 35–36
  imperative, 34–35
Disease management, 32–33
Disease process, 25, 53, 56–57
Donepezil, 74
Drug development, 32

E
Early-stage dementia. See Mild-stage
    dementia
Economic imperative, 36–37

Economics of dementia, 36
Education lack, 273
Education/training, 277–278
Empirical evidence, 162
Engagement, 25, 40
  in meaningful activities, 41
Environmental
  assessments, 181–186, 182t
  factors, 273–274
  gerontology, 171
  modifications, 187–188
    home modifications for safety and optimization of function, 187b
    principles for home environmental changes, 188b
    triggers for relocation to nursing home, 189b
Ethnicity, 32–33
Etiology, 7
Evidence-based approaches, 127–129
  average pooled effect sizes across reviews, 128t
  types of caregiver interventions, 127b
Evidence-based care, 30, 35–36
Evidence-based strategies, 258
Excess disability, 78
Exemplars, 129–142
Experience of dementia, 3, 37–38, 42, 60, 275–276
Experienced stigma, 36–37

F
Fall risk, 35–36
Families care and service, 34
Family caregivers, 30–31, 37–38, 97–100, 99t, 155–156, 219
Family caregiving, 114
Family member as care partner. *See also* Support families
  caregivers, 100–103, 101f
  caregivers need, 105–106
  consequences of caregiving, 103–105
  family caregivers, 98–100, 99t
  future of caregiving, 107
  research implications, 106
  Suzanne and Good Life Model, 97b
Family-based centered model, 250–251
Family-centered approaches, 258
Family-centered dementia, 126–127
Family-centered programs and models, 106
Family/friends/employers, disclosing diagnosis to, 39–40

"Felt" stigma. *See* Self-stigma
Fluid biomarkers, 11–12
Formal caregivers, 155–157
  case example, 155b
  dementia competencies across all practitioners, 165b
  interprofessional approach to, 158–160
  interprofessional care importants, 161–162
  requires to practice as part of interprofessional care team, 163–164
  dementia-specific interprofessional competencies, 163t
  discipline-specific core competencies in dementia care, 164t
  well-prepared dementia care workforce, 157b
Frontotemporal dementia (FTD), 4–5, 7
Function Focused Care, 78
Functional decline, 78–79

G
G8 Dementia Summit (2013), 230–231
Galantamine, 74
GDP. *See* Gross domestic product (GDP)
General caregiver program, 128
Global disease burden of dementia, 228–230
Global efforts for cure dementia
  dementia by numbers globally, 228
  gaps in global efforts, 241–242
    conversation with Dr. James Pickett, 243b
    missing pieces in national plans, 241b
  global disease burden, 228–230
Glutamate, 74
Good Life model, 26–27, 67–68, 97–98
  with dementia, 87–88
  Suzanne and, 97b
Gross domestic product (GDP), 229–230

H
Hazards, 179–180, 278
HBDC. *See* Home-based dementia care (HBDC)
Health and human services, 253–258
  strategies for implementing evidence, 253–256
  strategies for selecting evidence for implementation, 256–258, 257f
Health and Retirement Survey, 54–56

Health and social service systems, 257–258
Health care organization, 277–278
Health professionals, 177
Health provider perspective, 180–181
 challenges working in home for health and human service professionals, 181b
Heart disease, 228–229
High technology-outfitted experimental communities, 172–173
Hippocampus, 4–5
Home, 171
 environments impact on daily life, 174–176
 as epicenter for dementia care, 190–191
 conversation with Dr. Constantine (Kostas) Lyketsos, 190b
 safety, 33, 180
 considerations, 177–180, 178b
Home-based dementia care (HBDC), 191
Home-based Program, 136
Home-like arrangements, 172–173
Hospital at Home, 173–174
Hypertension, 275

I
ICHOM. *See* International Consortium for Health Outcomes (ICHOM)
Imaging biomarkers, 12–13
Imaging techniques, 12
Immunotherapies, 56
Individual level, 249–250
Institute of Medicine Report (IOM), 104
Integrating evidence-based strategies, 253
"Internalized" stigma. *See* Self-stigma
International Consortium for Health Outcomes (ICHOM), 67–68
Interprofessional care team
 dementia competencies across all practitioners, 165b
 formal caregivers requires to practice as part of, 163–164
 dementia-specific interprofessional competencies, 163t
 discipline-specific core competencies in dementia care, 164t
 interprofessional approach to formal caregiving, 158–160
 interdisciplinary team members in care of person with dementia, 159t
 interprofessional care team, 159f, 277–278
 interprofessional care importants, 161–162
 benefits of interprofessional team approach to dementia care, 162b
IOM. *See* Institute of Medicine Report (IOM)

K
Key transformative actions, 258

L
Laboratory evaluations, 136–138
Late-life smoking, 275
Late-stage dementia. *See* Severe-stage dementia
Leadership, 261
Lewy body dementia, 5–7
Lewy Body Dementia Association, 59
Lewy body disease, 6–7
Life course, 38–40, 274–275
Life expectancy, 45–46
Lived experiences of individuals with dementia, 23. *See also* Better life for individuals living with dementia; Quality of life
 case example, 26b
 conversation with Dr. Jason Karlowish, 45b
 daily challenges, 33–43
  disclosing diagnosis to family/friends/employers, 39–40
  maintaining sense of purpose, control, and agency, 41–43
  managing stigma, 34–39
  remaining engaged in meaningful activity, 40
  remaining safe at home, 33–34
 differential needs of people living with dementia, 27–33
  age of onset, 33
  needs by disease stage, 28–32
  race, ethnicity, and culture, 32–33
 good life model, 26–27
 key research gaps, 43b
 practical implications for dementia care, 43
 principles for, 25–26
 sectors of quality of life, 24f
Living environment, 251–252

Living in community, 197–198
  case examples, 197b
  community-based strategies, 199
  dementia-friendly communities, 200–208
  leading barriers to community involvement for persons with dementia, 200b
  need for security and belonging, 198–199
Long-term care setting, 215
"Longest Day" The event, 206

M

Maximizing independence at Home intervention (MIND at Home intervention), 221–222
MCI. *See* Mild cognitive impairment (MCI)
Medications, 74–75, 136–138
Memory cafes, 206
Memory Care Home Solutions, 145–146
Meta-analyses, 120–121
Middle-stage dementia. *See* Moderate-stage dementia
Midlife hearing loss, 275
Mild cognitive impairment (MCI), 45–46
Mild-stage dementia, 13–15, 218–219
MIND at Home intervention. *See* Maximizing independence at Home intervention (MIND at Home intervention)
Minimum viable product, 256
Mixed dementia, 5–6
Moderate-stage dementia, 15, 219
Moral distress, 37–38
Moral/ethical dimension of dementia care, 37
Motivational theory of life-span development, 41
MRI, 9, 12

N

National Dementia Strategy (England), 31
National Health and Aging Trends Study (NHATS), 40, 199
National Institute on Aging, 8–9, 139
National plans for dementia, 45
  and impacts of dementia, 230–241
    elements of national plans, 240f
    thirty-seven national dementia plans, 232t
  missing pieces in, 241b
Neighborhood, 252
Neocortex, 4–5

Neurodegenerative process, 15–16
Neuropsychiatric behaviors, 29–31
Neuropsychiatric Inventory (NPI), 79–80
NHATS. *See* National Health and Aging Trends Study (NHATS)
NMDA antagonists, 74
Nonpharmacological cognitive approaches, 77
Nonpharmacological options, 75–77
NPI. *See* Neuropsychiatric Inventory (NPI)
Numbers imperative, 33–34
Nursing homes, 220

O

Obesity, 275
Objective environment, 26–27, 29
Occupational therapist (OT), 126, 136
Olanzapine, 75
Olfactory identification test, 12
OT. *See* Occupational therapist (OT)

P

PACE. *See* Program of All-Inclusive Care for the Elderly (PACE)
Paradigm shift, 31
Parkinson's disease, 6–7
Pathophysiology, 273
  of dementia, 4–7
Payment models, 258
Peñalolén, 206
Perceived stigma, 37
Perceived valuation, 26
Person-and family-centered care, 215–217
Person-centered programming, 220–221
Person-centered service models, 221–223
  care coordination, 222
  care management models, 221–222
  PACE, 223
  Transitional Care Model, 222–223
Personal tool navigator, 140
Personhood movement, 38
PET. *See* Positron emission tomography (PET)
Pharmacological treatment options, 74–75
Philosophy of dementia care, 241
Physical environment, 278–279
Physical home environment, 42, 198–199
  case example, 175b
  critical drivers of home as epicenter for dementia care, 172–174
  environmental assessments, 181–186, 182t

environmental modifications, 187–188
health provider perspective, 180–181
home as epicenter for dementia care, 190–191
home environments impact on daily life, 174–176
home safety considerations, 177–180, 178b
staying and leaving, 189
unintended negative consequences of staying home, 189–190
Physical inactivity, 275
Pick's disease, 5, 7
Policies, 45, 277–278
Positron emission tomography (PET), 12
Preclinical Alzheimer's disease, 4–5
Prevention, 54
Preventive–curative research, 54
Primary desired outcome, 117
Prognosis, 45–46
Program of All-Inclusive Care for the Elderly (PACE), 223
Psychological distress, 29–31
Psychological well-being, 26

Q

Quality of life, 31–33, 35–36, 45, 69b. *See also* Better life for individuals living with dementia
dementia impacts and supporting caring about care, 32–37
challenges, 43–45
conceptual framework for dementia care, 38–43
roadmap, 45–46
feasible and interrelated treatment goals to support, 69b
individual's, 16
issues, 15
sectors, 24f
Quetiapine, 75

R

Race, 32–33
Randomized controlled trials (RCTs), 127
Rapid population aging, 99
RCTs. *See* Randomized controlled trials (RCTs)
REACH I initiative. *See* Resources for Enhancing Alzheimer's Caregiver Health initiative (REACH I initiative)

REACH II intervention, 255
REACH Risk Appraisal Measure, 127
Reliable transportation, 201–202
Research agenda, 241–242
Research and accurate dementia diagnosis, 17b
Residential care, 219
Resources for Enhancing Alzheimer's Caregiver Health initiative (REACH I initiative), 120–121
Respite care, 219
Risperidone, 75
Rivastigmine, 74

S

Safety, 177
home, 33, 180
considerations, 177–180, 178b
home modifications for, 187b
remaining safe at home, 33–34
and security, 27
Savvy Caregiver program, 128, 255
Scotland, national plans for dementia, 231–240, 232t
Self-stigma, 45–46
Sensory impairments, 35–36
Severe-stage dementia, 15, 220
Shared components, 129
Single photon emission tomography, 12
Smart homes, 172–173
Social ecological model, 253
Social isolation, 275
Social media, 270
Social policy, 258–259
advancing policies to support persons living with dementia and families, 259b
moving towards comprehensive dementia care, 259f
Social–ecological factors, 273–274
Social–ecological framework, 42, 45
Social–ecological model, 38–40, 267–269
for implementing care and services, 39f
Social–medical comprehensive dementia care model, 247–249
Spillover stigma, 45–46
Stereotyped threat, 46–47
Stigma, 35–36, 35b, 45–46
effects, 36–37, 37b
for individuals with dementia, 36
management, 33–39

Stigma (*Continued*)
  research needs, 37–38
  strategies to address stigma, 38–39, 38*b*
Structural brain imaging, 12
Support families, 113. *See also* Family member as care partner
  assessment, 121–127
  assumptions, 115*b*
    for providing care and services to families, 114–116
  caregiver interventions, 119 testing, 131*t*
  caregivers, 145–146
    core treatment principles of face-to-face programs, 144*t*
  common lessons caregivers, 140*t*
  discernable second wave of intervention studies, 119–120
  ethical considerations, 146–147
  evidence-based approaches, 127–129
  exemplars, 129–142
    caregiver assessments, 123*t*
  lessons learning, 142–145
    key principles, 143*t*
    modalities, 143*b*
  meta-analyses, 120–121
  novel approaches, 121
  pathways for supporting family caregivers, 116–119
    direct and indirect, 118*f*
    key outcomes, 117*b*
Supportive programs, 30
Supportive services, 60–61, 114, 145–146

T

Tailored Activity Program (TAP), 76–78, 81–85, 180, 189–190
Targeted program, 128
Three buckets of research, 54–57, 55*f*
Timely referral to hospice care, 220
Transformation, 31, 43. *See also* Dementia care—transformation
Transitional Care Model, 222–223

U

Unintended negative consequences of staying home, 189–190
United States, individual with dementia living in, 39
US Preventative Task Force, 8–9
Utilitarian framework, 37

V

Vascular dementia, 5–6
Vascular disease-related process, 5–6

W

Web-based Program, 139–140
WeCareAdvisor, 140, 142
WHO. *See* World Health Organization (WHO)
"Woman in the middle", 99
Workforce
  of formal caregivers, 156
  well-prepared dementia care workforce, 157*b*, 158
World Health Organization (WHO), 34, 230–231, 242

CPSIA information can be obtained
at www.ICGtesting.com
Printed in the USA
LVHW041431201118
597786LV00012B/1221/P